Advantages and Disadvantages of Electronic Cigarettes

Advantages and Disadvantages of Electronic Cigarettes

Editors

Andrzej Sobczak
Leon Kośmider

MDPI • Basel • Beijing • Wuhan • Barcelona • Belgrade • Manchester • Tokyo • Cluj • Tianjin

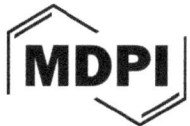

Editors
Andrzej Sobczak
Medical University of Silesia
Katowice
Poland

Leon Kośmider
Medical University of Silesia
Katowice
Poland

Editorial Office
MDPI
St. Alban-Anlage 66
4052 Basel, Switzerland

This is a reprint of articles from the Special Issue published online in the open access journal *Toxics* (ISSN 2305-6304) (available at: https://www.mdpi.com/journal/toxics/special_issues/e-cigarettes_harm).

For citation purposes, cite each article independently as indicated on the article page online and as indicated below:

LastName, A.A.; LastName, B.B.; LastName, C.C. Article Title. *Journal Name* **Year**, *Volume Number*, Page Range.

ISBN 978-3-0365-6503-3 (Hbk)
ISBN 978-3-0365-6504-0 (PDF)

© 2023 by the authors. Articles in this book are Open Access and distributed under the Creative Commons Attribution (CC BY) license, which allows users to download, copy and build upon published articles, as long as the author and publisher are properly credited, which ensures maximum dissemination and a wider impact of our publications.

The book as a whole is distributed by MDPI under the terms and conditions of the Creative Commons license CC BY-NC-ND.

Contents

About the Editors vii

Andrzej Sobczak and Leon Kośmider
Advantages and Disadvantages of Electronic Cigarettes
Reprinted from: *Toxics* **2023**, *11*, 66, doi:10.3390/toxics11010066 1

Greg Hartwell, Matt Egan, Jamie Brown, Triantafyllos Pliakas and Mark Petticrew
Use of e-Cigarettes and Attendance at Stop Smoking Services: A Population Survey in England
Reprinted from: *Toxics* **2022**, *10*, 593, doi:10.3390/toxics10100593 5

Thomas Nicholson, Lauren Davis, Edward T. Davis, Matthew Newton Ede, Aaron Scott and Simon W. Jones
e-Cigarette Vapour Condensate Reduces Viability and Impairs Function of Human Osteoblasts, in Part, via a Nicotine Dependent Mechanism
Reprinted from: *Toxics* **2022**, *10*, 506, doi:10.3390/toxics10090506 17

Yvonne C. M. Staal, Peter M. J. Bos and Reinskje Talhout
Methodological Approaches for Risk Assessment of Tobacco and Related Products
Reprinted from: *Toxics* **2022**, *10*, 491, doi:10.3390/toxics10090491 35

Thomas Lamb, Thivanka Muthumalage, Jiries Meehan-Atrash and Irfan Rahman
Nose-Only Exposure to Cherry- and Tobacco-Flavored E-Cigarettes Induced Lung Inflammation in Mice in a Sex-Dependent Manner
Reprinted from: *Toxics* **2022**, *10*, 471, doi:10.3390/toxics10080471 49

Shaiesh Yogeswaran and Irfan Rahman
Differences in Acellular Reactive Oxygen Species (ROS) Generation by E-Cigarettes Containing Synthetic Nicotine and Tobacco-Derived Nicotine
Reprinted from: *Toxics* **2022**, *10*, 134, doi:10.3390/toxics10030134 61

Alexandra Jităreanu, Irina Gabriela Cara, Alexandru Sava, Ioana Mârțu, Ioana-Cezara Caba and Luminița Agoroaei
The Impact of the Storage Conditions and Type of Clearomizers on the Increase of Heavy Metal Levels in Electronic Cigarette Liquids Retailed in Romania
Reprinted from: *Toxics* **2022**, *10*, 126, doi:10.3390/toxics10030126 73

Patryk Krystian Bebenek, Vinit Gholap, Matthew Halquist, Andrzej Sobczak and Leon Kośmider
E-Liquids from Seven European Countries–Warnings Analysis and Freebase Nicotine Content
Reprinted from: *Toxics* **2022**, *10*, 51, doi:10.3390/toxics10020051 89

Mariusz Duplaga and Marcin Grysztar
The Use of E-Cigarettes among High School Students in Poland Is Associated with Health Locus of Control but Not with Health Literacy: A Cross-Sectional Study
Reprinted from: *Toxics* **2022**, *10*, 41, doi:10.3390/toxics10010041 105

Dominika Cichońska, Oliwia Król, Ewa M. Słomińska, Barbara Kochańska, Dariusz Świetlik, Jolanta Ochocińska and Aida Kusiak
Influence of Electronic Cigarettes on Antioxidant Capacity and Nucleotide Metabolites in Saliva
Reprinted from: *Toxics* **2021**, *9*, 263, doi:10.3390/toxics9100263 119

Shaiesh Yogeswaran, Thivanka Muthumalage and Irfan Rahman
Comparative Reactive Oxygen Species (ROS) Content among Various Flavored Disposable Vape Bars, including Cool (Iced) Flavored Bars
Reprinted from: *Toxics* **2021**, *9*, 235, doi:10.3390/toxics9100235 . . . . **131**

Connor R. Miller, Hangchuan Shi, Dongmei Li and Maciej L. Goniewicz
Cross-Sectional Associations of Smoking and E-cigarette Use with Self-Reported Diagnosed Hypertension: Findings from Wave 3 of the Population Assessment of Tobacco and Health Study
Reprinted from: *Toxics* **2021**, *9*, 52, doi:10.3390/toxics9030052 . . . . **157**

Sebastien Soulet and Roberto A Sussman
Critical Review of the Recent Literature on Organic Byproducts in E-Cigarette Aerosol Emissions
Reprinted from: *Toxics* **2022**, *10*, 714, doi:10.3390/10.3390/toxics10120714 . . . . **171**

Sebastien Soulet and Roberto A Sussman
A Critical Review of Recent Literature on Metal Contents in E-Cigarette Aerosol
Reprinted from: *Toxics* **2022**, *10*, 510, doi:10.3390/toxics10090510 . . . . **221**

Paweł Szumilas, Aleksandra Wilk, Kamila Szumilas and Beata Karakiewicz
The Effects of E-Cigarette Aerosol on Oral Cavity Cells and Tissues: A Narrative Review
Reprinted from: *Toxics* **2022**, *10*, 74, doi:10.3390/toxics10020074 . . . . **257**

About the Editors

Andrzej Sobczak

Andrzej Sobczak is a Professor in the Faculty of Pharmaceutical Sciences at the Medical University of Silesia. He is graduate of the Gdańsk University of Technology (1974). He defended his doctoral dissertation in 1979. In 1983–1985, he completed a postdoctoral fellowship at the Institute of Organic Chemistry of the University of Hubland (Würzburg, West Germany). Since 1985, he has been associated with the Medical University of Silesia, initially with the Faculty of Medicine, and since 2001, with the Faculty of Pharmacy. In the years 2006–2020, he was the head of the Department of General and Inorganic Chemistry of the Faculty of Pharmacy with the Division of Laboratory Medicine. Additionally, he headed the Department of Chemical Harm and Genetic Toxicology at the Institute of Occupational Medicine and Environmental Health in Sosnowiec in 2008–2019. In the years 2018–2022, he was a member of the Council of the National Science Center. For over a dozen years, he has been dealing with the impact of tobacco smoke on smokers' bodies and the safety of using innovative tobacco products (smokeless cigarettes and electronic cigarettes) in the context of harm-reduction strategies caused by smoking. He is the author of over 180 publications. He has published in prestigious journals, e.g.: *Tobacco Control*; *Nicotine & Tobacco Research*; *Thorax*; *Cancer Epidemiology, Biomarkers & Prevention*; *Circulation Journal*; *European Journal of Public Health*; *International Journal of Public Health*; *Addiction Biology*; *Journal of Applied Toxicology*; *Atherosclerosis*, etc. His work has been cited more than 5,000 times. He has received two awards of the Minister of Health for scientific achievements (2009) and for overall teaching and research activity (2019).

Leon Kośmider

Leon Kośmider is an Assistant Professor in the Faculty of Pharmaceutical Sciences at the Medical University of Silesia. He obtained his Pharm. D. and Ph.D. in Pharmacy in 2012 and 2016 at the Medical University of Silesia, Poland. He has over 10 years of experience in toxicology research and a solid background in the analytical chemistry, biostatistics, and pharmacokinetic fields. He has conducted research regarding the toxicology of tobacco products involving various tobacco products (i.e., e-cigarettes and tobacco), focusing mainly on the yields of toxic agents in tobacco smoke generated in various smoking conditions and its influence on biomarkers of exposure.

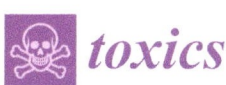

Editorial

Advantages and Disadvantages of Electronic Cigarettes

Andrzej Sobczak * and Leon Kośmider

Department of General and Inorganic Chemistry, Faculty of Pharmaceutical Sciences in Sosnowiec, Medical University of Silesia, 40-055 Katowice, Poland
* Correspondence: asobczak@sum.edu.pl

Despite nearly nine thousand publications on e-cigarettes (EC) in the PubMed database, there is still no consensus in the scientific community and among decision makers regarding the risks and benefits of using these products. As we emphasized in the call for papers, further research is needed to provide new evidence-based knowledge to better inform the public about the possible risks as well as the benefits for smokers related to the use of e-cigarettes. We proposed a wide range of topics, which included laboratory studies related to the presence of harmful substances in the liquid and aerosol, in vivo and in vitro health effects studies, the role of nicotine in addiction, and observational population studies on the use of EC.

The papers submitted for the Special Issue (SI) fit into the proposed topics. Two papers concern reactive oxygen species (ROS) generated during the use of an e-cigarette containing synthetic nicotine [1] and the influence of flavoring substances on the appearance of ROS in the aerosol [2]. Flavoring substances are also the subject of research by Bebenek et al. [3]. The authors analyze their influence on the content of free and protonated nicotine and the consequences associated with nicotine addiction. In turn, animal studies [4] have hypothesized that exposure to flavored e-cigarettes would cause lung inflammation in C57BL/6 J mice. This study revealed that flavor-based e-cigarette exposure elicited sex-specific alterations in lung inflammation, with cherry flavors/benzaldehyde eliciting female-specific and tobacco flavor resulting in male-specific increases in lung inflammation. Such studies indicate the potential toxicity of some flavorings added to e-liquid which should be taken into account when formulating regulations.

In in vivo studies, Cichońska et al. [5] conclude that e-cigarette usage adversely affects the antioxidant capacity of saliva, in comparison to non-smokers, to the same extent as smoking traditional cigarettes. This might present an important clinical risk of oral cavity disorders. Additionally, in their review paper, Szumilas et al. [6] review the literature in terms of the impact of e-cigarette aerosol on the cells and tissues of the oral cavity.

In turn, in vitro studies have shown that e-cigarette vapor condensate (ECVC) has a negative effect on both osteoblast viability and function, with these effects being mediated, in part, by nicotine-dependent mechanisms and also reactive carbonyl species derived from e-liquid humectants. Reduced osteoblast viability, coupled with a reduction in OPG secretion as observed following ECVC treatment, may lead to increased bone resorption following chronic exposure, in turn potentially impacting bone development in younger users, while increasing bone-associated disease progression and negatively impacting orthopedic and dental surgery outcomes [7].

Another article in this SI is devoted to the study of the storage conditions and type of clearomizers on the increase in heavy metal levels in e-cigarette liquids retailed in Romania [8]. It has been found that the long period and high storage temperature of e-liquids in the clearomizer have an effect on increasing the level of heavy metals in the generated aerosol. This is important information for users of these products, aiming to reduce the harmfulness of their use.

In many reports published by prestigious scientific institutions, special attention is paid to the threat that e-cigarettes may pose to young people. Therefore, we welcomed the

Citation: Sobczak, A.; Kośmider, L. Advantages and Disadvantages of Electronic Cigarettes. *Toxics* **2023**, *11*, 66. https://doi.org/10.3390/toxics11010066

Received: 28 December 2022
Accepted: 5 January 2023
Published: 11 January 2023

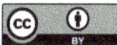

Copyright: © 2023 by the authors. Licensee MDPI, Basel, Switzerland. This article is an open access article distributed under the terms and conditions of the Creative Commons Attribution (CC BY) license (https://creativecommons.org/licenses/by/4.0/).

paper describing the results of a cross-sectional study conducted in Poland [9]. The main aim of this study was the assessment of the factors associated with the use of electronic cigarettes among high school students. Two parameters used to assess public health were used for this purpose: health literacy (HL) and the health locus of control (HLC). Personal health literacy is the degree to which individuals have the ability to find, understand, and use information and services to inform health-related decisions and actions for themselves and others. The health locus of control refers to the belief that health is in one's control (internal control) or is not in one's control (external control). Among adults, the external locus of control is associated with negative health outcomes, whereas the internal locus of control is associated with favorable outcomes. The obtained results showed that students smoking conventional cigarettes were more prone to using e-cigarettes. To sum up, it was an unexpected result that HL is not associated with the use of e-cigarettes. A greater likelihood of using e-cigarettes was positively associated with higher HLC scores, as in the case of traditional smoking.

There are currently ongoing debates about the relationship between e-cigarette use, NRT use, and the uptake and provision of other quit methods including behavioral support. It has been suggested, for instance, that widespread e-cigarette use may be reducing the need for stop smoking services (SSSs). Meanwhile, research by Harweell et al. [10] does not support this argument; some smokers participating in the study were still willing to receive additional support in quitting from SSSs, even if they were already using e-cigarettes.

Another paper [11] uses data from Wave 3 of The Population Assessment of Tobacco and Health (PATH) study which is a nationally representative longitudinal study of tobacco use and health in the United States. The authors assess associations between e-cigarette use and self-reported hypertension, a highly prevalent health condition and major contributor to cardiovascular disease burden. According to the authors, after adjusting for potential confounders, current vaping (OR = 1.31) and current smoking (OR = 1.27) were both associated with higher odds of hypertension; those odds were lower for respondents who were concurrently smoking and vaping (OR = 1.77). The results obtained make an important contribution to the evaluation of the association of e-cigarette use with major adverse cardiovascular endpoints (e.g., stroke and myocardial infarction).

Controversies around the risks posed by e-cigarettes are often due to the wide variety of products and user behavior, the underestimation or overestimation of risk, as well as the wrong methodological approach. In this context, we pay particular attention to two further works. Talhout et al. [12] used several approaches to quantify the health risk of tobacco products, either the absolute risk or that relative to a tobacco cigarette. The hazard index (HI) and relative potency factor (RPF) approaches may be used for the quantification of health risk, provided that sufficient and relevant hazard and exposure data are available. None of the methods are ready to be used in regulation yet due to a lack of relevant data on hazard and exposure, but also due to a variety of regulatory needs and wishes. However, the application of these methods may be possible in due time.

One of the reasons for the controversy surrounding e-cigarettes is the different, often contradictory results of studies covering the same research topic. The reasons may vary. However, the most important is the research methodology. This topic was discussed in two papers by Soulet and Sussman. In the first paper [13], the authors critically reviewed laboratory studies published after 2017 on the metal content of EC aerosol, focusing on the consistency between their experimental design, the actual use of the device, and the corresponding exposure risk assessment. The authors showed the most important reasons for the variation in results in the reviewed papers. They included inadequate BA test protocols unsuited to the power of the heater; miscalculation of exposure levels based on experimental results; devices manufactured many months before the experiment, which could be the cause of corrosion of the e-cigarette's metal components; and lack of sufficient information to allow repetition of the study.

Similar topics are addressed in the second paper [14]. They review the literature on laboratory studies quantifying the production of potentially toxic organic by-products (carbonyls, carbon monoxide, and free radicals) in e-cigarette aerosol emissions, focusing on the consistency between their experimental design and a realistic usage of the devices. The authors conclude that laboratory testing requires a much more flexible standard, not only providing appropriate technical guidelines, but facilitating the incorporation of end users to complement laboratory logistics.

We agree with the authors of these papers that an objective assessment of the risk of using e-cigarettes requires the elimination of incorrect research methodology and signals the necessity to upgrade current laboratory-testing standards.

The papers posted in the SI cover various research areas related to e-cigarettes. In our opinion, they show two important directions for further research. The first is the role of flavor additives in the overall assessment of the harmfulness of e-cigarettes, and the second is the need to take steps toward standardizing methods at least for areas of research in which we observe considerable variation in the results obtained, which at present makes it difficult to take rational regulatory action and recommendations.

Funding: This research received no external funding.

Conflicts of Interest: The authors declare no conflict of interest.

References

1. Yogeswaran, S.; Rahman, I. Differences in Acellular Reactive Oxygen Species (ROS) Generation by E-Cigarettes Containing Synthetic Nicotine and Tobacco-Derived Nicotine. *Toxics* **2022**, *10*, 134. [CrossRef] [PubMed]
2. Yogeswaran, S.; Muthumalage, T.; Rahman, I. Comparative Reactive Oxygen Species (ROS) Content among Various Flavored Disposable Vape Bars, including Cool (Iced) Flavored Bars. *Toxics* **2021**, *9*, 235. [CrossRef] [PubMed]
3. Bębenek, P.K.; Gholap, V.; Halquist, M.; Sobczak, A.; Kośmider, L. E-Liquids from Seven European Countries–Warnings Analysis and Freebase Nicotine Content. *Toxics* **2022**, *10*, 51. [CrossRef] [PubMed]
4. Lamb, T.; Muthumalage, T.; Meehan-Atrash, J.; Rahman, I. Nose-Only Exposure to Cherry- and Tobacco-Flavored E-Cigarettes Induced Lung Inflammation in Mice in a Sex-Dependent Manner. *Toxics* **2022**, *10*, 471. [CrossRef] [PubMed]
5. Cichońska, D.; Król, O.; Słomińska, E.M.; Kochańska, B.; Świetlik, D.; Ochocińska, J.; Kusiak, A. Influence of Electronic Cigarettes on Antioxidant Capacity and Nucleotide Metabolites in Saliva. *Toxics* **2021**, *9*, 263. [CrossRef] [PubMed]
6. Szumilas, P.; Wilk, A.; Szumilas, K.; Karakiewicz, B. The Effects of E-Cigarette Aerosol on Oral Cavity Cells and Tissues: A Narrative Review. *Toxics* **2022**, *10*, 74. [CrossRef] [PubMed]
7. Nicholson, T.; Davis, L.; Davis, E.T.; Ede, M.N.; Scott, A.; Jones, S.W. e-Cigarette Vapour Condensate Reduces Viability and Impairs Function of Human Osteoblasts, in Part, via a Nicotine Dependent Mechanism. *Toxics* **2022**, *10*, 506. [CrossRef]
8. Jităreanu, A.; Cara, I.G.; Sava, A.; Mârțu, I.; Caba, I.-C.; Agoroaei, L. The Impact of the Storage Conditions and Type of Clearomizers on the Increase of Heavy Metal Levels in Electronic Cigarette Liquids Retailed in Romania. *Toxics* **2022**, *10*, 126. [CrossRef] [PubMed]
9. Duplaga, M.; Grysztar, M. The Use of E-Cigarettes among High School Students in Poland Is Associated with Health Locus of Control but Not with Health Literacy: A Cross-Sectional Study. *Toxics* **2022**, *10*, 41. [CrossRef] [PubMed]
10. Hartwell, G.; Egan, M.; Brown, J.; Pliakas, T.; Petticrew, M. Use of e-Cigarettes and Attendance at Stop Smoking Services: A Population Survey in England. *Toxics* **2022**, *10*, 593. [CrossRef] [PubMed]
11. Miller, C.R.; Shi, H.; Li, D.; Goniewicz, M.L. Cross-Sectional Associations of Smoking and E-cigarette Use with Self-Reported Diagnosed Hypertension: Findings from Wave 3 of the Population Assessment of Tobacco and Health Study. *Toxics* **2021**, *9*, 52. [CrossRef] [PubMed]
12. Staal, Y.C.M.; Bos, P.M.J.; Talhout, R. Methodological Approaches for Risk Assessment of Tobacco and Related Products. *Toxics* **2022**, *10*, 491. [CrossRef] [PubMed]
13. Soulet, S.; Sussman, R.A. A Critical Review of Recent Literature on Metal Contents in E-Cigarette Aerosol. *Toxics* **2022**, *10*, 510. [CrossRef] [PubMed]
14. Soulet, S.; Sussman, R.A. Critical Review of the Recent Literature on Organic Byproducts in E-Cigarette Aerosol Emissions. *Toxics* **2022**, *10*, 714. [CrossRef] [PubMed]

Disclaimer/Publisher's Note: The statements, opinions and data contained in all publications are solely those of the individual author(s) and contributor(s) and not of MDPI and/or the editor(s). MDPI and/or the editor(s) disclaim responsibility for any injury to people or property resulting from any ideas, methods, instructions or products referred to in the content.

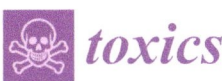

Article

Use of e-Cigarettes and Attendance at Stop Smoking Services: A Population Survey in England

Greg Hartwell [1,*], Matt Egan [1], Jamie Brown [2], Triantafyllos Pliakas [1,3] and Mark Petticrew [1]

1 Department of Public Health, Environments & Society, London School of Hygiene & Tropical Medicine, London WC1H 9SH, UK
2 Health Behaviour Research Centre, University College London, London WC1E 6BT, UK
3 Impact Epilysis, Taxiarchon 35, Kalamaria, 55 132 Thessaloniki, Greece
* Correspondence: gregory.hartwell@lshtm.ac.uk

Abstract: Little is known about whether e-cigarette use influences tobacco smokers' decisions around other smoking cessation options, including the most effective one available: stop smoking service (SSS) attendance. Our repeat cross-sectional survey therefore assessed associations between use of e-cigarettes with past and planned future uptake of SSSs. Nicotine replacement therapy (NRT) use was also assessed as a comparator. Participants were drawn from the Smoking Toolkit Study, a nationally representative, validated, face-to-face survey. Data were aggregated on 2139 English adults reporting current smoking of cigarettes or other tobacco products. Multivariable logistic regression was used to adjust for potential confounders. Results showed dual users of combustible tobacco and e-cigarettes were more likely than other smokers to report having accessed SSSs in the past (AOR 1.43, 95% CI 1.08 to 1.90) and intending to take up these services in future (AOR 1.51, 95% CI 1.14 to 2.00). Dual users of combustible tobacco and NRT showed similar associations. Secondary objectives provided evidence on key psychosocial factors that influenced smokers' decision-making in this area. In summary, despite speculation that e-cigarette use might deter smokers from accessing SSSs, our study found dual users of tobacco and e-cigarettes were more likely to report uptake of such services, compared to smokers not using e-cigarettes.

Keywords: electronic cigarettes; e-cigarettes; smoking; tobacco; addiction; addictive behavior; health services; access to healthcare

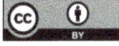

1. Introduction

The last decade has seen major shifts in smokers' behaviours relating to nicotine consumption and smoking cessation. Behavioural counselling, for instance (the most effective route known for quitting smoking when combined with licensed pharmacotherapy) [1,2], has experienced sustained declines in uptake. In England, the stop smoking services (SSSs) that provide such support to smokers have seen attendance rates drop year-on-year for almost a full decade [3], a decline mirrored in equivalent services across the EU [4]. Over a similar timeframe, the prevalence of regular e-cigarette use has increased in the UK from an estimated 700,000 people in 2012 to an estimated 3.6 million in 2021 [5], and it has been suggested these diverging trends in use of e-cigarettes and SSSs may be linked [6–8]. In other words, declines in service uptake could be related to increases in vaping prevalence. This hypothesis is the subject of recurrent debate given its important public health implications; after all, if e-cigarettes suppress uptake of behavioural support, this may exacerbate smoking-related health inequalities (SSSs are notably effective at supporting smokers from lower socioeconomic groups to quit) [1,9]. Similarly, although there is a growing evidence base about the relative level of effectiveness of using e-cigarettes in a smoking cessation attempt [10–13], researchers and policy-makers remain keen to monitor connected issues with potential public health impacts. Growing research has focused, for instance, on the prevalence of vaping amongst non-smoking adolescents, potential health harms posed by long-term use of e-cigarettes, or support for ex-smokers to quit ongoing vaping.

The role that e-cigarettes play within the smoking cessation sector thus remains highly topical and subject to wide differences internationally in terms of policy, guidance and regulations [14]. In England, SSSs are not permitted to prescribe e-cigarettes, so do not offer them to clients in the same way that they currently provide behavioural support and access to NRT as part of their standard provision. The English National Institute for Health and Care Excellence (NICE) recommends professionals advise that e-cigarettes, while substantially less harmful than smoking, are not risk-free [15]. Specific guidance for SSSs issued by key professional organisations has recognised that behavioural support is most crucial for improving odds of quitting and has recommended SSS practitioners can work with smokers who wish to use their own e-cigarettes alongside SSS support [10,16,17]. Yet, among smokers who vape, SSS attendance rates have been far lower than amongst other smokers [18]. Some smokers who would otherwise have accessed SSSs may therefore be choosing to try quitting through the less effective route of vaping alone, either out of personal preference or due to local services being reduced. Several councils have even posited the popularity of e-cigarettes as part of a rationale for decommissioning local SSSs entirely [19–21].

Qualitative studies in this area suggest that smokers, particularly from disadvantaged backgrounds, are influenced by both internal and external factors when deciding whether to attend SSSs [22–24]. Beliefs about the effectiveness of SSSs appear particularly influential, as well as fears about how smokers will be received or welcomed by the services (including their expectations of being judged by practitioners, for instance). Meanwhile, qualitative research on e-cigarettes has generally studied them in isolation from other quit methods. Little is known, for instance, about how smokers' knowledge and beliefs about vaping could relate to their decision-making around other smoking cessation options.

Similarly, research has only recently begun to explore whether vaping amongst smokers may be specifically affecting behavioural support uptake, with mixed findings. A recent UK prospective study suggested that, amongst smokers making a "serious quit attempt", use of e-cigarettes was associated with reduced likelihood of specifically using behavioural support or prescription medication [25]. Although conclusions that can be drawn from cross-sectional or ecological research are more limited, available studies have found different results. An earlier UK time series analysis found no clear evidence for population-level associations between e-cigarette use and behavioural support uptake [26]. A cross-sectional US survey meanwhile suggested that amongst dual users of combustible tobacco and e-cigarettes almost all age groups were as likely to access such support as other smokers [27].

None of these studies were designed to assess possible sociodemographic interactions, however, or mechanistic associations with related knowledge and beliefs. In fact, no studies outside the US have examined sociodemographic differences in behavioural support uptake amongst smokers using e-cigarettes. Furthermore, no studies anywhere have examined such smokers' intended future SSS use—a variable with clear implications for the long-term viability of these particularly effective services—or to control for important beliefs and knowledge that could also influence service uptake. Our study therefore aimed to examine whether e-cigarette use (and NRT use as a comparator) were associated with past and planned SSS uptake among smokers. Secondary objectives were to explore potential sociodemographic differences in these outcomes, as well as the kinds of knowledge and beliefs about e-cigarettes and SSSs that were associated with them.

2. Methods

2.1. Design

This repeat cross-sectional study's data were collected through the Smoking Toolkit Study (STS), a monthly survey dating back to 2006 [28]. STS sampling is a hybrid between random location and quota: small output areas of approximately 200 households are stratified by geodemographic ordering of the population and randomly selected. Trained interviewers are assigned pre-specified quotas to fulfil, tailored to the areas, before undertaking face-to-face interviews with single members of households. Recruitment is from the general population, with each monthly dataset involving approximately 1700 adults (16+). Previous research demonstrates the STS's national representativeness [28].

2.2. Study Population

This research was approved by the appropriate ethics committees (see 'Institutional Review Board Statement') and conformed to the principles embodied in the Declaration of Helsinki. Data were collected between February and November 2017 from 13,735 English adults, with each monthly dataset providing a unique sample of individuals (no repeat interviews occurred). The study sample was created from those 2313 respondents, pooled from the multiple months, who responded to the question "Which of the following best applies to you?" by selecting either "I smoke cigarettes (including hand-rolled) every day", "I smoke cigarettes (including hand-rolled), but not every day" or "I do not smoke cigarettes at all, but I do smoke tobacco of some kind (e.g., pipe, cigar or shisha)".

2.3. Measures

2.3.1. Measurement of e-Cigarette/NRT Use

All questions and response options are detailed in the study's questionnaire (Supplementary Material S1). Existing STS questions provided data on current use of e-cigarettes and/or NRT. As with previous studies incorporating STS data [26,29,30], these concepts were measured via three separate questions to capture all relevant smokers and maximise accuracy ("Do you regularly use any of the following in situations when you are not allowed to smoke?", "Are you using any of the following either to help you stop smoking, to help you cut down or for any other reason at all?", "Which, if any, of the following are you currently using to help you cut down the amount you smoke?"). Current e-cigarette use was defined as selecting 'Electronic cigarette' from the possible responses to any of these questions, with current NRT use defined as choosing any of the nicotine products listed: nicotine gum, nicotine lozenge, nicotine patch, nicotine inhaler\inhalator, another nicotine product or nicotine mouthspray. Respondents selected multiple products if relevant.

2.3.2. Measurement of Outcomes

Primary outcome variables were previous SSS use ('past uptake') and future intention to access services ('planned uptake'), measured by asking "Have you ever sought help from an NHS stop smoking service at any point in the past?" and "How likely or unlikely are you to consider seeking help from your NHS stop smoking service at any point in the future?". The latter was a single-item measure with five response options; for analysis and interpretation, data were dichotomised to reflect any intention to access services ("Very likely" or "Fairly likely") versus no intention ("Very unlikely", "Fairly unlikely" or "Neither likely nor unlikely").

2.3.3. Measurement of Potential Confounders

Our analysis plan specified confounders a priori, with the exception of two sensitivity analyses outlined below. Existing STS questions provided data on sociodemographics and smoking-related factors. Sociodemographics included age, gender, ethnicity (dichotomised into white versus non-white) and social grade (dichotomised into ABC1 versus C2DE). The established 'Motivation To Stop Scale' (MTSS) recorded intention to quit smoking ("Which of the following best describes you?", dichotomised into "I REALLY want to stop smoking and intend to in the next month", "I REALLY want to stop smoking and intend to in the next 3 months" or "I want to stop smoking and hope to soon" versus "I REALLY want to stop smoking but I don't know when I will", "I want to stop smoking but haven't thought about when", "I think I should stop smoking but don't really want to" or "I don't want to stop smoking") [31]. The established 'Heaviness of Smoking Index' (HSI) assessed nicotine dependence [32]. Past year quit attempts were assessed by asking "How many serious attempts to stop smoking have you made in the last 12 months?" (dichotomised into zero attempts versus 1+ attempts).

Data were also collected on knowledge and beliefs that could potentially influence SSS attendance or e-cigarette use. Participants were asked: "To what extent do you agree or disagree with each of the following statements?". Statements covered potential facilitators and barriers to uptake of the respective quit methods, including perceived ease of use/access and reporting of peer precedents who had tried them (see Supplementary Material S1 for comprehensive list of statements).

Responses, based on five-point Likert scales, were dichotomised into "Strongly agree" or "Tend to agree" versus "Neither agree nor disagree", "Tend to disagree" or "Strongly disagree". Responses to the question "Out of these two approaches for quitting smoking, which do you think would be more likely to help someone to quit?" were dichotomised into "Getting support from NHS SSSs" versus "Using e-cigarettes" or "Both equally likely". Finally, participants reporting previous SSS uptake were asked "Overall, to what extent did you find the NHS SSS you attended helpful or not for your efforts to quit smoking?" (responses dichotomised into "Very helpful" or "Fairly helpful", versus "Not very helpful" or "Not at all helpful").

2.4. Testing of Questions

Seventeen members of the public with varied experiences of smoking, using e-cigarettes/NRT and accessing SSSs were recruited purposively at the research's outset for face validity testing of the new survey questions proposed. These people reviewed draft questions by email and provided written feedback on their overall merits, as well as any specific wording within them that could be clearer. Seven subject matter experts (tobacco researchers, national policy-makers, survey specialists and SSS staff) were consulted in the same way.

2.5. Statistical Analyses

Our planned analyses and sample size calculation were pre-registered publicly on Open Science Framework (www.osf.io/ur3j8, accessed on 30 August 2022). Descriptive statistics were produced for sociodemographic and smoking-related variables, with chi-squared and t tests undertaken to examine potential differences in these by use of e-cigarettes or NRT (Table 1). Final analyses investigated the impact of dual use (of combustible tobacco and e-cigarettes or NRT respectively) on SSS uptake (past or planned respectively), adjusting for smoking-related and sociodemographic co-variables. These furthermore assessed interactions between the dual use variables and key sociodemographics (age, gender, social grade, ethnicity) on past or planned SSS uptake.

Analyses were structured as follows. First, multivariable logistic regression models (M1) were produced for exploratory analyses of knowledge and beliefs concerning e-cigarettes and SSSs. These examined the impact of each knowledge/belief variable in turn on SSS uptake (past and planned respectively), after adjusting for smoking-related and demographic co-variables. Secondly, we developed unadjusted logistic regression models (M2) examining the impact of the dual use variables on the SSS uptake variables to provide crude odds ratios (ORs). Thirdly, we developed fully adjusted models (M3) examining the impact of each dual use variable in turn on each SSS uptake variable, after adjusting for a priori variables and statistically significant knowledge/belief variables ($p < 0.05$) identified in M1, in order to produce final adjusted ORs with 95% CIs. In a further stage, we also examined interactions between each dual use variable and key sociodemographic variable (socioeconomic status, age, gender, ethnicity) on each SSS uptake variable. This involved developing a series of different 'interaction' models—each model having the interaction term in question (e.g., dual use of combustible tobacco and e-cigarettes x gender)—which adjusted for all a priori and other statistically significant variables (as in M3). Following these pre-registered analyses, some unplanned sensitivity analyses explored, in the M3 models, the impact of including two potentially relevant further variables: use of NRT (when examining dual combustible tobacco/e-cigarette use) or e-cigarettes (when examining dual combustible tobacco/NRT use), as well as past SSS uptake (when examining planned SSS uptake). Analyses were undertaken using SPSS v24.

Table 1. Sample characteristics by dual use of combustible tobacco/e-cigarettes or combustible tobacco/NRT.

	All Smokers	Dual e-Cig/Tobacco Use		p *	Dual NRT/Tobacco Use		p *	Tobacco Use Only		p *
		Yes	No		Yes	No		Yes	No	
All smokers	-	18.2%	81.8%	<0.001 *	10.2%	89.8%	<0.001 *	74.1%	25.9%	<0.001 *
			Demographic characteristics							
Age, Mean (SD)	43.5 (17.3)	43.0 (16.5)	43.6 (17.5)	0.555	47.0 (16.9)	43.1 (17.3)	0.001 *	43.1 (17.4)	44.6 (16.9)	0.086
Female	49.7%	50.9%	49.4%	0.590	54.3%	49.1%	0.147	48.6%	52.6%	0.109
White	90.0%	93.2%	89.3%	0.019 *	90.1%	90.0%	0.961	89.1%	92.6%	0.018 *
Social grade C2DE	56.7%	54.6%	57.2%	0.359	54.3%	57.0%	0.439	57.3%	55.0%	0.352
No 16+ qualifications	60.9%	61.7%	60.8%	0.747	60.5%	61.0%	0.896	60.6%	61.9%	0.585
With disability	17.4%	18.9%	17.1%	0.381	22.4%	16.9%	0.038 *	16.5%	20.0%	0.058
Heterosexual	87.4%	89.4%	87.0%	0.191	82.5%	88.0%	0.020 *	87.6%	86.9%	0.653
Region: North	32.2%	36.8%	31.1%	0.027 *	25.6%	32.9%	0.026 *	32.2%	32.1%	0.971
Central	29.7%	29.1%	29.8%	0.764	29.1%	29.8%	0.851	29.7%	29.6%	0.969
South	38.1%	34.1%	39.1%	0.065	45.3%	37.3%	0.020 *	38.1%	38.3%	0.943
			Smoking characteristics							
Intent to quit smoking	33.1%	51.6%	29.0%	<0.001 *	58.3%	30.3%	<0.001 *	25.9%	53.8%	<0.001 *
Past year quit attempt	29.9%	50.9%	25.2%	<0.001 *	59.2%	26.6%	<0.001 *	21.7%	53.3%	<0.001 *
HSI Index, Mean (SD)	1.72 (1.51)	1.78 (1.43)	1.71 (1.53)	0.382	1.79 (1.49)	1.71 (1.51)	0.484	1.71 (1.52)	1.77 (1.47)	0.374

NRT: nicotine replacement therapy; SD: Standard deviation; C2DE: small employers and own account workers, lower supervisory and technical occupations, semi-routine and routine occupations, never workers and long-term unemployed (ABC1: managerial, professional and intermediate occupations); North: North East, North West, Yorkshire and Humber; Central: East Midlands, West Midlands, East of England; South: London, South East, South West; HSI: Heaviness of Smoking Index (index ranges from 0 to 6: the higher the score, the higher the dependence on nicotine); Tobacco use only: current smokers of combustible tobacco with no current use of e-cigarettes or NRT. *: statistically significant ($p < 0.05$).

3. Results

3.1. Sample Characteristics

Out of 2313 smokers interviewed, complete data on key co-variables (HSI, age and gender) was provided by 2189 (94.5%). Those excluded due to missing data (5.0% HSI, 0.4% age, 0.1% gender) were significantly less likely to be white or female ($p < 0.05$) than those remaining. Both groups of dual users were likelier than other smokers to report a quit smoking attempt within the previous year and a future quit intention. Dual users of combustible tobacco/e-cigarettes were similar to other smokers in most sociodemographic characteristics (Table 1), but were significantly likelier to be white or Northern England residents. Dual users of combustible tobacco/NRT were significantly older than other smokers and likelier to have a disability or to be Southern England residents, but less likely to be heterosexual or Northern England residents.

18.2% of participants (399/2189) were currently using e-cigarettes, 10.2% (223/2189) were using NRT and 74.1% were using neither (1622/2189). 21.6% of participants (472/2189) had accessed SSSs previously and 23.2% (508/2189) planned to do so in future.

3.2. Knowledge and Beliefs Regarding e-Cigarettes and SSSs (M1)

In the M1 analyses of knowledge and belief variables (see Supplementary Material S2 for comprehensive findings), having accessed SSSs in the past and planning to do so in future were associated with knowing people who used e-cigarettes (AOR = 1.79, 95% CI: 1.35–2.38 for past uptake and AOR = 1.43, 95% CI: 1.09–1.88 for planned uptake) and thinking that e-cigarettes were less effective than SSSs (AOR = 1.33, 95% CI: 1.06–1.65 for past uptake and AOR = 2.35, 95% CI: 1.89–2.93 for planned uptake). Past use of SSSs was also associated with knowing how to use e-cigarettes (AOR = 2.01, 95% CI: 1.54–2.63).

Furthermore, having accessed SSSs in the past and planning to do so in future were associated with: knowing people who had used SSSs (AOR = 3.39, 95% CI: 2.71–4.24 for past uptake and AOR = 1.59, 95% CI: 1.27–1.99 for planned uptake); thinking that SSSs were a convenient way to quit smoking (AOR = 1.73, 95% CI: 1.39–2.16 for past uptake and AOR = 3.07, 95% CI: 2.43–3.87 for planned uptake); knowing how to access SSSs (AOR = 4.66, 95% CI: 3.25–6.69 for past uptake and AOR = 2.00, 95% CI: 1.49–2.68 for planned uptake); and thinking they would be made to feel welcome by SSSs (AOR = 1.99, 95% CI: 1.53–2.58 for past uptake and AOR = 2.91, 95% CI: 2.19–3.87 for planned uptake). Planned uptake was also associated with having found past use of SSSs helpful (AOR = 5.61, 95% CI: 3.57–8.82); thinking dual users of e-cigarettes and combustible tobacco were eligible for SSSs (AOR = 1.32, 95% CI: 1.06–1.63); and thinking lots of time was needed to access SSSs (AOR = 0.61, 95% CI: 0.47–0.79; NB: inversely associated, unlike the others).

3.3. Past and Planned Uptake of SSSs (M2&3)

In the M2 unadjusted analyses (Tables 2 and 3), dual users of combustible tobacco/e-cigarettes were more likely than other smokers to report past (OR 1.93, 95% CI: 1.51–2.45) and planned SSS uptake (OR 1.53, 95% CI: 1.20–1.95). Dual users of combustible tobacco/NRT were also more likely than other smokers to report past (OR 2.93, 95% CI: 2.20–3.91) and planned SSS uptake (OR 3.04, 95% CI: 2.28–4.04). After adjustment for demographic, smoking-related, and knowledge/belief variables in M3, these associations all remained statistically significant (Tables 2 and 3).

Table 2. E-cigarette or NRT use and past uptake of SSSs amongst current smokers of combustible tobacco.

		Past Uptake of SSSs		
		% [n]	OR [95% CI]	AOR [95% CI]
Dual e-cig/tobacco use	No	19.3% (346/1790)	1.00	1.00
	Yes	31.6% (126/399)	1.93 (1.51–2.45)	1.43 (1.08–1.90)
Dual NRT/tobacco use	No	19.3% (380/1966)	1.00	1.00
	Yes	41.3% (92/223)	2.93 (2.20–3.91)	2.10 (1.51–2.93)

Table 3. E-cigarette or NRT use and planned uptake of SSSs amongst current smokers of combustible tobacco.

		Planned Uptake of SSSs		
		% [n]	OR [95% CI]	AOR [95% CI]
Dual e-cig/tobacco use	No	21.7% (389/1790)	1.00	1.00
	Yes	29.8% (119/399)	1.53 (1.20–1.95)	1.51 (1.14–2.00)
Dual NRT/tobacco use	No	20.8% (409/1966)	1.00	1.00
	Yes	44.4% (99/223)	3.04 (2.28–4.04)	2.30 (1.66–3.18)

There were no interactions between use and social grade, age or ethnicity for any outcomes. A significant interaction was observed for gender with dual combustible tobacco/NRT use on planned SSS uptake. For females, dual combustible tobacco/NRT use was associated with significantly increased odds of intending to access SSSs (OR 3.40, 95% CI: 2.19–5.28), which was not observed with males (OR 1.45, 95% CI: 0.90–2.35). Similar gender interactions were not evident with other outcomes. In sensitivity analyses further adjusted for NRT use, e-cigarette use or past SSS uptake, results were very similar: dual combustible tobacco/e-cigarette users remained likelier than other smokers to have accessed SSSs previously (AOR 1.43, 95% CI: 1.08–1.91) and to plan future uptake (AOR 1.40, 95% CI: 1.05–1.88), as did dual combustible tobacco/NRT users (past SSS uptake: AOR 2.10, 95% CI: 1.51–2.93; planned uptake: AOR 2.03, 95% CI: 1.45–2.84).

4. Discussion

Amongst current smokers, those also using either e-cigarettes or NRT were more likely to report having accessed SSSs in the past and intending to access services in future. To our knowledge, this research is the first of its kind to combine data on e-cigarette use with data about both past and planned behavioural support uptake. It therefore has particular relevance to current debates around the popularity of e-cigarettes and their potential impact on smokers' decisions regarding cessation services. Another key strength is its use of a representative sample of the English population. Through our secondary objectives, we also generated evidence on what knowledge and beliefs influence smokers when deciding whether or not to access behavioural support, the most effective route available to quitting smoking.

Limitations of our study include the need for some caution when generalising our findings to other populations. Many countries regulate e-cigarettes differently to England, while models of behavioural support available to smokers also vary internationally [14]. Although cross-sectional associations can still be indicative and important for guiding future research, they need to be interpreted with caution given the potential for biases and unknown confounders. For example, we relied—in part—on data gathered using novel questions as there were no relevant established questionnaires from which to take our new questions regarding SSS uptake (though face validity was tested beforehand with a range of smokers reporting varying uptake of different quit routes). It is thus possible that our finding of a positive association between the different dual use variables and planned SSS uptake reflects residual confounding—e.g., it may be caused by smokers' general motivation to quit smoking more than anything particularly related to SSSs, or by other unidentified confounders. The 'intention to quit' concept was, however, captured by the MTSS—an established, validated tool used regularly for broader published analyses of STS data—and was also adjusted for within all our analyses [26,29–31]. Finally, social desirability bias may have influenced reported future actions. Larger studies could attempt to tackle this by following up respondents over time and assessing how far intentions to access services translate into genuine uptake. Similarly, sociodemographic differences in choice of quit routes, including behavioural support, remain a valuable area for further research.

This study nonetheless provides important new evidence in an area—associations between e-cigarette use and behavioural support uptake—where a clear understanding has yet to be established. Our findings suggest a modest positive association, with smokers using e-cigarettes or NRT significantly more likely than other smokers to have accessed services previously and to plan future use of them. A plausible explanation is that, given most smokers using e-cigarettes or NRT do so in an attempt to quit smoking [12], the increased reports of past and planned SSS uptake among these groups may reflect willingness to consider other quit methods beyond e-cigarettes/NRT. It also likely reflects that some previous SSS attenders will have been introduced to e-cigarettes or NRT by services directly, and given advice by practitioners, leading to more sustained use of such products compared to non-attenders. Indeed, further research could usefully examine how often such e-cigarette use following English SSS attendance is continuing long-term, given the conclusion of a recent systematic review in this area that "use of e-cigarettes as a therapeutic intervention for smoking cessation may lead to permanent nicotine dependence" [33]. Future intentions to access services in current users of e-cigarettes or NRT may similarly reflect at least in part the fact that some of these smokers will have been introduced to these products through previous use of such services. Cross-sectional research is inevitably limited in conclusions it can draw regarding the temporal or causal nature of such relationships. Our sensitivity analyses did however adjust for past use of services when examining future use (as outlined in 'Results'), with very similar results to main analyses. Alternatively, experiences with other satisfying nicotine products may stimulate thoughts about quitting and boost self-efficacy. Finally, this phenomenon may link to financial considerations. In numerous studies, smokers report lower costs of e-cigarettes, compared to combustible cigarettes, as a major incentive for use, while it has also been shown that subsidised NRT offered by SSSs is positively associated with quit attempts [34,35]. It is thus plausible that smokers motivated to attempt switching from combustible tobacco to e-cigarettes or NRT for economic reasons may be attracted to this SSS offer of subsidised pharmacotherapy. Our findings align with some aforementioned studies that have not found e-cigarette use to be associated with depressed uptake of behavioural support [26,27]. Conversely, an English study found in an unplanned analysis that dual users of tobacco/e-cigarettes were significantly less likely than dual users of tobacco/NRT to specifically use behavioural support or prescription medication, though the two groups did not differ in their overall use of evidence-based cessation aids [25]. This mixed evidence base could result from differences in study designs, since Beard et al. employed a prospective cohort design [25]. Alternatively, it could reflect the fact that this previous study combined prescription medication with behavioural support, whereas our own isolated the latter. Either way, further studies in other settings directly comparing dual e-cigarette/tobacco use against dual tobacco/NRT use would be valuable given such statistical analyses were not a primary focus of our own. Our study does concur though with Beard et al.'s assertion that a clearer picture in this area requires a greater understanding of the perceptions and motivations of smokers in relation to e-cigarettes and other quit routes.

Our own study provides some further early insights in relation to that specific need, marking an important quantitative contribution to the largely qualitative evidence base on what factors motivate smokers' choices of quit routes. Despite the earlier caveat regarding the challenges of investigating temporal relationships via cross-sectional research, this study to our knowledge, still constitutes the only quantitative study to date to examine how knowledge and beliefs about e-cigarettes may be influencing uptake of behavioural support. This is particularly salient given the aforementioned ongoing debate as to whether e-cigarettes' popularity could be depressing uptake of more effective routes to quitting combustible tobacco [4,6,18]. Smokers in our adjusted analyses who reported having acquaintances who used e-cigarettes were more likely to have accessed SSSs in the past and to plan to do so in future, while past SSS use was also associated with reported knowledge of how to use e-cigarettes oneself. This result aligns with recent survey findings that exposure to other people's e-cigarette use may have some effects on smokers' quitting motivation and behaviour [36]—perhaps by normalising attempts to quit—as well as with broader research suggesting e-cigarettes are not viewed by smokers as being in competition with, or mutually exclusive from behavioural support [26,27]. Indeed, recent studies have indicated that both current and ex-smoking vapers have an appetite to access other forms of treatment such as behavioural support [37,38]. Our findings further show that reported knowledge and beliefs about vaping have significant associations with planned SSS uptake, including the perception that dual users of e-cigarettes and tobacco are eligible for SSS support. Future research could therefore consider exploring whether or not changing these beliefs about eligibility for SSSs—for instance, through the provision of clearer information to the public about SSS eligibility criteria—may potentially influence intentions to access these services. Similarly, further studies could consider investigating whether or not social connections with other vapers potentially influence knowledge of different quit routes and normalise quitting behaviour, perhaps through discussions with these friend and family 'precedents'.

5. Conclusions

Our study has clear relevance for ongoing debates about the relationship between e-cigarette use, NRT use and the uptake and provision of other quit methods including behavioural support. It has been suggested, for instance, that widespread e-cigarette use may be reducing the need for SSSs, an argument that has formed part of the rationale for cutting such services in a number of English local authorities [19–21]. Our findings do not support this argument; rather than wanting to 'go it alone', a proportion of smokers in our sample remained keen to receive additional support to quit from SSSs even when already using e-cigarettes. Instead of assuming that long-term declines in SSS attendance are primarily linked to e-cigarette use, alternative explanations should thus also be considered. Future research should explore, for example, the potential role that may be being played by significant cuts in recent years to the local authority public health budgets that fund such services.

Supplementary Materials: The following supporting information can be downloaded at: https://www.mdpi.com/article/10.3390/toxics10100593/s1, Supplementary Material S1: full list of questions and response options; Supplementary Material S2: full model 1 results.

Author Contributions: Conceptualization and design, G.H., M.E., J.B. and M.P.; methodology, all authors; data curation and analysis, G.H.; writing—original draft preparation, G.H.; writing—review and editing, all authors. All authors have read and agreed to the published version of the manuscript.

Funding: G.H. was supported by a Health Education England (HEE) and National Institute for Health Research (NIHR) ICA Programme Clinical Doctoral Research Fellowship (ICA-CDRF-2015-01-017). M.P. and M.E.'s research was funded by the NIHR School for Public Health Research (SPHR). This paper presents independent research funded by the National Institute for Health Research (NIHR) and NIHR School for Public Health Research (SPHR). Cancer Research UK funded additional data collection and J.B.'s salary (C1417/A22962).

Institutional Review Board Statement: Ethical approval for the Smoking Toolkit Study was granted originally by the UCL Ethics Committee (ID 0498/001). This project received further ethical approval from the LSHTM Observational Research Ethics Committee (reference 11672). The data were not collected by UCL or LSHTM and were anonymised when received by LSHTM.

Informed Consent Statement: Informed consent was obtained from all subjects involved in the study.

Data Availability Statement: The datasets used and analysed during the current study are available from the corresponding author on reasonable request.

Conflicts of Interest: All authors have completed the Unified Competing Interest form (available on request from the corresponding author) and declare that: JB has received unrestricted research funding from Pfizer, who manufacture smoking cessation medications, but declares no financial links with tobacco companies or e-cigarette manufacturers or their representatives. All authors declare there are no other relationships or activities that could appear to have influenced the submitted work. The funders had no role in the design of the study; in the collection, analyses, or interpretation of data; in the writing of the manuscript; or in the decision to publish the results. The views expressed are those of the authors and not necessarily those of the NHS, the NIHR or the Department of Health and Social Care.

References

1. West, R.; May, S.; West, M.; Croghan, E.; McEwen, A. Performance of English stop smoking services in first 10 years: Analysis of service monitoring data. *BMJ* **2013**, *347*, f4921. [CrossRef]
2. West, R. *Stop Smoking Services: Increased Chances of Quitting*; NCSCT: London, UK, 2012. Available online: http://www.ncsct.co.uk/publication_Stop_smoking_services_impact_on_quitting.php (accessed on 30 August 2022).
3. NHS Digital. Statistics on NHS Stop Smoking Services in England—April 2020 to March 2021. Available online: https://digital.nhs.uk/data-and-information/publications/statistical/statistics-on-nhs-stop-smoking-services-in-england/april-2020-to-march-2021 (accessed on 30 August 2022).
4. Filippidis, F.T.; Laverty, A.A.; Mons, U.; Jimenez-Ruiz, C.; Vardavas, C.I. Changes in smoking cessation assistance in the European Union between 2012 and 2017: Pharmacotherapy versus counselling versus e-cigarettes. *Tob. Control* **2019**, *28*, 95. [CrossRef] [PubMed]
5. Action on Smoking and Health. Use of E-Cigarettes among Adults in Great Britain. 2021. Available online: https://ash.org.uk/information-and-resources/fact-sheets/statistical/use-of-e-cigarettes-among-adults-in-great-britain-2021/ (accessed on 30 August 2022).
6. Britton, J. Electronic cigarettes and smoking cessation in England. *BMJ* **2016**, *354*, i4819. [CrossRef] [PubMed]
7. Iacobucci, G. Stop smoking services: BMJ analysis shows how councils are stubbing them out. *BMJ* **2018**, *362*, k3649. [CrossRef] [PubMed]
8. McNeill, A.; Brose, L.S.; Calder, R.; Bauld, L.; Robson, D. *Vaping in England: An Evidence Update February 2019*; Public Health England: London, UK, 2019. Available online: https://assets.publishing.service.gov.uk/government/uploads/system/uploads/attachment_data/file/781748/Vaping_in_England_an_evidence_update_February_2019.pdf (accessed on 30 August 2022).

9. Smith, C.E.; Hill, S.E.; Amos, A. Impact of specialist and primary care stop smoking support on socio-economic inequalities in cessation in the United Kingdom: A systematic review and national equity analysis. *Addiction* 2020, *115*, 34–46. [CrossRef]
10. Cancer Research UK; RCGP. *Joint Position Statement on E-Cigarettes*; CRUK: London, UK, 2017. Available online: https://www.cancerresearchuk.org/health-professional/awareness-and-prevention/e-cigarette-hub-information-for-health-professionals/e-cigarette-statement (accessed on 30 August 2022).
11. National Academies of Sciences. *Public Health Consequences of E-Cigarettes*; National Academies: Washington, DC, USA, 2018. [CrossRef]
12. McNeill, A.; Brose, L.S.; Calder, R.; Simonavicius, E.; Robson, D. *Vaping in England: 2021 Evidence Update Summary*; Public Health England: London, UK, 2021. Available online: https://www.gov.uk/government/publications/vaping-in-england-evidence-update-february-2021/vaping-in-england-2021-evidence-update-summary (accessed on 30 August 2022).
13. Hartmann-Boyce, J.; McRobbie, H.; Butler, A.R.; Lindson, N.; Bullen, C.; Begh, R.; Theodoulou, A.; Notley, C.; Rigotti, N.A.; Turner, T.; et al. Electronic cigarettes for smoking cessation. *Cochrane Database Syst. Rev.* 2021, *9*, CD010216. [CrossRef]
14. Kennedy, R.D.; Awopegba, A.; De León, E.; Cohen, J.E. Global approaches to regulating electronic cigarettes. *Tob. Control* 2017, *26*, 440. [CrossRef]
15. NICE. Tobacco: Preventing Uptake, Promoting Quitting and Treating Dependence. 2021. Available online: https://www.nice.org.uk/guidance/ng209/chapter/recommendations-on-treating-tobacco-dependence (accessed on 30 August 2022).
16. National Centre for Smoking Cessation and Training. Electronic Cigarettes: A Briefing for Stop Smoking Services. 2016. Available online: http://www.ncsct.co.uk/publication_electronic_cigarette_briefing.php (accessed on 30 August 2022).
17. Public Health England. *E-Cigarettes: A Developing Public Health Consensus*; Public Health England: London, UK, 2016.
18. Public Health England. Seizing the Opportunity: E-Cigarettes and Stop Smoking Services—Linking the Most Popular with the Most Effective. Available online: https://publichealthmatters.blog.gov.uk/2018/03/21/seizing-the-opportunity-e-cigarettes-and-stop-smoking-services-linking-the-most-popular-with-the-most-effective/ (accessed on 30 August 2022).
19. *Feeling the Heat: The Decline of Stop Smoking Services in England*; CRUK & ASH: London, UK, 2018. Available online: https://www.cancerresearchuk.org/sites/default/files/la_survey_report_2017.pdf (accessed on 30 August 2022).
20. Pulse. Councils Cut Hundreds of Thousands of Pounds from Stop Smoking Services. 2016. Available online: http://www.pulsetoday.co.uk/clinical/clinical-specialties/respiratory-/councils-cuthundreds-of-thousands-of-pounds-from-stop-smoking-services/20030905.article (accessed on 30 August 2022).
21. Hopkinson, N.S. The prominence of e-cigarettes is a symptom of decades of failure to tackle smoking properly. *BMJ* 2019, *364*, l647. [CrossRef]
22. Benson, F.E.; Stronks, K.; Willemsen, M.C.; Bogaerts, N.M.; Nierkens, V. Wanting to attend isn't just wanting to quit: Why some disadvantaged smokers regularly attend smoking cessation behavioural therapy while others do not: A qualitative study. *BMC Public Health* 2014, *14*, 695. [CrossRef]
23. Roddy, E.; Antoniak, M.; Britton, J.; Molyneux, A.; Lewis, S. Barriers and motivators to gaining access to smoking cessation services amongst deprived smokers—A qualitative study. *BMC Health Serv. Res.* 2006, *6*, 147. [CrossRef]
24. Murray, R.L.; Bauld, L.; Hackshaw, L.E.; McNeill, A. Improving access to smoking cessation services for disadvantaged groups: A systematic review. *J. Public Health* 2009, *31*, 258–277. [CrossRef]
25. Jackson, S.E.; Farrow, E.; Brown, J.; Shahab, L. Is dual use of nicotine products and cigarettes associated with smoking reduction and cessation behaviours? A prospective study in England. *BMJ Open* 2020, *10*, e036055. [CrossRef] [PubMed]
26. Beard, E.; West, R.; Michie, S.; Brown, J. Association between electronic cigarette use and changes in quit attempts, success of quit attempts, use of smoking cessation pharmacotherapy, and use of stop smoking services in England: Time series analysis of population trends. *BMJ* 2016, *354*, i4645. [CrossRef]
27. Salloum, R.G.; Lee, J.H.; Porter, M.; Dallery, J.; McDaniel, A.M.; Bian, J.; Thrasher, J. Evidence-based tobacco treatment utilization among dual users of cigarettes and E-cigarettes. *Prev. Med.* 2018, *114*, 193–199. [CrossRef] [PubMed]
28. Fidler, J.A.; Shahab, L.; West, O.; Jarvis, M.J.; McEwen, A.; Stapleton, J.A.; Vangeli, E.; West, R. "The smoking toolkit study": A national study of smoking and smoking cessation in England. *BMC Public Health* 2011, *11*, 479. [CrossRef] [PubMed]
29. Beard, E.; Brown, J.; McNeill, A.; Michie, S.; West, R. Has growth in electronic cigarette use by smokers been responsible for the decline in use of licensed nicotine products? Findings from repeated cross-sectional surveys. *Thorax* 2015, *70*, 974. [CrossRef] [PubMed]
30. Beard, E.; Brown, J.; Michie, S.; West, R. Is prevalence of e-cigarette and nicotine replacement therapy use among smokers associated with average cigarette consumption in England? A time-series analysis. *BMJ Open* 2018, *8*, e016046. [CrossRef] [PubMed]
31. Kotz, D.; Brown, J.; West, R. Predictive validity of the Motivation To Stop Scale (MTSS): A single-item measure of motivation to stop smoking. *Drug Alcohol Depend.* 2013, *128*, 15–19. [CrossRef] [PubMed]
32. Borland, R.; Yong, H.H.; O'Connor, R.J.; Hyland, A.; Thompson, M.E. The reliability and predictive validity of the Heaviness of Smoking Index and its two components: Findings from the International Tobacco Control Four Country study. *Nicotine Tob. Res.* 2010, *12*, S45–S50. [CrossRef] [PubMed]
33. Hanewinkel, R.; Niederberger, K.; Pedersen, A.; Unger, J.B.; Galimov, A. E-cigarettes and nicotine abstinence: A meta-analysis of randomised controlled trials. *Eur. Respir. Rev.* 2022, *31*, 210215. [CrossRef]

34. Romijnders, K.A.G.J.; van Osch, L.; de Vries, H.; Talhout, R. Perceptions and reasons regarding e-cigarette use among users and non-users: A narrative literature review. *Int. J. Environ. Res. Public Health* **2018**, *15*, 1190. [CrossRef] [PubMed]
35. van den Brand, F.A.; Nagelhout, G.E.; Hummel, K.; Willemsen, M.C.; McNeill, A.; van Schayck, O.C.P. Does free or lower cost smoking cessation medication stimulate quitting? Findings from the International Tobacco Control (ITC) Netherlands and UK surveys. *Tob. Control* **2019**, *28*, s61. [CrossRef] [PubMed]
36. Jackson, S.E.; Beard, E.; Michie, S.; Shahab, L.; Raupach, T.; West, R.; Brown, J. Are smokers who are regularly exposed to e-cigarette use by others more or less motivated to stop or to make a quit attempt? A cross-sectional and longitudinal survey. *BMC Med.* **2018**, *16*, 206. [CrossRef] [PubMed]
37. Etter, J.-F. Are long-term vapers interested in vaping cessation support? *Addiction* **2019**, *114*, 1473–1477. [CrossRef]
38. Hajek, P.; Phillips-Waller, A.; Przulj, D.; Pesola, F.; Myers Smith, K.; Bisal, N.; Li, J.; Parrott, S.; Sasieni, P.; Dawkins, L.; et al. A Randomized Trial of E-Cigarettes versus Nicotine-Replacement Therapy. *N. Engl. J. Med.* **2019**, *380*, 629–637. [CrossRef] [PubMed]

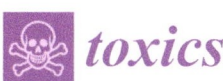

Article

e-Cigarette Vapour Condensate Reduces Viability and Impairs Function of Human Osteoblasts, in Part, via a Nicotine Dependent Mechanism

Thomas Nicholson [1], Lauren Davis [2], Edward T. Davis [3], Matthew Newton Ede [3], Aaron Scott [2,†] and Simon W. Jones [1,*,†]

1. Institute of Inflammation and Ageing, MRC-ARUK Centre for Musculoskeletal Ageing Research, Institute of Inflammation and Ageing, University of Birmingham, Birmingham B15 2TT, UK
2. Birmingham Acute Care Research Group, Institute of Inflammation and Ageing, University of Birmingham, Birmingham B15 2TT, UK
3. Royal Orthopaedic Hospital, Bristol Road South, Birmingham B15 2TT, UK
* Correspondence: s.w.jones@bham.ac.uk; Tel.: +44-121-371-3224
† Joint senior authorship.

Abstract: Cigarette consumption negatively impacts bone quality and is a risk-factor for the development of multiple bone associated disorders, due to the highly vascularised structure of bone being exposed to systemic factors. However, the impact on bone to electronic cigarette (e-cigarette) use, which contains high doses of nicotine and other compounds including flavouring chemicals, metal particulates and carbonyls, is poorly understood. Here, we present the first evidence demonstrating the impact of e-cigarette vapour condensate (replicating changes in e-cigarette liquid chemical structure that occur upon device usage), on human primary osteoblast viability and function. 24 h exposure of osteoblasts to e-cigarette vapour condensate, generated from either second or third generation devices, significantly reduced osteoblast viability in a dose dependent manner, with condensate generated from the more powerful third generation device having greater toxicity. This effect was mediated in-part by nicotine, since exposure to nicotine-free condensate of an equal concentration had a less toxic effect. The detrimental effect of e-cigarette vapour condensate on osteoblast viability was rescued by co-treatment with the antioxidant N-Acetyl-L-cysteine (NAC), indicating toxicity may also be driven by reactive species generated upon device usage. Finally, non-toxic doses of either second or third generation condensate significantly blunted osteoblast osteoprotegerin secretion after 24 h, which was sustained for up to 7 days. In summary we demonstrate that e-cigarette vapour condensate, generated from commonly used second and third generation devices, can significantly reduce osteoblast viability and impair osteoblast function, at physiologically relevant doses. These data highlight the need for further investigation to inform users of the potential risks of e-cigarette use on bone health, including, accelerating bone associated disease progression, impacting skeletal development in younger users and to advise patients following orthopaedic surgery, dental surgery, or injury to maximise bone healing.

Keywords: electronic cigarettes; osteoblast; e-cigarette; vaping; viability; bone; osteoprotegerin; human primary cells

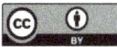

1. Introduction

Multiple meta-analyses have reported that a history of cigarette smoking is associated with significantly reduced bone mineral density (BMD), increased risk of fracture and reduced fracture healing, in comparison to age, sex and BMI-matched non-smokers [1]. It is also apparent that such smoking-associated effects are cumulative, demonstrating a positive correlation with pack year history [2–4]. Furthermore, fracture risk in smoking cohorts is greater than in non-smokers when corrected for BMD, indicating that smoking may directly impact bone architecture and quality. Indeed, a decrease in trabecular bone mass and increased trabecular separation has been reported in older smokers [5], while in younger individuals smoking is associated with a reduction in trabecular bone volume, independent of age, BMI, activity level and calcium intake [6]. Recent studies have also demonstrated that smoking is independently associated with increased post-surgery complications such as infection and aseptic loosening following arthroplasty [7–10].

While cigarette consumption has declined over the past decade, the use of electronic cigarettes (e-cigarettes) or vaping has risen dramatically, partly due to being regarded as a safer alternative to smoking, although, 8% of current EC users in the UK have never smoked a cigarette [11–13]. Increased use of e-cigarettes will undoubtedly make a significant contribution towards harm reduction in comparison to cigarettes. However, e-cigarette usage still results in systemic exposure to numerous and potentially harmful vapour constituents, particularly to highly vascularised tissues such as the bone. In support of this, Agoons et al. recently reported that e-cigarette users have a 46% higher prevalence of fractures, in comparison to those who have never used e-cigarettes based on a cohort of 4519 individuals [14].

E-cigarette vapour is much less complex than cigarette smoke, yet many harmful constituents of cigarette smoke are found in e-cigarette vapour. Upon thermal decomposition, e-liquid humectants propylene glycol (PG) and vegetable glycerine (VG) form products such as acrolein and formaldehyde, commonly termed reactive carbonyl species (RCS), which are causatively linked to systemic harm [15,16]. Furthermore, since their invention in 2003, e-cigarette device technology has developed rapidly with current 3rd generation devices capable of delivering vapour at a much higher temperature than earlier models due to larger battery sizes. Consequently, this enables greater delivery of nicotine [17–19], increasing user satisfaction but also delivering much greater amounts of harmful RCS [20–22].

As to be expected, the majority of research on e-cigarettes to date has been carried out in models relevant to the lungs. Importantly, we and others have investigated the effect of vaping constituents on lung immune cells, reporting cytotoxic, proinflammatory and anti-phagocytic effects in alveolar macrophages [15,23]. Similar reductions in neutrophil function have also been reported, including reduced neutrophil migration and phagocytosis, suppression of NETosis and increased ROS production [24]. Additionally, dysfunctional cilia beat frequency and motility has been reported in human airway epithelial cells and normal human bronchial epithelial (NHBE) cells following cigarette vapour exposure [25–28].

However, there has been limited investigation into the impact of e-cigarette usage on bone physiology, particularly following long-term use [29,30]. There are also limited in vitro data, particularly utilising human osteoblasts. Typically exhibiting a large, cuboidal morphology, osteoblasts are the primary cell type responsible for bone formation, through secretion of collagenous and non-collagenous proteins and proteoglycans that in turn become mineralised.

Utilising a novel system previously described by our group [23], we have performed the first investigation into the effect of e-cigarette vapour condensate on human primary osteoblast viability and function. Importantly, we report the comparative effects of vaping constituents generated by 2nd generation and 3rd generation devices, which together account for 77% of devices used in the UK [31]. Finally, we have utilised both nicotine containing and nicotine-free vapour condensate, in addition to the antioxidant, N-acetyl cysteine (NAC) to investigate the contribution of the vapour constituents nicotine and RCS, respectively, on osteoblast viability.

2. Materials and Methods
2.1. Ethical Approval and Subject Recruitment

Femoral heads were collected from hip osteoarthritis (OA) patients undergoing orthopaedic joint replacement surgery at the Royal Orthopaedic Hospital (Birmingham, UK).

All patient participants were recruited on a volunteer basis, after being fully informed of the study requirements by the clinical research staff, and providing written consent (NRES 16/SS/0172).

2.2. Primary Human Osteoblast Cell Culture

Trabecular bone chips (<100 mm^3) were obtained from the OA patient femoral heads using a Friedman Rongeur, washed three times in phosphate-buffered saline (PBS) [Life Technologies Ltd., Renfrew, UK] and once with high-glucose Dulbecco's Modified Eagle Medium (DMEM) to remove excess fat, blood, marrow, and connective tissue. Bone chips were then cut into small pieces (<5 mm^3) and transferred to a 25 cm^2 vented flask containing primary human osteoblast media (DMEM, 10% FBS, 100 Units/mL Penicillin Streptomycin, 2 mM L-Glutamine, 1% NEAA, 2 mM β-glycerophosphate disodium salt hydrate, 50 ug/mL L-Ascorbic Acid, 10 nM Dexamethasone). Bone chips were incubated at 37 °C and 5% CO_2 for 5 days before the initial media change. Following 5 days, differentiation media was changed every 3 days, and bone chips were removed once primary osteoblast cell coverage reached approximately 50% confluency. Upon reaching confluency, cells were passaged into a 75 cm^2 flask. For all experiments primary human osteoblasts were limited to passage 5.

2.3. e-Cigarette Devices

Two popular devices in the UK were chosen for condensate generation, a 2nd generation device and 3rd generation device from Kanger tech Ltd., (Shenzhen, China). The 2nd generation device was fitted with a standard 650 mAh battery with a fresh 1.8 Ohm atomiser for each preparation, generating 7.6 W. The 3rd generation device, the most powerful of the devices, was fitted with a 3000 mAh battery with a fresh 0.15 Ohm atomizer fitted for each preparation, generating 75 W. The same devices were used for each condensate preparation.

2.4. e-Cigarette Vapour Condensate Collection

e-cigarette vapour condensate (ECVC) or nicotine-free e-cigarette vapour condensate (nfECVC) was collected from 2nd and 3rd generation e-cigarette devices, as previously described by Scott et al. [23]. Prior to use, e-Cigarette devices were cleaned and prepared with either 36 mg/mL nicotine flavourless liquid (Durasmoke® Unflavored e-Liquid (50% PG/50% VG Base), American e-liquid Store, (Wauwatosa, WI, USA) or nicotine-free flavourless liquid (Durasmoke® Unflavored eLiquid (50% PG/50% VG Base), American e-liquid Store, (Wauwatosa, WI, USA). Next, six tracheal suction taps (Unomedical, UK) were arranged in sequence and sealed with parafilm. EC devices were attached to the open end of tap 1, while tap 6 was connected to a vacuum tap by plastic tubing. Taps 2–6 were sealed inside 30 mL universal tubes with parafilm, to provide insulation and prevent cracking upon cooling. Next insulated taps were suspended in a dry ice/methanol bath and allowed to cool, tap 1 was kept outside the bath for observation of vapour production. The optimum puff duration of 3 s (previously determined by Scott et al.) was performed every 30 s until EC liquid was exhausted. Taps were then allowed to warm to room temperature, before centrifugation (2755× g, 5 min) to collect condensate. Condensate was pooled into a single 1.5 mL Eppendorf and stored at −40 °C for a maximum of 24 h before use.

2.5. Osteoblast Challenge and Intervention

Challenge with ECVC, nfECVC, PG, VG and N-Acetyl-Cysteine (Sigma-Aldrich, St. Louis, MO, USA) were diluted in osteoblast differentiation media to concentrations detailed in individual Figure legends. Incubation periods are described per experiment as appropriate.

2.6. Primary Human Osteoblast Viability and Cellular Morphology

Osteoblast viability was determined using CellTiter 96® AQueous One Solution Cell Proliferation Assay (CTA) (Promega, UK) following the manufacturers protocol. Following addition of CTA reagent, cells were incubated in the dark for 3 h at 37 °C and 5% CO_2. Absorbance at 490 nm was then immediately measured using a Synergy HT (BioTek, Santa Clara, CA, USA) plate reader. Additionally, in order to assess cell morphology, osteoblasts were imaged at 20× magnification using an SP8 Lightning confocal microscope (Leica Microsystems, UK).

2.7. Quantification of OPG and RANK-L Secretion from Primary Human Osteoblasts

OPG and RANK-L protein in primary human osteoblast supernatants were quantified in duplicate using commercially available ELISAs (Osteoprotegerin/TNFRSF11B (R&D Systems, Minneapolis, MN, USA), Human TRANCE/RANK L/TNFSF11 (R&D Systems, 29, Minneapolis, MN, USA) following the manufacturer's instructions. Absorbance was measured at 450 nm and 570 nm on a Synergy HT (BioTek, USA) plate reader.

2.8. Statistical Analysis

Data analysis was carried out using GraphPad Prism v8 statistical package. For data sets with 2 variables, significance was determined by 2-way ANOVA followed by Tukey's multiple comparisons test where appropriate. For data sets with one variable, data was analysed using a non-parametric Kruskal–Wallis test, followed by post hoc Dunn's multiple comparison tests. Data is presented as mean ± S.E.M with a p value < 0.05 considered statistically significant.

3. Results

3.1. ECVC from either 2nd or 3rd Generation e-Cigarette Devices Reduces Human Osteoblast Viability and Alters Cellular Morphology

Osteoblast viability was quantified and cellular morphology observed following 24 h exposure to increasing doses of ECVC (0.25% to 10%), generated from either 2nd or 3rd generation devices. ECVC at 0.25% or 0.5%, generated from either 2nd or 3rd generation devices, had no significant effect on osteoblast viability (Figure 1A) or cellular morphology (Figure 1C,G). However, in contrast to the 2nd generation device, 1% ECVC generated by the 3rd generation device resulted in a significant reduction in osteoblast viability (46.6% ± 10.0% p = 0.002), compared to untreated control cells (Figure 1A). At ECVC concentrations of 2.5% and greater, condensate generated by either 2nd or 3rd generation devices significantly reduced osteoblast viability ($p < 0.0001$, Figure 1A). Furthermore, osteoblasts exposed to 2nd or 3rd generation ECVC at concentrations of 2.5% or greater, showed clear signs of altered cellular morphology, with loss of spindle cell shape (Figure 1C,G).

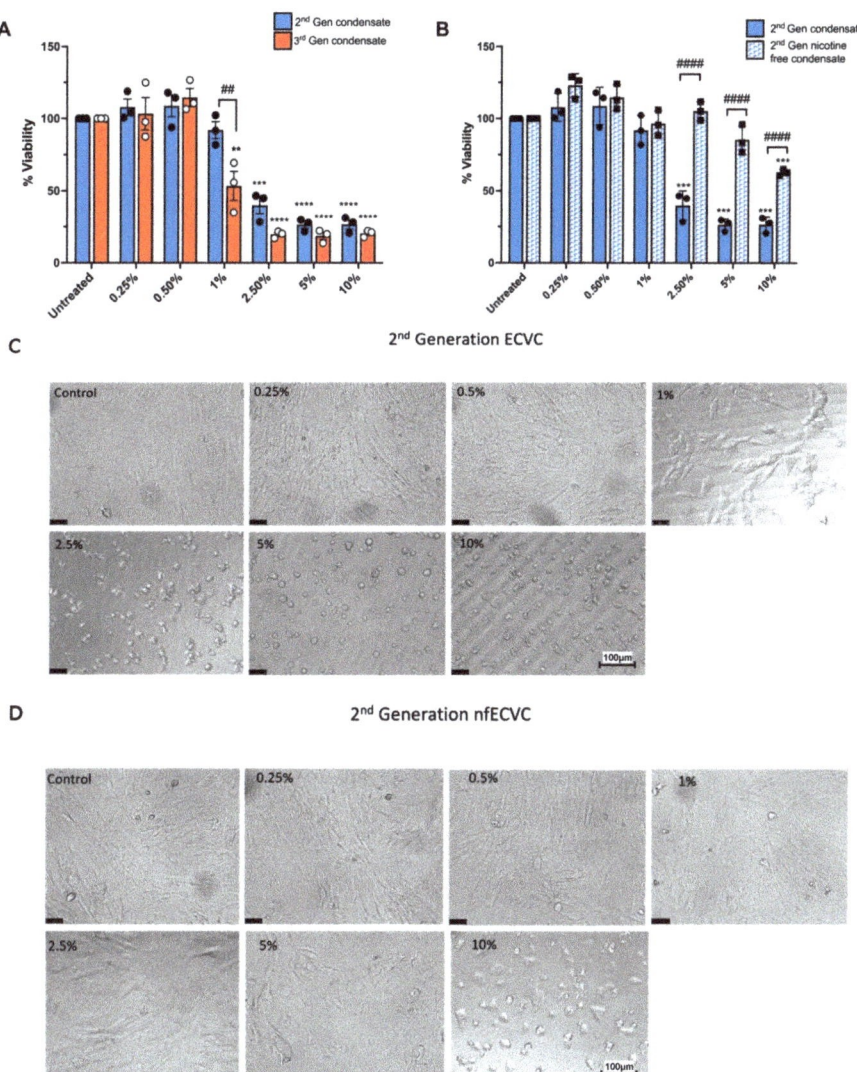

Figure 1. *Cont.*

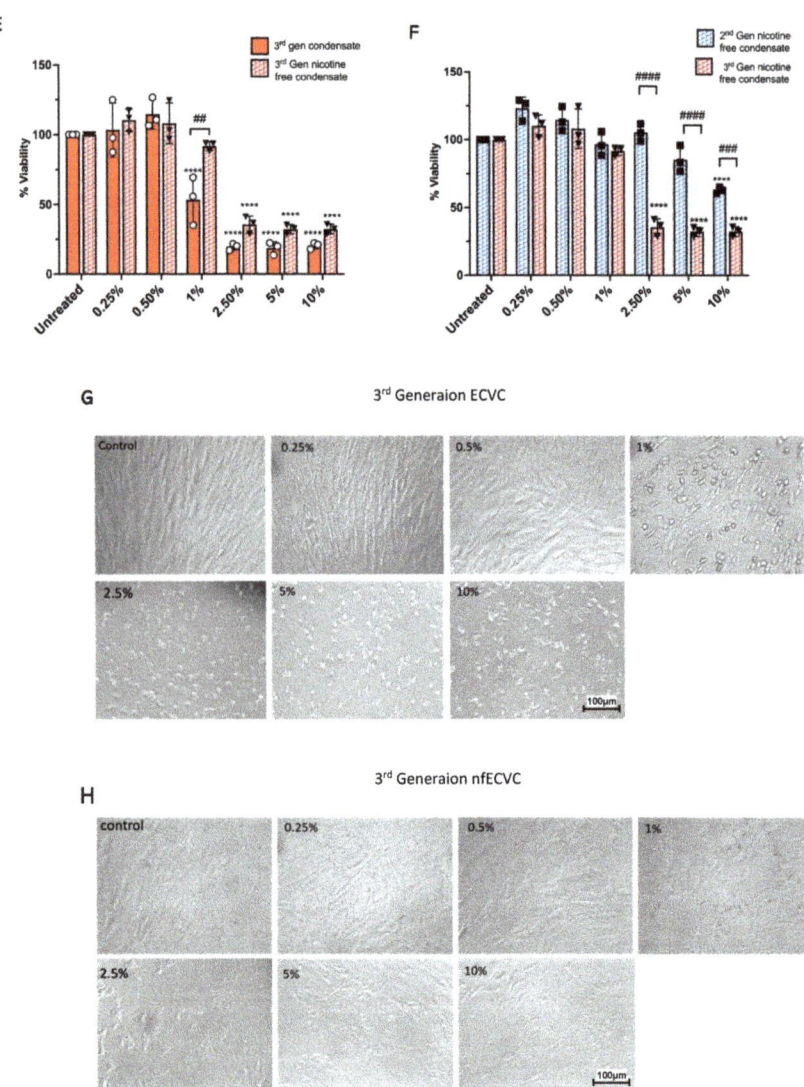

Figure 1. The effect of 2nd and 3rd generation ECVC and contribution of nicotine on human Primary osteoblast viability. (**A**) Osteoblast viability following 24 h exposure to 2nd or 3rd generation nicotine-

containing ECVC (0.25–10%). (**B**) Osteoblast viability following 24 h exposure to either nicotine-containing or nicotine-free 2nd generation ECVC (0.25–10%). (**C,D**) Representative images of primary human osteoblasts treated with 2nd gen ECVC or nfECVF (0–10%). (**E**) Osteoblast viability following 24 h exposure to either nicotine-containing or nicotine-free 3rd generation ECVC (0.25–10%). (**F**) Osteoblast viability following 24 h exposure nicotine-free ECVC from either 2nd or 3rd generation devices (0.25–10%). (**G,H**) Representative images of primary human osteoblasts treated with 3rd generation ECVC or nfECVC (0–10%). Viability was inferred by 4 h incubation with cell titre aqueous assay. Images captured at 20× magnification. $n = 3$ patient replicates, with 5 biological replicates performed per patient. ** $p < 0.01$, *** $p < 0.001$, **** $p < 0.0001$ denoting a significant denoting a significant difference to relevant untreated control. ## $p < 0.01$, ### $p < 0.001$, #### $p < 0.0001$, denoting a significant difference between treatment groups.

3.2. ECVC from Nicotine-Free 3rd Generation Devices Has a Greater Effect on Reducing Osteoblast Viability than Nicotine-Free 2nd Generation e-Cigarette Devices

To determine the extent that the observed reduction in osteoblast viability was attributable to nicotine content in the condensate, we compared the effects of nicotine-containing and nicotine-free ECVC (Figure 1B,E,F). As expected, from the 2nd generation devices, nicotine-containing ECVC at 2.5%, 5% and 10% induced a significant reduction in osteoblast viability ($p > 0.0001$) (Figure 1B,D). However, osteoblasts exposed to the nicotine-free 2nd generation condensate experienced a significantly lower loss in viability after; 10% nfECVC (37.2% ± 1.27% loss in viability), vs. just 2.5% ECVC $p =< 0.0001$) (Figure 1B,D). Exposure to 3rd generation condensate did not follow this pattern. 1% nfECVC challenge caused significantly less osteoblast toxicity than 1% nicotine containing ECVC ($p = 0.001$, Figure 1E,H). However, at higher concentrations, both nicotine-containing and nicotine-free condensate elicited a significant reduction in osteoblast viability, compared to untreated controls (Figure 1E,H). Whilst this effect was more pronounced with nicotine-containing condensate there was no significant difference between nicotine containing and nicotine free challenge at these doses (Figure 1E). Directly comparing nfECVC generated by 2nd generation and 3rd generation devices confirmed a greater toxic effect on osteoblasts when exposed to 3rd generation nfECVC at concentrations of 2.5% and above ($p > 0.0001$, Figure 1F).

3.3. Sub-Cytotoxic Doses of e-Cigarette Condensate Alters Human Osteoblast Function

Next, we investigated the potential for e-cigarette condensate to impact primary human osteoblast function, by assessing the secretion of the pro-osteogenic protein Osteoprotegerin (OPG) after low dose condensate exposure. In untreated cells, OPG secretion increased with each timepoint (Figure 2A). Following incubation with either 2nd generation or 3rd generation ECVC for 24 h, OPG secretion declined in a dose dependent manner (Figure 2A,B). Notably, OPG secretion was significantly reduced after exposure to 0.5% ECVC from either 2nd generation (33% ± 1.43% reduction, $p = 0.015$) or 3rd generation (52% ± 0.08% reduction, $p =< 0.0001$) devices (Figure 2A,B), despite this dosage having no effect on osteoblast viability, or morphology (Figure 1).

Furthermore, over 7 days, OPG secretion continued to increase significantly in untreated osteoblasts in a time dependent manner (Figure 2C). However, continuous exposure to either 0.25% or 0.5% ECVC for 7 days, significantly blunted OPG secretion at each timepoint for both 2nd and 3rd generation devices. By day 7, OPG secretion was approximately 2-fold or 4-fold less than that of untreated control cells for 2nd and 3rd generation devices, respectively, ($p < 0.0001$) (Figure 2C,D), whilst cellular viability and morphology remained unaffected (Figure 2E,F and Figure A1 in Appendix A).

3.4. The Antioxidant N-Acetyl Cysteine Rescues the ECVC-Induced Reduction in Osteoblast Viability

To elucidate the mechanism by which ECVC may interact with and affect osteoblast function, we challenged osteoblasts with a toxic dose (2.5%) of ECVC, previously identified to negatively impact osteoblast viability for both 2nd and 3rd generation devices (Figure 1A). These experiments assessed the efficacy of the antioxidant and antialdehyde, NAC to rescue osteoblast viability when given concurrently with condensate challenge. NAC alone had no significant effect on osteoblast viability (Figure 3A,B). However, NAC treatment was able to partially mitigate the toxic effects of ECVC challenge, offering a significant protective effect after the 3rd generation condensate challenge (48.5% restoration, $p < 0.0001$). NAC intervention also mitigated effects on osteoblast morphology following treatment with 2.5% ECVC (Figure 3C).

Having observed this NAC mediated rescue effect, we next performed a series of experiments in which we treated osteoblasts with the humectants propylene glycol and vegetable glycerine in isolation, to further validate whether e-cigarette vapour components other than nicotine may reduce osteoblast viability (Figure 4). A significant treatment effect of PG on osteoblast viability was observed ($p < 0.05$, Kruskal–Wallace test), with 10% PG decreasing viability up to 80% (Figure 4A) and clearly altered cellular morphology observed with 5–10% dosages (Figure 4C). VG had no significant effect on osteoblast viability or morphology (Figure 4B,D).

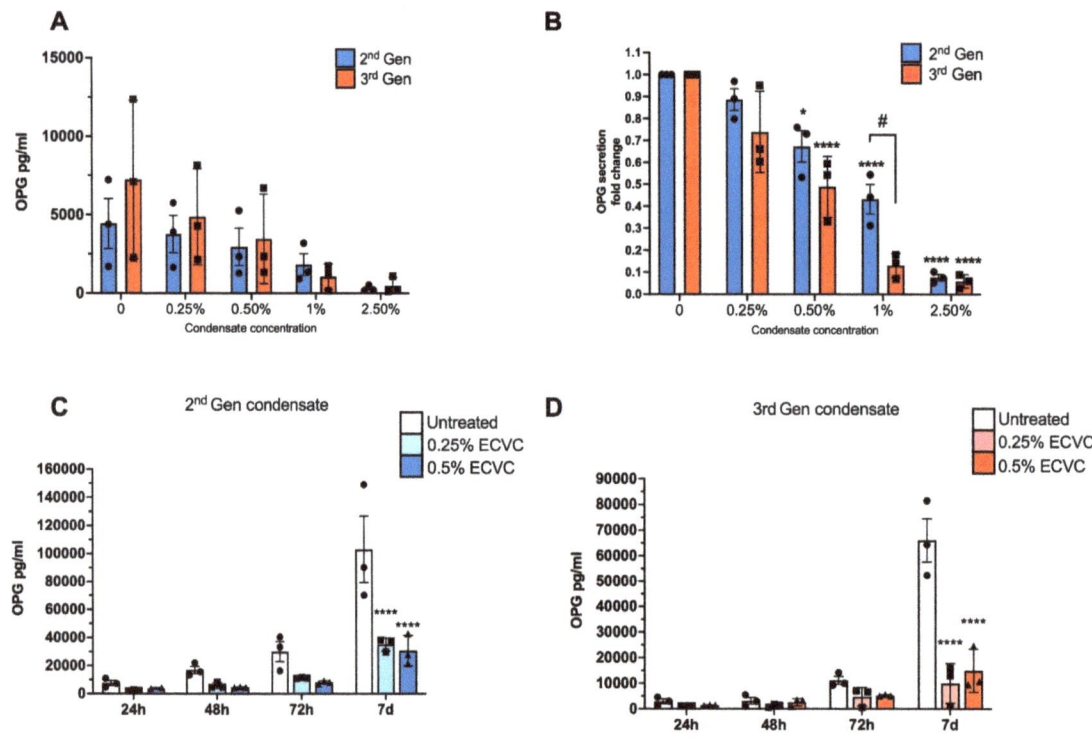

Figure 2. Cont.

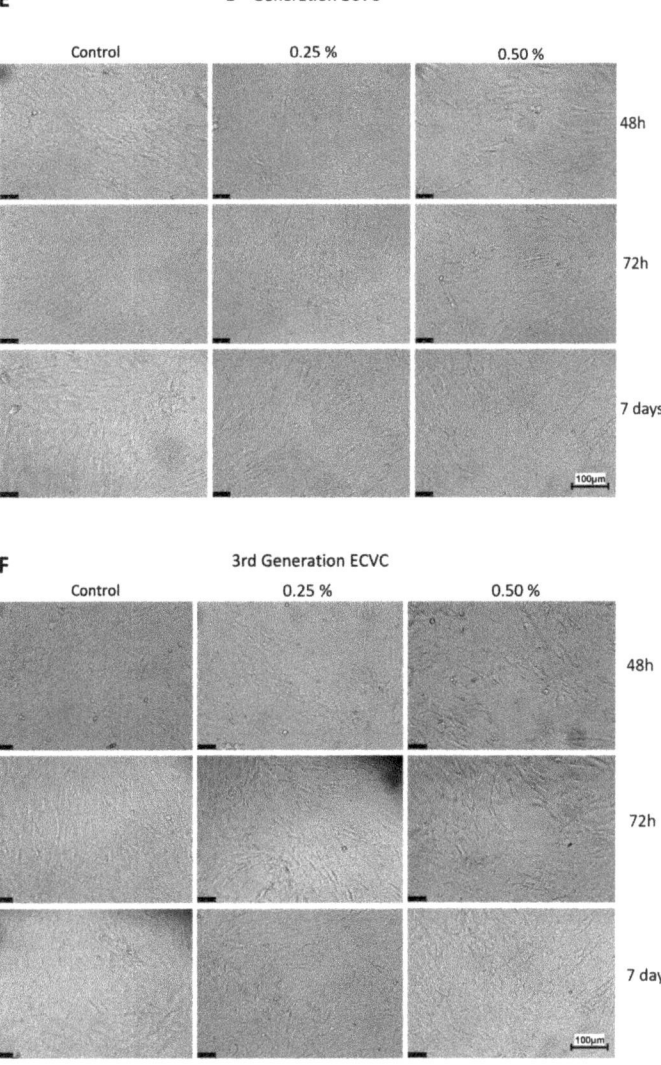

Figure 2. The impact of 2nd and 3rd generation ECVC on human primary osteoblast function. (**A**) Effect of 24 h exposure to 2nd and 3rd generation ECVC at concentrations from 0.25–2.5% on human primary osteoblast OPG secretion. (**B**) Effect of 24 h exposure to 2nd and 3rd generation ECVC at concentrations from 0.25–2.5% on human primary osteoblast OPG secretion expressed as fold change from untreated control. (**C**) Effect of 24–168 h (7d) exposure to 2nd generation ECVC at concentrations from 0.25–0.5% on human primary osteoblast OPG secretion. (**D**) Effect of 24–168 h (7d) exposure to 3rd generation ECVC at concentrations from 0.25–0.5% on human primary osteoblast OPG secretion. (**E,F**) Representative images of primary human osteoblasts treated with 0–0.5% 2nd and 3rd generation ECVC for up to 7 days. $n = 3$ patient replicates, with 3 biological replicates performed per patient. * $p < 0.05$, **** $p < 0.0001$ denoting a significant difference to relevant untreated control. # $p < 0.05$, denoting a significant difference between treatment groups.

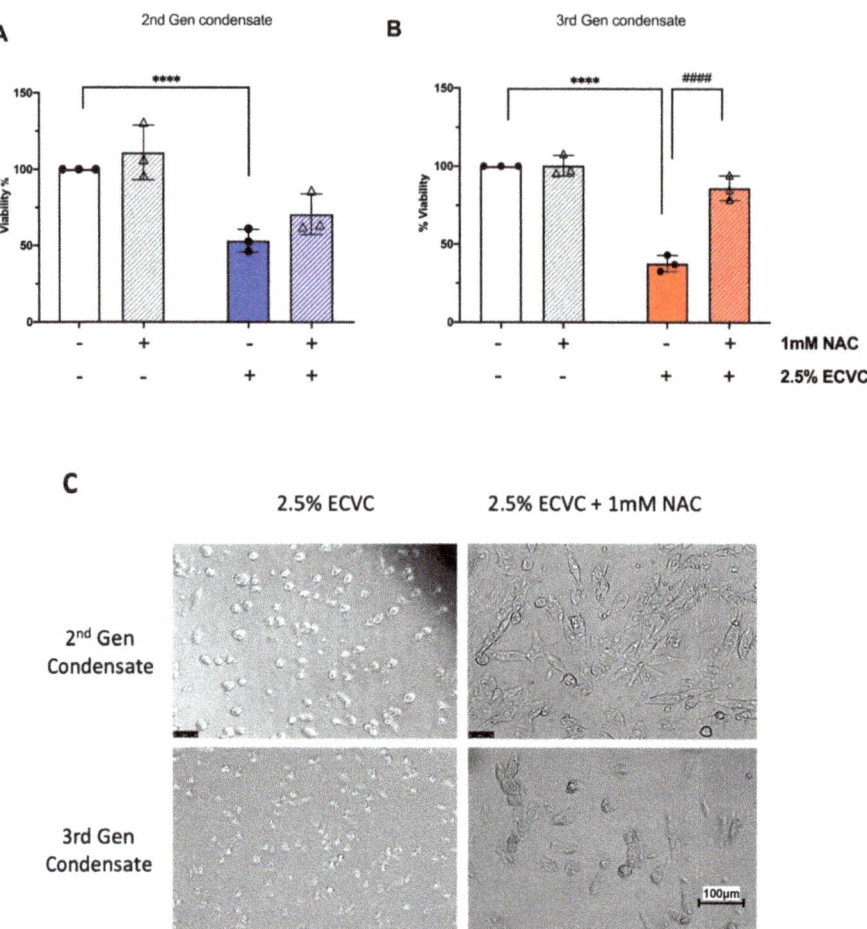

Figure 3. Pharmacological rescue of ECVC induced reductions in human osteoblast viability. (**A**) Effect of 1 mM NAC on human primary osteoblast viability in the absence or presence of 2.5% 2nd generation ECVC for 24 h. (**B**) Effect of 1 mM NAC on human primary osteoblast viability in the absence or presence of 2.5% 3rd generation ECVC for 24 h. (**C**) Representative images of human primary osteoblasts following 24 h exposure to 2nd or 3rd generation ECVC in the presence or absence of 1 mM NAC. Images captured at 20× magnification. Viability was inferred by 4 h incubation with cell titre aqueous assay. $n = 3$ patient replicates, with 3 biological replicates performed per patient. **** $p < 0.0001$ denoting a significant difference to relevant untreated control. #### $p < 0.05$ denoting a significant difference between treatment groups.

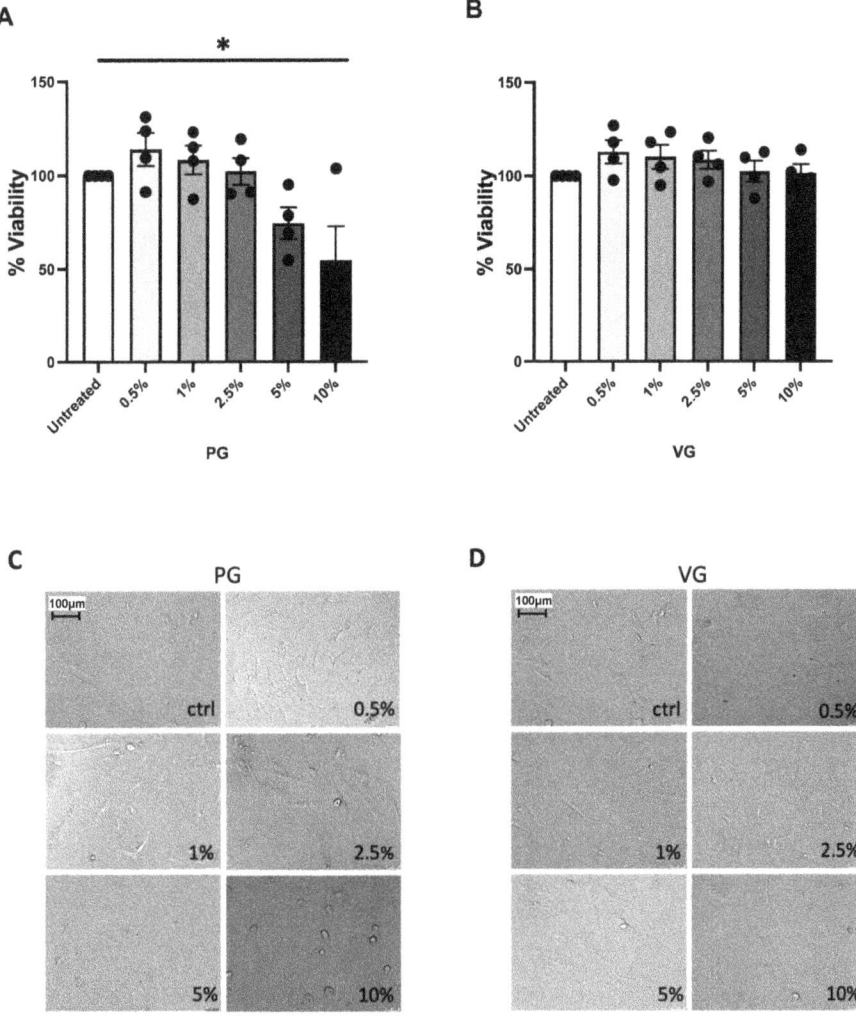

Figure 4. The effect of treatment with e-cigarette constituents on human osteoblast viability. (**A**,**B**) Effect of 24 h treatment of increasing dosages of PG and VG human primary osteoblast viability. (**C**,**D**) Representative images of human primary osteoblasts following 24 h exposure to increasing dosages of PG and VG, images captured at 20× magnification. n = 4 Patient replicates with 4 biological replicates performed per patient. * signifies $p < 0.05$ denoting a significant treatment effect by a Kruscal-Wallace test.

4. Discussion

This is the first study to demonstrate that e-cigarette condensate exposure reduces human primary osteoblast viability and function in a dose-dependent manner, utilising a model system that accounts for changes in the chemical composition of e-cigarette liquids that occur during vaping.

Treatment of osteoblasts with concentrations of 2.5% ECVC and above, was cytotoxic from both 2nd generation and 3rd generation devices, reducing viability to less than 30% compared to untreated controls. Although there is a lack of data regarding the concentration of nicotine and other vapour constituents delivered to bone following e-cigarette usage, a concentration of 2.5% ECVC (15.5 µM, 3rd generation) as used here is within a physiologically relevant systemic concentration based on reported levels after e-cigarette usage [32]. In concordance with these results, previous studies have demonstrated that cigarette smoke is toxic to human osteoblasts, reducing osteoblast viability in both a concentration and time-dependent manner [33]. More recently, a toxic effect of e-cigarette vapour on a variety of cell types, including alveolar macrophages and epithelial cells has been reported [23,34]. Additionally, Shaito et al. observed both reduced proliferation and impaired osteoblastic differentiation of bone marrow derived mesenchymal stem cells (MSCs) following exposure to e-cigarette aerosol extract [34]. Therefore, e-cigarette use may not only reduce osteoblast viability directly, as observed in this study, but could also reduce MSC-mediated bone repair. Together, these data suggest long-term e-cigarette use could have significant implications for individuals following chronic use and especially individuals with disorders of the skeletal system such as osteoarthritis [35,36], osteoporosis [36] and scoliosis [37], where there is evidence of abnormal bone and/or osteoblast pathology. In addition, this is also likely to impact skeletal remodelling during bone healing following injury, orthopaedic surgery and oral surgery such as dental implants, where exposure to e-cigarette vapour will be in very close proximity to the wounded site. Furthermore, it is also very important to consider the impact of e-cigarettes on adolescent and young adults, who comprise one of the largest cohort of e-cigarette users. Sustained e-cigarette use in such individuals may impair ongoing bone development, leading to reduced bone mineral density into adulthood. Harmful effects of conventional cigarettes and e-Cigarettes have been attributed, at least in part, to nicotine [38]. Our data supports a role for nicotine in driving osteoblast dysfunction, as the impact of nfECVC on osteoblast viability was significantly less than following exposure to ECVC of the same concentration. This effect was particularly apparent for second-generation device condensate. However, it should be noted that although osteoblast viability was greater following 10% 2nd gen nfECVC exposure in comparison to the 3rd generation device, cellular morphology appeared abnormal. This could be explained due to the viability assay fundamentally being based on cellular metabolism, therefore it is possible that although stressed and so losing typical morphology, the cells treated with the 2nd generation condensate were still more metabolically active. Whereas those treated with the 3rd gen condensate, quickly began to die after treatment. The considerable sustained impact of 3rd generation nfECVC on osteoblast viability may be attributable to differences in vapour constituent content. In addition to nicotine, e-Cigarette vapour also contains carrier agents/humectants including propylene glycol and vegetable glycerine. Thermal degradation of these carrier compounds generates reactive carbonyl species at similar concentrations to those seen in cigarettesmoke (~5 µg·puff^{-1}) [39] and in some cases, in excess of cigarette smoke (200 ug·puff^{-1}) [21]. Importantly, reactive carbonyl species have been demonstrated to reduce proliferation, increase cell death and inhibit both osteoblast alkaline phosphatase activity and mineralisation [40–42]. Additionally, e-cigarette liquids also generate a considerable amount of short-lived, highly reactive free radicals (>10^{13} molecules/puff) [21,43–45] upon vapourising. ROS are reported to induce apoptosis of osteoblasts, as well as inhibit osteoblastic differentiation, reducing osteoblast number and impairing function [45–47]. Furthermore, Bai et al. present evidence that increased intracellular ROS can stimulate the expression of RANKL in human osteoblast-like cells, which would be expected to promote osteoclast activity and bone resorption [48]. Collectively, these findings suggest that ROS not only reduces osteoblast mediated bone formation, but may also increase bone resorption through activation of osteoclasts, ultimately resulting in reduced bone density. Critically, increasing battery size and decreased coil resistance result in increased amounts of both ROS and RCS being generated per puff by newer generation e-cigarette devices, such as the 3rd generation device used in this study [20,22,45]. Unlike previous studies that treat cells with e-cigarette liquids directly from the bottle, our model system accounts for changes in chemical composition that occur upon vaping. Therefore, it is possible that the nicotine free ECVC from the 3rd generation device used in this study contained a greater amount of reactive species compared to 2nd generation devices, in turn mediating a greater impact on osteoblasts. To investigate this possibility, we treated osteoblasts with ECVC in the presence of NAC, an antioxidant that has been reported to protect against ROS and reactive aldehydes [49]. Following treatment with 3rd generation ECVC, NAC provided a significant protective effect, restoring viability to the level of control osteoblasts. This suggests that the toxic effects of ECVC may indeed be mediated in part by increased levels of reactive species. We also demonstrate that components of e-cigarette condensate other than nicotine, including the humectant PG, also significantly impaired osteoblast viability and altered cellular morphology. Emerging data in gingival and airway epithelial cells has also shown cytotoxic, inflammatory and metabolic effects of such compounds, widely regarded as inert carrier agents [50,51]. It should be noted that repeated exposure to vapour generated from humectants alone over a 6 month period had no significant effect on bone morphology in mice [52]. However, the potential impact of such humectant exposure on osteoblast/osteoclast function and bone turnover remains to be determined and therefore potential implications to processes such as bone healing still need to be considered. Indeed, although we observed no reduction in viability following VG treatment, recent work has demonstrated that VG exposure can impact chloride channel expression [53]. Therefore, non-toxic doses of VG and PG may still have considerable effects on osteoblast function, similarly to the effect non-toxic doses of ECVC had on OPG secretion as we report in this study. Collectively these data emphasise that further studies are necessary to understand the effect of chronic exposure to humectants and other components of e-cigarettes on human bone, especially following chronic use. Additionally the need for such studies is paramount, as e-cigarette devices are continually innovating, leading to ever greater power output and therefore increasing burden of RCS per puff and so in turn potential harm is only likely to increase

In line with the detrimental effect of ECVC on osteoblast viability, we also found that ECVC impaired the functional ability of osteoblasts by reducing their secretion of OPG, the decoy receptor for RANK ligand and a key regulator of bone turnover. Previous studies have examined the impact of conventional cigarette smoking on serum OPG levels, concluding that levels were significantly reduced in smokers [54]. In addition, OPG:RANKL is significantly reduced in patients who smoke, suggesting smoking may drive bone resorption [54]. Here, we also observed that OPG production by osteoblasts was significantly reduced following treatment with ECVC at 24 h, suggesting that the effects of e-Cigarette use and conventional cigarette smoking on osteoblast function maybe comparable. We did attempt to measure RANKL protein content in osteoblast supernatants by ELISA, however protein concentrations were below the lower limit of detection of our assay. Critically, as e-cigarette use is typically chronic, we also found that stimulation using concentrations of ECVC from either 2nd or 3rd generation devices, that did not impair osteoblast viability (0.25% and 0.50%) was sufficient to elicit a sustained reduction in OPG secretion for up to 7 days. This suggests long term use of e-cigarettes could lead to chronic suppression of OPG, promoting greater bone resorption Such non-toxic effects could also extend to suppression of other critical cellular functions of osteoblasts, such as alkaline phosphatase activity, or expression of genes such as COL1A1, in turn reducing extracellular matrix secretion. This carries clear clinical implications for a number cohorts including; adolescent users still undergoing bone development, in addition to individuals with bone associated disease such as osteoporosis, and those recovering from injury and surgery as discussed above. In line with this, it may also be important to consider chronic e-cigarette use in the context of DNA damage and ageing. Although e-cigarettes are widely thought to produce fewer carcinogenic compounds relative to cigarettes, nicotine nitrosation does indeed occur following e-cigarettes use, inducing the formation of the DNA adducts O(6)-methyl-deoxyguanosines and cyclic γ-hydroxy-1, N2–propano-dG [55]. Additionally, the presence of DNA adducts associated with reactive carbonyl species, such as acrolein, have also been reported following e-cigarette use in humans [56–58]. Therefore, it seems reasonable to assume that chronic systemic delivery of such compounds following e-cigarette use could reduce DNA repair in bone, in turn driving an accelerated bone ageing phenotype as described by Chen et al. [59]. Consequently, this may compound dysfunctional bone remodelling and further contribute to reduced bone mass and increased fracture risk, particularly in older users.

Due to the difficulty in replicating e-cigarette use in vitro, this study does have limitations. Firstly, although we have used a range of does in this study, concentrations of nicotine and other metabolites in the vapour condensate may not represent localised interstitial concentrations. Smoker and vaper plasma nicotine will of course vary greatly dependent on personal addiction level. However, ex-smokers will vape to meet their individual nicotine addiction needs [18] and as such, it is likely tissue exposure will remain comparable between these groups. Smoker urinary nicotine and nicotine metabolites (assessing chronic exposure) have been quantified in a range from 7–338 µM [60]. Here, we have delivered non-toxic nicotine doses of 0.82 µM (0.5% 2nd generation challenge); and 3.1 µM (0.5% 3rd generation challenge) [32]. Whilst lacking definitive data for comparison, these low dose challenges are well within a feasible physiological range [32]. Secondly, osteoblasts were only stimulated with one dose of ECVC, and therefore we can only speculate that repeated daily usage of chronic e-cigarette use would have a similarly detrimental effect on osteoblast viability.

5. Conclusions

In summary, we have demonstrated that ECVC has a negative effect on both osteoblast viability and function, with these effects being mediated, in part, by nicotine-dependent mechanisms and also reactive carbonyl species derived from e-liquid humectants as summarised in Table 1. Reduced osteoblast viability, coupled with a reduction in OPG secretion as observed following ECVC treatment, may lead to increased bone resorption following chronic exposure, in turn potentially impacting bone development in younger users, while increasing bone associated disease progression and negatively impacting orthopaedic and dental surgeryoutcomes.

Table 1. A summary of key findings.

	2nd Generation Device		3rd Generation Device		Humectants	
	ECVC	nfECVC	ECVC	nfECVC	PG	VG
Dose to significantly reduce osteoblast viability (24 h)	2.5%	10%	1%	2.5%	Significant treatment effect 0.5–10%	No significant effect
Dose to significantly reduce osteoblast OPG secretion (24 h)	0.5%	-	0.5%	-	-	-

Author Contributions: Conceptualization, S.W.J., A.S., M.N.E. and T.N. Methodology T.N., L.D., A.S. and S.W.J. Formal analysis, T.N.; S.W.J and A.S. Investigation T.N., L.D., S.W.J. and A.S. Resources, S.W.J., A.S., M.N.E. and E.T.D. Data curation, T.N., L.D. and S.W.J. Writing—original draft preparation, T.N., L.D., A.S. and S.W.J. Writing—review and editing, T.N., S.W.J. and A.S. Visualization, T.N., S.W.J. and A.S. Supervision, S.W.J. and A.S. project administration, S.W.J. and A.S. Funding acquisition, S.W.J. and A.S. All authors have read and agreed to the published version of the manuscript.

Funding: AS is Supported by Asthma + Lung UK (MCFPHD20F\2), the NIHR Health technology assessment (NIHR129593), NIHR EME programme (NIHR131600) and Medical Research Council (MR/L002736/1). SWJ is supported by Versus Arthritis, UK (21530; 21812).

Institutional Review Board Statement: Not applicable.

Informed Consent Statement: Informed consent was obtained from all subjects involved in the study (NRES 16/SS/0172).

Data Availability Statement: Not applicable.

Acknowledgments: We gratefully acknowledge the contributions of Grace Shattock and Hollie Cooke to the collection of data. We also wish to acknowledge the research nurses and research healthcare practitioners at the Royal Orthopaedic Hospital, Birmingham, UK, for their efforts in recruiting patients and collecting tissue samples. Finally, we thank the patients who participated in this study, without which, this work would not have been possible.

Conflicts of Interest: The authors declare no conflict of interest.

Appendix A

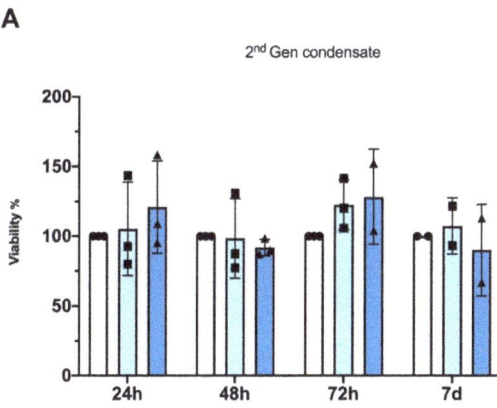

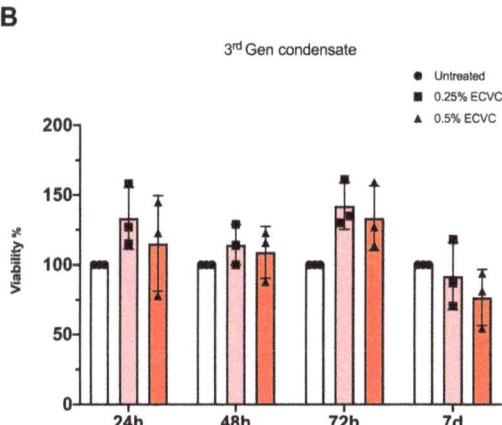

Figure A1. Low dose stimulation of Primary human osteoblasts for up to 7 days does not affect viability. Effect of treating primary human osteoblasts either 2nd (**A**) or 3rd generation (**B**) ECVC at either 0.25% or 0.5% for 24 h-7d on primary human osteoblasts. n = 3 patient replicates with 4 biological replicates performed per patient.

References

1. Patel, R.A.; Wilson, R.F.; Patel, P.A.; Palmer, R.M. The effect of smoking on bone healing: A systematic review. *Bone Jt. Res.* **2013**, *2*, 102–111. [CrossRef] [PubMed]
2. Law, M.R.; Hackshaw, A.K. A meta-analysis of cigarette smoking, bone mineral density and risk of hip fracture: Recognition of a major effect. *BMJ* **1997**, *315*, 841–846. [CrossRef] [PubMed]
3. Tamaki, J.; Iki, M.; Sato, Y.; Kajita, E.; Kagamimori, S.; Kagawa, Y.; Yoneshima, H. Smoking among premenopausal women is associated with increased risk of low bone status: The JPOS Study. *J. Bone Min. Metab.* **2010**, *28*, 320–327. [CrossRef]
4. Ward, K.D.; Klesges, R.C. A meta-analysis of the effects of cigarette smoking on bone mineral density. *Calcif. Tissue Int.* **2001**, *68*, 259–270. [CrossRef] [PubMed]
5. Szulc, P.; Debiesse, E.; Boutroy, S.; Vilauphiou, N.; Chapurlat, R. Poor trabecular microarchitecture in male current smokers: The cross-sectional STRAMBO study. *Calcif. Tissue Int.* **2011**, *89*, 303–311. [CrossRef] [PubMed]

6. Rudang, R.; Darelid, A.; Nilsson, M.; Nilsson, S.; Mellstrom, D.; Ohlsson, C.; Lorentzon, M. Smoking is associated with impaired bone mass development in young adult men: A 5-year longitudinal study. *J. Bone Min. Res.* **2012**, *27*, 2189–2197. [CrossRef] [PubMed]
7. Singh, J.A.; Schleck, C.; Harmsen, W.S.; Jacob, A.K.; Warner, D.O.; Lewallen, D.G. Current tobacco use is associated with higher rates of implant revision and deep infection after total hip or knee arthroplasty: A prospective cohort study. *BMC Med.* **2015**, *13*, 283. [CrossRef] [PubMed]
8. Matharu, G.S.; Mouchti, S.; Twigg, S.; Delmestri, A.; Murray, D.W.; Judge, A.; Pandit, H.G. The effect of smoking on outcomes following primary total hip and knee arthroplasty: A population-based cohort study of 117,024 patients. *Acta Orthop.* **2019**, *90*, 559–567. [CrossRef]
9. Teng, S.; Yi, C.; Krettek, C.; Jagodzinski, M. Smoking and risk of prosthesis-related complications after total hip arthroplasty: A meta-analysis of cohort studies. *PLoS ONE* **2015**, *10*, e0125294. [CrossRef]
10. Abrahamsen, B.; Brask-Lindemann, D.; Rubin, K.H.; Schwarz, P. A review of lifestyle, smoking and other modifiable risk factors for osteoporotic fractures. *BoneKey Rep.* **2014**, *3*, 574. [CrossRef]
11. Rom, O.; Pecorelli, A.; Valacchi, G.; Reznick, A.Z. Are E-cigarettes a safe and good alternative to cigarette smoking? *Ann. N.Y. Acad. Sci.* **2015**, *1340*, 65–74. [CrossRef] [PubMed]
12. McNeill, A.; Brose, L.S.; Calder, R.; Bauld, L.; Robson, D. *Evidence Review of E-Cigarettes and Heated Tobacco Products 2018*; Public Health England: London, UK, 2018.
13. Cornish, D.; Brookman, A.; Horton, M.; Scanlon, S. *Adult Smoking Habits in the UK: 2018*; Office for National Statistics, Ed.; Office for National Statistics: Newport, UK, 2019.
14. Agoons, D.D.; Agoons, B.B.; Emmanuel, K.E.; Matawalle, F.A.; Cunningham, J.M. Association between electronic cigarette use and fragility fractures among US adults. *Am. J. Med. Open* **2021**, *1*, 100002. [CrossRef]
15. Davis, L.C.; Sapey, E.; Thickett, D.R.; Scott, A. Predicting the pulmonary effects of long-term e-cigarette use: Are the clouds clearing? *Eur. Respir. Rev.* **2022**, *31*, 210121. [CrossRef]
16. Jasper, A.E.; McIver, W.J.; Sapey, E.; Walton, G.M. Understanding the role of neutrophils in chronic inflammatory airway disease. *F1000Research* **2019**, *8*, F1000 Faculty Rev-55. [CrossRef]
17. Son, Y.; Wackowski, O.; Weisel, C.; Schwander, S.; Mainelis, G.; Delnevo, C.; Meng, Q. Evaluation of E-Vapor Nicotine and Nicotyrine Concentrations under Various E-Liquid Compositions, Device Settings, and Vaping Topographies. *Chem. Res. Toxicol.* **2018**, *31*, 861–868. [CrossRef]
18. Hiler, M.; Karaoghlanian, N.; Talih, S.; Maloney, S.; Breland, A.; Shihadeh, A.; Eissenberg, T. Effects of electronic cigarette heating coil resistance and liquid nicotine concentration on user nicotine delivery, heart rate, subjective effects, puff topography, and liquid consumption. *Exp. Clin. Psychopharmacol.* **2020**, *28*, 527–539. [CrossRef]
19. Kosmider, L.; Spindle, T.R.; Gawron, M.; Sobczak, A.; Goniewicz, M.L. Nicotine emissions from electronic cigarettes: Individual and interactive effects of propylene glycol to vegetable glycerin composition and device power output. *Food Chem. Toxicol.* **2018**, *115*, 302–305. [CrossRef]
20. Geiss, O.; Bianchi, I.; Barrero-Moreno, J. Correlation of volatile carbonyl yields emitted by e-cigarettes with the temperature of the heating coil and the perceived sensorial quality of the generated vapours. *Int. J. Hyg. Envrion. Health* **2016**, *219*, 268–277. [CrossRef]
21. Uchiyama, S.; Noguchi, M.; Sato, A.; Ishitsuka, M.; Inaba, Y.; Kunugita, N. Determination of Thermal Decomposition Products Generated from E-Cigarettes. *Chem. Res. Toxicol.* **2020**, *33*, 576–583. [CrossRef]
22. Gillman, I.G.; Kistler, K.A.; Stewart, E.W.; Paolantonio, A.R. Effect of variable power levels on the yield of total aerosol mass and formation of aldehydes in e-cigarette aerosols. *Regul. Toxicol. Pharm.* **2016**, *75*, 58–65. [CrossRef] [PubMed]
23. Scott, A.; Lugg, S.T.; Aldridge, K.; Lewis, K.E.; Bowden, A.; Mahida, R.Y.; Grudzinska, F.S.; Dosanjh, D.; Parekh, D.; Foronjy, R.; et al. Pro-inflammatory effects of e-cigarette vapour condensate on human alveolar macrophages. *Thorax* **2018**, *73*, 1161–1169. [CrossRef] [PubMed]
24. Corriden, R.; Moshensky, A.; Bojanowski, C.M.; Meier, A.; Chien, J.; Nelson, R.K.; Crotty Alexander, L.E. E-cigarette use increases susceptibility to bacterial infection by impairment of human neutrophil chemotaxis, phagocytosis, and NET formation. *Am. J. Physiol. Cell Physiol.* **2020**, *318*, C205–C214. [CrossRef] [PubMed]
25. Garcia-Arcos, I.; Geraghty, P.; Baumlin, N.; Campos, M.; Dabo, A.J.; Jundi, B.; Cummins, N.; Eden, E.; Grosche, A.; Salathe, M.; et al. Chronic electronic cigarette exposure in mice induces features of COPD in a nicotine-dependent manner. *Thorax* **2016**, *71*, 1119–1129. [CrossRef] [PubMed]
26. Carson, J.L.; Zhou, L.; Brighton, L.; Mills, K.H.; Zhou, H.; Jaspers, I.; Hazucha, M. Temporal structure/function variation in cultured differentiated human nasal epithelium associated with acute single exposure to tobacco smoke or E-cigarette vapor. *Inhal. Toxicol.* **2017**, *29*, 137–144. [CrossRef]
27. Higham, A.; Bostock, D.; Booth, G.; Dungwa, J.V.; Singh, D. The effect of electronic cigarette and tobacco smoke exposure on COPD bronchial epithelial cell inflammatory responses. *Int. J. Chronic Obstr. Pulm. Dis.* **2018**, *13*, 989–1000. [CrossRef]
28. Shen, Y.; Wolkowicz, M.J.; Kotova, T.; Fan, L.; Timko, M.P. Transcriptome sequencing reveals e-cigarette vapor and mainstream-smoke from tobacco cigarettes activate different gene expression profiles in human bronchial epithelial cells. *Sci. Rep.* **2016**, *6*, 23984. [CrossRef]

29. Nicholson, T.; Scott, A.; Newton Ede, M.; Jones, S.W. The impact of E-cigarette vaping and vapour constituents on bone health. *J. Inflamm.* **2021**, *18*, 16. [CrossRef]
30. Nicholson, T.; Scott, A.; Newton Ede, M.; Jones, S.W. Do E-cigarettes and vaping have a lower risk of osteoporosis, nonunion, and infection than tobacco smoking? *Bone Jt. Res.* **2021**, *10*, 188–191. [CrossRef]
31. ASH. *Use of E-Cigarettes (Vapes) among Adults in Great Britain*; Action on Smoking and Health: London, UK, 2021.
32. Ghosh, A.; Coakley, R.D.; Ghio, A.J.; Muhlebach, M.S.; Esther, C.R., Jr.; Alexis, N.E.; Tarran, R. Chronic E-Cigarette Use Increases Neutrophil Elastase and Matrix Metalloprotease Levels in the Lung. *Am. J. Respir. Crit. Care Med.* **2019**, *200*, 1392–1401. [CrossRef]
33. Braun, K.F.; Ehnert, S.; Freude, T.; Egaña, J.T.; Schenck, T.L.; Buchholz, A.; Schmitt, A.; Siebenlist, S.; Schyschka, L.; Neumaier, M.; et al. Quercetin protects primary human osteoblasts exposed to cigarette smoke through activation of the antioxidative enzymes HO-1 and SOD-1. *Sci. World J.* **2011**, *11*, 2348–2357. [CrossRef] [PubMed]
34. Shaito, A.; Saliba, J.; Husari, A.; El-Harakeh, M.; Chhouri, H.; Hashem, Y.; Shihadeh, A.; El-Sabban, M. Electronic Cigarette Smoke Impairs Normal Mesenchymal Stem Cell Differentiation. *Sci. Rep.* **2017**, *7*, 14281. [CrossRef] [PubMed]
35. Philp, A.M.; Collier, R.L.; Grover, L.M.; Davis, E.T.; Jones, S.W. Resistin promotes the abnormal Type I collagen phenotype of subchondral bone in obese patients with end stage hip osteoarthritis. *Sci. Rep.* **2017**, *7*, 4042. [CrossRef] [PubMed]
36. Tonge, D.P.; Pearson, M.J.; Jones, S.W. The hallmarks of osteoarthritis and the potential to develop personalised disease-modifying pharmacological therapeutics. *Osteoarthr. Cartil.* **2014**, *22*, 609–621. [CrossRef] [PubMed]
37. Newton Ede, M.M.; Jones, S.W. Adolescent idiopathic scoliosis: Evidence for intrinsic factors driving aetiology and progression. *Int. Orthop.* **2016**, *40*, 2075–2080. [CrossRef]
38. Kallala, R.; Barrow, J.; Graham, S.M.; Kanakaris, N.; Giannoudis, P.V. The in vitro and in vivo effects of nicotine on bone, bone cells and fracture repair. *Expert Opin. Drug Saf.* **2013**, *12*, 209–233. [CrossRef]
39. Samburova, V.; Bhattarai, C.; Strickland, M.; Darrow, L.; Angermann, J.; Son, Y.; Khlystov, A. Aldehydes in Exhaled Breath during E-Cigarette Vaping: Pilot Study Results. *Toxics* **2018**, *6*, 46. [CrossRef]
40. Pereira, M.L.; Carvalho, J.C.; Peres, F.; Fernandes, M.H. Simultaneous effects of nicotine, acrolein, and acetaldehyde on osteogenic-induced bone marrow cells cultured on plasma-sprayed titanium implants. *Int. J. Oral Maxillofac. Implant.* **2010**, *25*, 112–122.
41. Hoshi, H.; Hao, W.; Fujita, Y.; Funayama, A.; Miyauchi, Y.; Hashimoto, K.; Miyamoto, K.; Iwasaki, R.; Sato, Y.; Kobayashi, T.; et al. Aldehyde-stress resulting from Aldh2 mutation promotes osteoporosis due to impaired osteoblastogenesis. *J. Bone Min. Res.* **2012**, *27*, 2015–2023. [CrossRef]
42. Mittal, M.; Pal, S.; China, S.P.; Porwal, K.; Dev, K.; Shrivastava, R.; Raju, K.S.; Rashid, M.; Trivedi, A.K.; Sanyal, S.; et al. Pharmacological activation of aldehyde dehydrogenase 2 promotes osteoblast differentiation via bone morphogenetic protein-2 and induces bone anabolic effect. *Toxicol. Appl. Pharm.* **2017**, *316*, 63–73. [CrossRef]
43. Uchiyama, S.; Ohta, K.; Inaba, Y.; Kunugita, N. Determination of carbonyl compounds generated from the E-cigarette using coupled silica cartridges impregnated with hydroquinone and 2,4-dinitrophenylhydrazine, followed by high-performance liquid chromatography. *Anal. Sci.* **2013**, *29*, 1219–1222. [CrossRef] [PubMed]
44. Goel, R.; Durand, E.; Trushin, N.; Prokopczyk, B.; Foulds, J.; Elias, R.J.; Richie, J.P., Jr. Highly reactive free radicals in electronic cigarette aerosols. *Chem. Res. Toxicol.* **2015**, *28*, 1675–1677. [CrossRef] [PubMed]
45. Domazetovic, V.; Marcucci, G.; Iantomasi, T.; Brandi, M.L.; Vincenzini, M.T. Oxidative stress in bone remodeling: Role of antioxidants. *Clin. Cases Min. Bone Metab.* **2017**, *14*, 209–216. [CrossRef] [PubMed]
46. Mody, N.; Parhami, F.; Sarafian, T.A.; Demer, L.L. Oxidative stress modulates osteoblastic differentiation of vascular and bone cells. *Free Radic. Biol. Med.* **2001**, *31*, 509–519. [CrossRef]
47. Bai, X.C.; Lu, D.; Bai, J.; Zheng, H.; Ke, Z.Y.; Li, X.M.; Luo, S.Q. Oxidative stress inhibits osteoblastic differentiation of bone cells by ERK and NF-kappaB. *Biochem. Biophys. Res. Commun.* **2004**, *314*, 197–207. [CrossRef]
48. Bai, X.C.; Lu, D.; Liu, A.L.; Zhang, Z.M.; Li, X.M.; Zou, Z.P.; Zeng, W.S.; Cheng, B.L.; Luo, S.Q. Reactive oxygen species stimulates receptor activator of NF-kappaB ligand expression in osteoblast. *J. Biol. Chem.* **2005**, *280*, 17497–17506. [CrossRef]
49. Ezerina, D.; Takano, Y.; Hanaoka, K.; Urano, Y.; Dick, T.P. N-Acetyl Cysteine Functions as a Fast-Acting Antioxidant by Triggering Intracellular H(2)S and Sulfane Sulfur Production. *Cell Chem. Biol.* **2018**, *25*, 447–459.e444. [CrossRef]
50. Beklen, A.; Uckan, D. Electronic cigarette liquid substances propylene glycol and vegetable glycerin induce an inflammatory response in gingival epithelial cells. *Hum. Exp. Toxicol.* **2021**, *40*, 25–34. [CrossRef]
51. Woodall, M.; Jacob, J.; Kalsi, K.K.; Schroeder, V.; Davis, E.; Kenyon, B.; Khan, I.; Garnett, J.P.; Tarran, R.; Baines, D.L. E-cigarette constituents propylene glycol and vegetable glycerin decrease glucose uptake and its metabolism in airway epithelial cells in vitro. *Am. J. Physiol. Cell Mol. Physiol.* **2020**, *319*, L957–L967. [CrossRef]
52. Reumann, M.K.; Schaefer, J.; Titz, B.; Aspera-Werz, R.H.; Wong, E.T.; Szostak, J.; Häussling, V.; Ehnert, S.; Leroy, P.; Tan, W.T.; et al. E-vapor aerosols do not compromise bone integrity relative to cigarette smoke after 6-month inhalation in an ApoE(-/-) mouse model. *Arch. Toxicol.* **2020**, *94*, 2163–2177. [CrossRef]
53. Lin, V.Y.; Fain, M.D.; Jackson, P.L.; Berryhill, T.F.; Wilson, L.S.; Mazur, M.; Barnes, S.J.; Blalock, J.E.; Raju, S.V.; Rowe, S.M. Vaporized E-Cigarette Liquids Induce Ion Transport Dysfunction in Airway Epithelia. *Am. J. Respir. Cell Mol. Biol.* **2019**, *61*, 162–173. [CrossRef] [PubMed]
54. Lappin, D.F.; Sherrabeh, S.; Jenkins, W.M.; Macpherson, L.M. Effect of smoking on serum RANKL and OPG in sex, age and clinically matched supportive-therapy periodontitis patients. *J. Clin. Periodontol.* **2007**, *34*, 271–277. [CrossRef] [PubMed]

55. Lee, H.W.; Park, S.H.; Weng, M.W.; Wang, H.T.; Huang, W.C.; Lepor, H.; Wu, X.R.; Chen, L.C.; Tang, M.S. E-cigarette smoke damages DNA and reduces repair activity in mouse lung, heart, and bladder as well as in human lung and bladder cells. *Proc. Natl. Acad. Sci. USA* **2018**, *115*, E1560–E1569. [CrossRef] [PubMed]
56. Tang, M.S.; Wang, H.T.; Hu, Y.; Chen, W.S.; Akao, M.; Feng, Z.; Hu, W. Acrolein induced DNA damage, mutagenicity and effect on DNA repair. *Mol. Nutr. Food Res.* **2011**, *55*, 1291–1300. [CrossRef] [PubMed]
57. Yang, J.; Balbo, S.; Villalta, P.W.; Hecht, S.S. Analysis of Acrolein-Derived 1, N(2)-Propanodeoxyguanosine Adducts in Human Lung DNA from Smokers and Nonsmokers. *Chem. Res. Toxicol.* **2019**, *32*, 318–325. [CrossRef]
58. Cheng, G.; Guo, J.; Carmella, S.G.; Lindgren, B.; Ikuemonisan, J.; Niesen, B.; Jensen, J.; Hatsukami, D.K.; Balbo, S.; Hecht, S.S. Increased acrolein-DNA adducts in buccal brushings of e-cigarette users. *Carcinogenesis* **2022**, *43*, 437–444. [CrossRef]
59. Chen, Q.; Liu, K.; Robinson, A.R.; Clauson, C.L.; Blair, H.C.; Robbins, P.D.; Niedernhofer, L.J.; Ouyang, H. DNA damage drives accelerated bone aging via an NF-κB-dependent mechanism. *J. Bone Min. Res.* **2013**, *28*, 1214–1228. [CrossRef]
60. Russell, M.A.; Wilson, C.; Patel, U.A.; Feyerabend, C.; Cole, P.V. Plasma nicotine levels after smoking cigarettes with high, medium, and low nicotine yields. *Br. Med. J.* **1975**, *2*, 414–416. [CrossRef]

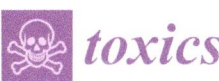 *toxics*

Article

Methodological Approaches for Risk Assessment of Tobacco and Related Products

Yvonne C. M. Staal *, Peter M. J. Bos and Reinskje Talhout

National Institute for Public Health and the Environment, P.O. Box 1, 3720 BA Bilthoven, The Netherlands
* Correspondence: yvonne.staal@rivm.nl

Abstract: Health risk assessment of tobacco and related products (TRPs) is highly challenging due to the variety in products, even within the product class, the complex mixture of components in the emission and the variety of user behaviour. In this paper, we summarize methods that can be used to assess the health risks associated with the use of TRPs. The choice of methods to be used and the data needed are dependent on the aim. Risk assessment can be used to identify the emission components of highest health concern. Alternatively, risk assessment methods can be used to determine the absolute risk of a TRP, which is the health risk of a product, not related to other products, or to determine the relative risk of a TRP, which is the health risk of a TRP compared to, for example, a cigarette. Generally, health risk assessment can be based on the effects of the complete mixture (whole smoke) or based on the (added) effects of individual components. Data requirements are dependent on the method used, but most methods require substantial data on identity and quantity of components in emissions and on the hazards of these components. Especially for hazards, only limited data are available. Currently, due to a lack of suitable data, quantitative risk assessment methods cannot be used to inform regulation.

Keywords: tobacco products; risk assessment; mixtures

Citation: Staal, Y.C.M.; Bos, P.M.J.; Talhout, R. Methodological Approaches for Risk Assessment of Tobacco and Related Products. *Toxics* **2022**, *10*, 491. https://doi.org/10.3390/toxics10090491

Academic Editors: Andrzej Sobczak and Leon Kośmider

Received: 19 July 2022
Accepted: 18 August 2022
Published: 24 August 2022

Publisher's Note: MDPI stays neutral with regard to jurisdictional claims in published maps and institutional affiliations.

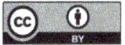

Copyright: © 2022 by the authors. Licensee MDPI, Basel, Switzerland. This article is an open access article distributed under the terms and conditions of the Creative Commons Attribution (CC BY) license (https://creativecommons.org/licenses/by/4.0/).

1. Introduction

Tobacco use is the major cause of premature death worldwide. Each year, about 8 million people die from tobacco-related diseases, including an estimated 1.2 million non-smokers who were exposed to second-hand smoke [1]. Although cigarettes are the most common tobacco product, especially in developed countries, other tobacco products also pose serious health risks. In India, more than 350,000 deaths are attributed to use of chewing and oral tobacco each year [2].

The toxic effects associated with the high mortality rate associated with tobacco consumption are due to carcinogenic and otherwise hazardous tobacco constituents and combustion products. The contributions of individual components to the carcinogenicity of tobacco use have been estimated [3,4], leading to identification of the major carcinogens and ranking of smoke constituents by their potency in inducing tumours. Similar approaches may also be used for cardiovascular and other health risks.

Strategies have been proposed to reduce the exposure of smokers to toxicants, including mandatory limits on the most relevant toxicants in cigarette smoke [5–7]. In addition, new tobacco and related products (TRPs) have been developed which have lower quantities of specific toxicants in their emission, such as heated tobacco products (HTPs) and e-cigarettes. These products may also contain other components than cigarettes, such as specific flavourings. We have defined TRPs as all tobacco products and all other products that may be used as alternatives to tobacco products; this includes both nicotine- and non-nicotine-containing products but excludes nicotine replacement products, as such products are not intended for replacing TRP use.

A smoker switching to a product that is potentially less harmful may experience a reduction in health risk, whereas the same product will lead to an increased health risk for a non-smoker compared to no TRP use at all. Quantitative hazard characterization, which includes a dose- or concentration–response relation, will give information on the health impact of a TRP. When information is available on the number of users and their use patterns, such hazard data can be used to obtain information on quantitative health impacts to determine the potential health effects at population level. Ideally, risk assessment of TRPs should be conducted separately for groups of devices or even for individual products [8]. As there is a wide variety in individual puff topography, a wide range of topographies must also be considered in estimating human exposure. This includes using relevant smoking topographies in smoking machines to characterize emissions. Practically, this ideal approach is not feasible since the variation in topographies is huge. A pragmatic solution would be to define extremes in the composition of the emission, using extreme (high and low), but realistic smoking topographies to define ranges for concentration of components in the emissions and whether the composition changes with topography. Such extremes in emission can be used to group TRPs or use scenarios and to select TRPs for a product-specific risk assessment. In such cases, generalization of risk assessment to product classes may be scientifically justified and a more pragmatic way to proceed.

This paper gives an overview of risk assessment methods that can be applied to get insight into the health impact of TRPs. The methods are described with their respective pros and cons when applied to assess the risk of a TRP. With this paper we aim to provide guidance for deciding which risk assessment method is relevant to apply in a specific case based on the information needed, the outcome and the limitations of the method. Risk assessment on population level comes with more challenges, such as the role of marketing in product initiation, addictive potential and attractiveness of the product [9,10]. Our paper focusses on toxicological risk assessment of a product as such and therefore does not discuss these other important aspects, although it should be realized that their role should not be ignored.

2. Methods for Quantifying Risk

Health risk assessment of TRP use is generally aimed either at assessing the relative (to another product) or absolute health risk of a TRP or to identify components in the emission that have a relatively large contribution to the TRPs' health risk. This could be used, for example, to set upper limits for specific constituents. The methods used and the data needed are dependent on the aim. Figure 1 gives an overview of risk assessment methods that can be used for these aims in relation to the data demand. These methods will be briefly discussed.

2.1. Evaluation Frameworks

Assessment of the health effects of TRPs could be based on an appropriate evaluation framework. In this approach, expert judgement is used to score aspects of a product in order to identify the most important risks of, for example, drugs [11,12]. Such aspects can be predefined properties of a product, such as composition of a product and user-specific characteristics like quantity of use. Each of these aspects is scored based on expert judgement on a scale running from not harmful to extremely harmful. Altogether this results in identification of the aspects of most concern to health. A non-quantitative evaluation framework has also been developed for tobacco products which summarizes all the factors that may influence the attractiveness, addictiveness and toxicity of a product and can be used to identify knowledge gaps or prioritize research on a specific product [9]. Input for such evaluation frameworks is information on product aspects that influence attractiveness and addictiveness in addition to data on the composition of emissions. These models allow evaluation of a product even when limited data are available but can be used to identify possible health risks. In addition, such models can also be used for product scoring, resulting in a quantitative outcome that can be used to compare health risks of TRPs.

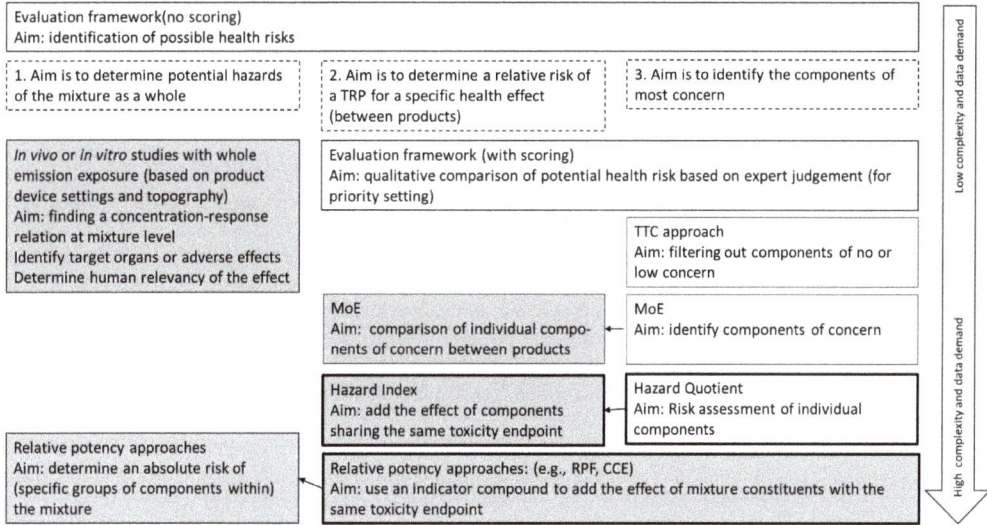

Figure 1. Overview of risk assessment methods for health risk assessment of TRPs. The choice of the method is dependent on the aim. Dashed boxes: the three different aims of the risk assessment methods. The methods that can be used for this aim are in the same column. White boxes: Methods resulting in an assessment for the individual compounds in the emission. Grey boxes: methods resulting in an assessment for the mixture of components. Interaction between components is not considered, except for experimental studies with whole emission. All methods, except experimental studies with whole smoke, are dependent on the available data on emission composition and on hazard for individual components. Black-lined boxes: these methods allow quantification of risk of single components. The arrows between boxes indicate a follow-up of that method; for example, the MoE approach first needs to be applied to identify components of concern before it can be used to compare these components between products. The arrow on the right indicates the complexity and data requirements of the methods.

2.2. Risk Assessment Based on Individual Components

Information on exposure and the hazard of individual components could be used to estimate the risk of a product as a whole, while ignoring the interaction of components in a mixture. For cigarettes, priority components have been identified based on their hazardous potential [6,13,14]. Compared to tobacco cigarette smoke, e-cigarette emissions contain a lower number of components. However, there may be other components in the emission than known tobacco toxicants, such as flavorants [15]. The data on hazards used in this approach are derived from studies providing information on the relationship between exposure and toxicity, including human epidemiological studies and animal experiments. If this relationship can be quantified sufficiently, safe levels of human exposure can be derived. In emissions from TRPs, the concentrations can be above the safe level of exposure, but the concentration and exposure regime (see Section 3) in emission is not the same as the exposure concentration reaching the lower respiratory tract due to dilution of the air by breathing. This should be accounted for and the final concentration in inhaled air should be used for risk assessment rather than the concentration in the emission. Therefore, information on emission composition and concentrations may be used as an indicator of potential concern or can be used to compare products but not directly for quantifying risks. A method based on health risk evaluation of individual components in order to estimate the risk of a complex mixture may result in underestimates of health risks, as interactive effects among components in the mixture are ignored. To compare the severity of effects of components in TRPs, detailed information is necessary on the relationships between exposure and health effects and how they can be extrapolated to effects in humans.

Below we discuss four methods for risk assessment of individual components, the threshold of toxicological concern, the margin of exposure approach, the hazard-quotient/hazard-index and relative potency approach.

2.2.1. Threshold of Toxicological Concern

One approach to evaluate the potential risk of exposure to complex mixtures is the threshold of toxicological concern (TTC) [16]. In this approach, originally developed for preventing risks, the components of potential toxicological concern in a mixture are identified from structure–activity relations and read-across. TTC values (in µg/person or µg/kg body weight per day) have been defined for three classes (Cramer classes I–III) according to structural elements, but only for oral exposure. Cramer class III indicates the highest health risk and consequently the lowest TTC value [17]. The TTC approach cannot be used to quantify health effects and is only designed to identify components for which there is no or low concern.

The risk of a mixture is then assessed by comparing exposure to each of the components in the mixture, with the appropriate TTC value. This results in identification of components with low or no concern and of components with a potential concern. This approach has been applied to complex mixtures such as botanical extracts [18], flavour complexes [19] and, although intended for oral exposure, it has also been applied to inhaled toxicants [20–22]. The TTC method might be used when no hazard data are available for the product as a whole or to identify components of potential concern in complex mixtures. This method does not indicate a risk to health but indicates that further testing is required if a component exceeds a TTC threshold; otherwise, the probability of a health risk is low. Although components below a TTC threshold could in combination result in a health risk, this will be limited in comparison with components exceeding the TTC. The TTC method relies on data of known toxicants to identify a possible health risk, which means that sufficient information of comparable components should be available. For TRPs, this method might be used to identify the components in the emission that potentially pose the highest health risk and to prioritize them for further testing. However, as the TTC method and the respective thresholds are based on oral toxicity data, and use a dose relative to body weight, this is quite different from assessments based on inhalation exposure, in which both concentration and exposure duration are important determinants of toxicity [23]. A TTC for inhaled components should be derived from inhalation toxicity data, among other factors, because toxicity is determined by the specific combination of both the exposure concentration and duration, and not just the (inhaled) dose. This is especially important for TRPs as users are throughout the day regularly exposed to peaks of high concentrations of components. Furthermore, an oral toxicity database does not contain information about adverse effects on the respiratory tract which is an important endpoint in inhalation exposure.

2.2.2. Hazard Quotient and Hazard Index

The hazard index (HI) can be used to estimate the potential risks of a chemical mixture and is defined as the sum of component-specific hazard quotients (HQ) [24,25]. An HQ relates the exposure to a component to a reference value (or limit value) and is calculated as the ratio of exposure and reference value. Assessment factors, for example to correct for differences between animals and humans, have already been considered in these reference values. Therefore, an HQ > 1 indicates a potential health risk for that component. The HI for a mixture of components, as for TRPs, can be calculated as the sum of the HQ for the individual components. An HI > 1 indicates a potential for health risk of exposure to the mixture, and the component(s) which add(s) the most to the HI can be evaluated. However, the HI approach can only be applied to a group of components if the reference levels for the individual components are based on the same health endpoint, i.e., the components need to share a common mechanism of action. For components with a different mechanism of action or a different target organ, subgroups of components should be identified to allow estimation of the effects of a mixture. A further disadvantage may be that reference values may not only reflect the toxicity of a component, since assessment factors applied may not only be health-based but may also be policy-driven or driven by the quality of the database [24].

2.2.3. Margin of Exposure Approach

The margin of exposure (MOE) approach is based on the ratio of the exposure at which no effects occur or the dose at which a predefined adverse effect occurs (e.g., a benchmark dose level) and the exposure level. This approach has been applied to compare components between tobacco products based on potential health risks [26–28] and can be used to prioritize components for reduction in tobacco smoke emissions or to assess individual components in the emissions of TRPs. An MOE is calculated for each component from information on hazard and data on inhaled emissions (corrected for inhaled total volume of air, i.e., final concentration in inhaled air). The approach requires relevant hazard and exposure data but does not result in a quantification of the health risks. Its main goal is to determine whether or not an exposure to a specific component is of concern. The magnitude of the margin of exposure is not a measure of risk and can therefore not be used to compare (the chance of) health risks between components. Furthermore, MOEs of individual components cannot be added straightforwardly to estimate the risk of the combination of components [23]. The MOE approach is a pragmatic approach to compare mixtures consisting of the same components while incorporating differences in exposure. Differences between the exposure pattern on which the hazard information is based and that of the TRP user can be weighed in the evaluation of the magnitude of the margin of exposure (see also Figure 3 in [23] on the application of the MOE approach)). For instance, the impact of differences in the exposure of a TRP user (i.e., frequent high peak exposures during a day) and that of a daily 6 h animal experiment on the health outcome needs to be considered.

2.2.4. Comparison of the HI/HQ Approach and the Margin of Exposure Approach

The main advantage of the HI/HQ approach as compared to the MOE approach is that HQs for different components can be added, provided the aforementioned conditions are met, whereas MOEs cannot be added. However, an important difference between the HI/HQ approach and the MOE approach is the comparator, i.e., a reference value or a point of departure (such as a BMD or NOAEL), respectively. It should be realized that for the HQ (and thus for the HI), issues such as the quality of the data and practical feasibility may have been accounted for in the derivation process of the reference value. Also, the point of departure underlying the reference value may not be the optimal point for evaluation of TRPs as, for example, the exposure scenario may be considerably different. Without verification of the derivation of each reference value, the impact of these issues on the outcome remains uncertain. For the MOE approach the best available data for each component can be used, whereas the HI/HQ approach is dependent on the availability of reference values and these should therefore be based on use comparable data for each component. In addition, the MOE approach has more flexibility and possibilities to account for differences between the exposure patterns of the hazard data and that of the user. This is especially important for TRPs as the reference values or limit values are based on exposure conditions that are highly different from TRP exposure scenarios (see Section 3.2).

2.2.5. Relative Potency Approaches

Relative potency approaches are based on expression of the potency of all components in a mixture with similar toxicity in relation to a reference component. This allows addition of the hazards of individual components to estimate total risk. Such approaches have been applied for components with related structures such as polycyclic aromatic hydrocarbons, dioxines and cholinesterase inhibitors (organophosphates and carbamates) [29–32]. In addition, studies have been conducted to estimate the carcinogenic potency of a tobacco product as a whole and relative to a (reference) tobacco cigarette [3,33]. In this approach, data from carcinogenicity studies are used to determine the carcinogenic potency of every component by using a modelled linear relation between exposure level and the number of tumours induced. The carcinogenic potential can be compared to a reference value of the index component to calculate the relative carcinogenic potency of each component. This is expressed as a Relative Potency Factor (RPF), which is 1 for the index component and can be higher or lower for the other components. The total relative carcinogenic potency of mixtures or aerosols can then be calculated by adding the concentration values for individual components multiplied by their relative potency and comparing the outcome with the toxicological reference value of the index component. This approach is used for components from different chemical classes and is based on the formation of tumours in general, as opposed to being organ-specific. However, components should show similar toxicity, and the mixture components show similar dose–response curves on a log scale (i.e., only differ in potency) and it is assumed the mixture components do not interact (i.e., do not show synergism or antagonism) [32]. Stephens (24) modelled the carcinogenic potency of aerosols from cigarettes, e-cigarettes and HTPs, and comparative modelling approaches have since been refined [3] to determine the relative cancer potency of individual components and product emissions, with confidence intervals. The ratio of cumulative exposure can then be calculated with a probabilistic approach for two products. For HTPs, the ratio of cumulative exposure to selected components was 10–25 times lower than from smoking cigarettes [3]. With relevant information on human dose responses, the change in cumulative exposure can be translated into an associated health impact for each device. This approach was initially used for eight carcinogens that occur in the aerosol of HTP and in cigarette smoke but should be extended to carcinogenic components that are found at higher levels in HTP aerosols than in cigarette smoke. This relative potency approach depends on the availability of either substance- or product-specific data on both emissions and carcinogenicity [34].

2.3. Risk Assessment of the Product as a Whole

Hazard assessment of the product as a whole can be done using epidemiological data, in vivo studies or in vitro models, which will give information on (adverse) effects in response to an exposure. Epidemiological studies might be preferred, but also have their limitations. For example, human studies with TRP users often involve former smokers, for which delayed effects of former smoking complicate the hazard assessment of the new TRP. In addition, many TRP users are also dual users (i.e., parallel use with tobacco cigarettes or other tobacco products). Unfortunately, epidemiological studies of the health effects of consistent exclusive e-cigarette use (or other TRP use) without a previous smoking history are difficult to conduct because of the relatively small population of non-former smokers and current e-cigarette users [35]. In addition, there are many confounders for TRP use, such as other life-style factors, as well as social and economic status, which make interpretation of the effect of TRP use challenging. In contrast to epidemiological studies, clinical studies assessing the effect of TRP use in a defined population are less impacted by these confounders.

On the other hand, bioassays in experimental animals may have disadvantages due to interspecies differences and ethical objections, and the results of cellular assays are difficult to translate into effects in humans. In addition, not only should the effects (read-out parameters) be extrapolated to human effects, but the exposure should resemble human exposure. This includes smoking topography and, in the case of a lung model, deposition in the airways. As the exposure in in vitro and in vivo differs largely from human exposure to TRPs, as explained above, such methods can be used for hazard assessment and can provide input for risk assessment, but only in combination with appropriate exposure information to bridge these differences. In vitro and in vivo studies can be used to determine an exposure

-elated response, for identifying relevant target organs or modes of action for adverse effects or for determining the human relevancy of an effect.

2.4. Possibilities and Limitations of Risk Assessment Methods

The methods described above can be used to compare the health risks of different products. Table 1 summarizes the methods, their data requirements and their applications. The relevancy of applying the methods is determined by the information available. In some methods, a weight-of-evidence approach can be used for data of different quality. All methods for risk quantification also require data on emissions, an indicator of human exposure. It should be noted that all the methods are described to assess health risks of users. Similar methods could be used to assess the risk of bystanders (second or third hand smoke exposure), provided that information is available on their exposure. In such cases, the exposure route may not be limited to the inhalation route of exposure, but oral and dermal exposure should be considered as well.

Table 1. Main limitations and advantages of each method for quantifying the health risk of TRPs.

	Potential Application for TRPs	Main Limitations	Main Advantages
Evaluation frameworks (with or without scoring)	Qualitative health risk assessment based on scores, can be used for setting priorities	Most subjective method No quantification of risks	Requires limited data; more data will improve outcomes
Threshold of toxicological concern (TTC)	Identification of components for further assessment/testing	Cannot assess risk of complete product. No quantification of risks	Identification of components of no concern
Hazard quotient (HQ)/Hazard index (HI)	Health risk assessment based on available data Health risk assessment of groups of components sharing the same toxicity endpoint	High data requirement. Only for groups with reference value based on similar toxicity endpoint Assessment factors may be based on non-scientific considerations	Considers target organ in the evaluation
Margin of exposure approach (MoE)	Identification of risks of components of concern Comparison between products on risks from individual components	High data requirement Cannot sum risks of different substances	Identification of individual components of (potential) concern
Relative potency approaches	Health risk assessment based on total risk of groups of components sharing the same toxicological endpoint Comparison between products based on groups of components	High data requirement for all components within a group. Components should share the same toxicological endpoint	Allows comparison of risks between products for groups of components
In vivo or in vitro studies with whole emission exposure	Hazard assessment based on dose–response data of mixture as a whole	Extensive testing required and extrapolation of exposure and results to humans Only information on one composition	Does not require data on emissions or hazard of individual components as the model is exposed to the emission as a whole Includes agonistic and antagonistic effects of all components

3. Challenges to Quantifying Risk

Quantification of the risks of chemical mixtures is inherently difficult, because of the interaction that may occur between components and because the effects of single components need to be factored in. In the case of TRPs, there are some additional topics that determine the exposure of the user and need to be accounted for: product variation, user-related factors and the complex composition of the emission. There is large variation in the product itself. For example, in heated tobacco differences between sticks of the same brand, and devices used to heat them, will lead to different emission profiles. Such differences will become even larger when one considers not one brand, but an entire product class. To complicate things further, this differs per consumer due to variation in the way the product is used, which affects the identity and quantity of the emission profile and the exposure pattern. Finally, health risk assessment of TRPs involves some complexities due to the complex mixture of components in the emission which may not be constant. These three topics are briefly discussed separately in the next three sections, although it should be noted that these topics may be interrelated.

3.1. Product Variation

The TRPs with currently the widest variation in heating devices and fillings (and their combinations) is the e-cigarette or electronic nicotine delivery systems (ENDS). The vapour that is inhaled by a user is dependent on the system itself, the possibilities to adapt the system, the adaptations by the user and the composition of the e-liquid. There are over 20,000 varieties of e-liquids notified in The Netherlands [36]. In the case of refillable e-cigarettes, endless combinations of devices and e-liquids can be made, which allow the user to adapt and choose the settings and the e-liquids he/she prefers. Some of these product variations are also applicable to other TRPs than e-cigarettes, such as different flavours of tobacco stick for HTPs. Variations in the product lead to changes in presence as well as the quantity of the components in emission.

3.2. User-Related Factors

A major complexity in using exposure information for risk assessment is that the exposure scenario that is used to determine hazard is substantially different between hazard assessment studies and TRP users. Inhalation studies are preferred over oral studies, since the exposure route is more relevant for TRPs and health risks will be related to the specific inhalation exposure characteristics (concentration, duration, frequency). However, exposure in experimental inhalation studies in animals is generally for 6 h/day, 5 days/week, which is not representative for the use of TRPs, as TRP use generally results in irregular peak exposure for 7 days/week. Therefore, studies in experimental animals may not provide meaningful results for assessing the risks that the complex exposure scenario of TRPs poses to humans [23]. The development and use of alternative models, such as cell models, are increasing rapidly, and may help to apply more relevant exposure scenarios in the near future [37,38]. Exposure scenarios for cell models would be based on local concentrations at the site of the cell and allow more rapid assessment of different exposure scenarios in relation to their effect. In vitro read-outs will, however, need to be extrapolated on the basis of effects at the organism level [39,40].

3.3. Complex Mixture of Components in the Emission

Tobacco smoke consists of a mixture of over 7000 chemicals, while the emission of many TRPs is less complex. The complexity of the product emissions is dependent on the product itself (as mentioned in Section 3.1) and the user (as mentioned in Section 3.2). For risk assessment methods that rely on the effects of individual components, the components in emissions must be characterized and quantified in order to assess the risk of these products [41]. Unfortunately, information on ingredients (contents) alone is insufficient, as they may not completely transfer into the emissions, they may degrade or burn during aerosolization or as components in the emissions may originate from the device (such as metals). Information on the chemical composition of the emissions is necessary to identify the components to which users are exposed. This mixture of components in the emissions varies both in presence and in quantity for the individual constituents. As this mixture is dependent on the user behaviour, this makes a risk assessment of TRP emission specific for a combination of a product and user or, to reduce complexity, a user group. Generalization of risk assessment to a group of products, for example e-cigarettes, relies on assumptions about limited variation or representative product choice, which are difficult to substantiate, and it is difficult to define their impact on health risk. Insight into the drivers of the variations in emission will help to group products according to their emissions, which can be used to substantiate grouping of TRPs for risk assessment purposes, to, ultimately, assess the risk of this group of TRPs.

Some work has been conducted on the toxicological effects of mixtures [42] to determine whether the effect of the mixture was different from those of the sum of the individual components [43]. For such purposes, components are often classified according to their target organ and their mechanism of action. Most mixture assessments have focused on binary mixtures, but risk assessment of the complex emissions of TRPs is even more complicated and is similar to the assessment of other complex mixtures, such as petroleum-derived products and air pollution [44,45].

To add to this complexity, TRP emissions are dynamic. Emissions cool as they pass to the exit of the device or the cigarette on their way to the respiratory tract and get humidified along the way, resulting in condensation of volatile components, agglomeration of particles, reactions of components with each other (aerosol aging) or binding to water in the humidified air. These processes occur simultaneously and determine local deposition in the airways, which can result in high doses at specific locations in the airways, which could have site-specific adverse effects. Models are being developed to estimate airway deposition of tobacco smoke and e-cigarette emissions to allow assessment of local dose; however, most models focus on a few components, not on complete emissions [46,47].

A summary of the factors affecting the exposure of a user is shown in Table 2.

Table 2. Factors that determine exposure and deposition in the respiratory tract of TRP emissions, while using the e-cigarette as an example.

	Factor	Effect on
Product-related	Settings of the device	Identity and quantity of components in emission, particle size distribution
Product-related	Product itself (such as brand)	Identity and quantity of components in emission, particle size distribution
User-related	Topography	Identity and quantity of components in the emission, user exposure
User-related	Number of items consumed per day	Quantity inhaled of each component, user exposure
User-related	Breathing volume	Quantity of air inhaled with a puff dilutes the emission and therefore determines the concentrations inhaled
Complex mixtures	Burning and degradation	Identity and quantity of components in emission
Complex mixtures	Emissions from other sources, such as the device	Identity and quantity of components in emission
Complex mixtures	Aerosol aging, humidification in the airways	Particle size distribution

4. Discussion

4.1. Overview and Applications

This paper provides an overview of methods that can be used to assess the health risks associated with the use of TRPs. Several models are available that could assess the risk of mixtures in TRPs, although most address carcinogenic effects. The methods described in this paper can be used for assessing the risks of TRPs, each aimed at answering a different question (Table 1). Moreover, probably more than one model will be required for a full assessment, which is dependent on the regulatory or scientific question to be answered. This question includes, amongst others, the group that is exposed (smokers, non-smokers or bystanders, for example). Methods based on the risk associated with components in emissions can be used to obtain an indication of the absolute or relative health risk of a product. At this time, not enough scientific data are available to make full health risk assessments of a TRP, but whether that is needed depends on the aim of performing TRP risk assessment. When more hazard information is available, only chemical analysis of the emissions of a novel TRP would be required, which, combined with models of deposition and risk assessment, would allow determination of the health effects.

4.2. Risk Characterization

Risk characterization requires information on the relation between actual human exposure and the occurrence of adverse effects. Such a relation is important to validate the methods for TRP risk assessment, and to ultimately apply risk assessment methods for novel TRPs prior to their market launch, when only limited information is available. A causal relation between TRP use and acute effects (short-term health risk) is generally easier to identify than the effects on the longer term, as the time between exposure and effect is short. In many cases, when users stop using the product the adverse effects may be mitigated. Assessment of the health risk of TRPs would benefit from data on health effects in long-time users; unfortunately, such data are not yet available, as novel TRPs have not been available for the time necessary to develop chronic health effects such as cancer. In addition, current TRP users are often former smokers. Thus, if a user develops a disease, it may be a delayed effect of smoking and not necessarily related to TRP use. The most robust data for assessing health risk would be for TRP users who are not former smokers and not dual users. The lack of long-term data and of information on non-smokers may change over time as the products remain on the market for longer. This is exactly why the methods to characterize TRP risk described in this paper are needed, since these can be applied before products are launched into the market.

4.3. Risks at Population Level

A quantified health risk of a TRP can be used to provide information on health risk at a population level of that TRP, when combining this with information on the number of users and the quantity of the TRP used. Although this has not yet been applied in practice, the feasibility of modelling population health effects has been explored [48]. When quantitative information on health risk and product use across the population is available, the health impact of TRPs in smokers, non-smokers and former smokers can be estimated when monitoring the popularity of the TRP (number of users) and how the TRP is used. The outcomes can be used to inform legislative measures to, for example, regulate contents and emissions or establish a basis for public education. It should be noted that quantification of health risks is not a static outcome but remains an estimation based on the available knowledge and is always influenced by the user and frequency of use. Information on novel TRPs is increasing, as is, probably even more important for e-cigarettes, the wide variety of devices, user settings and e-liquids, which will influence health risks.

4.4. Implications for Regulation

The risk assessment approaches described in this paper could inform policymakers on the health effects of a product or could be considered for use in regulation. However, there is insufficient data to reliably quantify the health risk of TRPs, and there is no uniformly used method to quantify risks of complex mixtures. Whether such information is needed, also depends on the regulatory aim, as most tobacco product legislations do not require detailed information on absolute risk of a TRP. As a first step, the conceptual model can be used to identify whether there are any health concerns to be expected, but the decision to apply subsequent models is dependent on the question that needs to be answered and the data that is available.

4.5. Recommendations

Development of risk assessment models should continue and, at some point, they should be validated with human data. Models of airway deposition should also be developed for application in risk assessment, as this is a crucial step between emission quantification and hazard characterization. From a scientific perspective, further development and ultimately implementation is currently limited by lack of data, which also implies that the models cannot yet be validated with data on human use. For a meaningful application of quantitative methods of risk assessment, data should be collected on the emissions, toxicity, use and effects of TRPs on exposed populations. Characterization of toxicants should include non-targeted screening approaches to identify product-specific components that are not usually measured in tobacco smoke.

It is recommended to evaluate the suitability of a framework published by Meek et al. [49] for combined exposures for the risk assessment of TRPs, in which the methods discussed come together. As follow-up of a WHO/IPCS Workshop on Aggregate/Cumulative risk assessment, Meek et al. [49] published a framework designed to aid in identifying priorities for risk management for exposure scenarios with combined exposures. Evaluation is done using a tiered approach which combines exposure assessment and hazard assessment. Along the evaluation, more refined tools are used. At any tier, the evaluation is made by calculating an MOE and the outcome of the analysis can be risk management, no further action, or further assessment. The assessment stops if an adequate assessment can be made. The framework helps to identify potential data gaps that need to be filled before the step to a next higher tier can be made. In addition to the MOE approach, the other methods also discussed in the present paper can be used in this framework, including the TTC approach, the Hazard Quotient and Hazard Index, and the use of relative potency factors, as is illustrated by the two example cases described in the paper by Meek et al. This framework, therefore, may provide useful guidance for the evaluation of combined exposure to multiple chemicals, as occurs when using TRPs.

From a regulatory perspective, these risk assessment methods can be selected based on regulatory needs, and based on these needs, address the requirements for data. These data requirements could be provided by the producers of TRPs, while following quality criteria [34] and using human-relevant scenarios to ensure its reliability and applicability. Such data would not only benefit risk assessment of TRPs but may also help to select ingredients, emissions and technical features that have the strongest contribution to health risks.

5. Conclusions

Several approaches have been used to quantify the health risk of tobacco products, either the absolute risk or that relative to a tobacco cigarette. The HI and RPF approaches may be used for quantification of health risk, provided that sufficient and relevant hazard and exposure data is available. None of the methods are ready to be used in regulation yet due to a lack of relevant data on hazard and exposure, but also due to a variety of regulatory needs and wishes. Nevertheless, application of these methods may be possible in due time.

Author Contributions: Conceptualization, Y.C.M.S., P.M.J.B. and R.T.; methodology, Y.C.M.S. and P.M.J.B.; writing—original draft preparation, Y.C.M.S. and P.M.J.B.; writing—review and editing, Y.C.M.S., P.M.J.B. and R.T.; project administration, Y.C.M.S. and R.T. All authors have read and agreed to the published version of the manuscript.

Funding: This work was funded by the Netherlands Food and Consumer Product Safety Authority (NVWA), Utrecht, the Netherlands. Project number 9.7.1.

Institutional Review Board Statement: Not applicable.

Informed Consent Statement: Not applicable.

Data Availability Statement: Not applicable.

Acknowledgments: The authors thank Aafje van der Burght, Peter Keizers and Marjolijn Woutersen for their review of the manuscript.

Conflicts of Interest: The authors declare no conflict of interest.

References

1. WHO. Tobacco. 2019. Available online: https://www.who.int/news-room/fact-sheets/detail/tobacco (accessed on 4 March 2020).
2. Sinha, D.N.; Palipudi, K.M.; Gupta, P.C.; Singhal, S.; Ramasundarahettige, C.; Jha, P.; Indrayan, A.; Asma, S.; Vendhan, G. Smokeless tobacco use: A meta-analysis of risk and attributable mortality estimates for India. *Indian J. Cancer* **2014**, *51* (Suppl. S1), S73–S77. [CrossRef] [PubMed]
3. Slob, W.; Soeteman-Hernández, L.G.; Bil, W.; Staal, Y.C.M.; Stephens, W.E.; Talhout, R. A method for comparing the impact on carcinogenicity of tobacco products: A case study on heated tobacco versus cigarettes. *Risk Anal.* **2020**, *40*, 1355–1366. [CrossRef] [PubMed]
4. Fowles, J.; Dybing, E. Application of toxicological risk assessment principles to the chemical constituents of cigarette smoke. *Tob. Control* **2003**, *12*, 424–430. [CrossRef] [PubMed]
5. Ashley, D.L.; Burns, D.; Djordjevic, M.; Dybing, E.; Gray, N.; Hammond, S.K.; Henningfield, J.; Jarvis, M.; Reddy, K.S.; Robertson, C.; et al. *The scientific Basis Of Tobacco Product Regulation*; World Health Organization Technical Report Series; World Health Organization: Geneva, Switzerland, 2008; pp. 1–277.
6. Burns, D.M.; Dybing, E.; Gray, N.; Hecht, S.; Anderson, C.; Sanner, T.; O'Connor, R.; Djordjevic, M.; Dresler, C.; Hainaut, P.; et al. Mandated lowering of toxicants in cigarette smoke: A description of the World Health Organization TobReg proposal. *Tob. Control* **2008**, *17*, 132–141. [CrossRef]
7. WHO. *Work in Progress in Relation to Articles 9 and 10 of the WHO FCTC*; World Health Organization: Geneva, Switzerland, 2014. Available online: http://apps.who.int/gb/fctc/PDF/cop6/FCTC_COP6_14-en.pdf (accessed on 15 April 2022).
8. U.S. Department of Health and Human Services; CDC. Smoking Cessation: A Report of the Surgeon General. 2020. Available online: https://www.hhs.gov/sites/default/files/2020-cessation-sgr-full-report.pdf (accessed on 15 April 2022).
9. Staal, Y.C.M.; Havermans, A.; van Nierop, L.; Visser, W.; Wijnhoven, S.; Bil, W.; Talhout, R. Conceptual model for the evaluation of attractiveness, addictiveness and toxicity of tobacco and related products: The example of JUUL e-cigarettes. *Regul Toxicol Pharmacol.* **2021**, *127*, 105077. [CrossRef]
10. Berman, M.L.; El-Sabawi, T.; Shields, P.G. Risk Assessment for Tobacco Regulation. *Tob. Regul. Sci.* **2019**, *5*, 36–49. [CrossRef]
11. van Amsterdam, J.; Nutt, D.; Phillips, L.; van den Brink, W. European rating of drug harms. *J. Psychopharmacol.* **2015**, *29*, 655–660. [CrossRef]
12. van Amsterdam, J.; Opperhuizen, A.; Koeter, M.; van den Brink, W. Ranking the harm of alcohol, tobacco and illicit drugs for the individual and the population. *Eur. Addict. Res.* **2010**, *16*, 202–207. [CrossRef]
13. WHO. *The Scientific Basis of Tobacco Product Regulation*; World Health Organization: Geneva, Switzerland, 2007; Volume 945.
14. Wagner, K.A.; Flora, J.W.; Melvin, M.S.; Avery, K.C.; Ballentine, R.M.; Brown, A.P.; McKinney, W.J. An evaluation of electronic cigarette formulations and aerosols for harmful and potentially harmful constituents (HPHCs) typically derived from combustion. *Regul Toxicol Pharmacol* **2018**, *95*, 153–160. [CrossRef]
15. Margham, J.; McAdam, K.; Cunningham, A.; Porter, A.; Fiebelkorn, S.; Mariner, D.; Digard, H.; Proctor, C. The Chemical Complexity of e-Cigarette Aerosols Compared With the Smoke From a Tobacco Burning Cigarette. *Front. Chem.* **2021**, *9*, 743060. [CrossRef]
16. Leeman, W.R.; Krul, L.; Houben, G.F. Complex mixtures: Relevance of combined exposure to substances at low dose levels. *Food Chem. Toxicol.* **2013**, *58*, 141–148. [CrossRef] [PubMed]
17. EFSA Scientific Committee. Scientific Opinion on Exploring options for providing advice about possible human health risks based on the concept of Threshold of Toxicological Concern (TTC). *EFSA J.* **2012**, *10*, 2750. [CrossRef]
18. Kawamoto, T.; Fuchs, A.; Fautz, R.; Morita, O. Threshold of Toxicological Concern (TTC) for Botanical Extracts (Botanical-TTC) derived from a meta-analysis of repeated-dose toxicity studies. *Toxicol. Lett.* **2019**, *316*, 1–9. [CrossRef]

19. Rietjens, I.; Cohen, S.M.; Eisenbrand, G.; Fukushima, S.; Gooderham, N.J.; Guengerich, F.P.; Hecht, S.S.; Rosol, T.J.; Davidsen, J.M.; Harman, C.L.; et al. FEMA GRAS assessment of natural flavor complexes: Cinnamomum and Myroxylon-derived flavoring ingredients. *Food Chem Toxicol* **2020**, *135*, 110949. [CrossRef] [PubMed]
20. Tluczkiewicz, I.; Kuhne, R.; Ebert, R.U.; Batke, M.; Schuurmann, G.; Mangelsdorf, I.; Escher, S.E. Inhalation TTC values: A new integrative grouping approach considering structural, toxicological and mechanistic features. *Regul. Toxicol. Pharm.* **2016**, *78*, 8–23. [CrossRef] [PubMed]
21. Schuurmann, G.; Ebert, R.U.; Tluczkiewicz, I.; Escher, S.E.; Kuhne, R. Inhalation threshold of toxicological concern (TTC)—Structural alerts discriminate high from low repeated-dose inhalation toxicity. *Environ. Int.* **2016**, *88*, 123–132. [CrossRef]
22. Talhout, R.; Schulz, T.; Florek, E.; van Benthem, J.; Wester, P.; Opperhuizen, A. Hazardous compounds in tobacco smoke. *Int. J. Environ. Res. Public Health* **2011**, *8*, 613–628. [CrossRef]
23. Bos, P.M.J.; Soeteman-Hernández, L.G.; Talhout, R. Risk assessment of components in tobacco smoke and e-cigarette aerosols: A pragmatic choice of dose metrics. *Inhal. Toxicol.* **2021**, *33*, 81–95. [CrossRef]
24. Sarigiannis, D.A.; Hansen, U. Considering the cumulative risk of mixtures of chemicals—A challenge for policy makers. *Environ. Health* **2012**, *11* (Suppl. S1), S18. [CrossRef]
25. Wilkinson, C.F.; Christoph, G.R.; Julien, E.; Kelley, J.M.; Kronenberg, J.; McCarthy, J.; Reiss, R. Assessing the risks of exposures to multiple chemicals with a common mechanism of toxicity: How to cumulate? *Regul. Toxicol. Pharmacol.* **2000**, *31*, 30–43. [CrossRef]
26. Visser, W.F.; Klerx, W.N.; Cremers, H.; Ramlal, R.; Schwillens, P.L.; Talhout, R. The Health Risks of Electronic Cigarette Use to Bystanders. *Int. J. Environ. Res. Public Health* **2019**, *16*, 1525. [CrossRef] [PubMed]
27. Cunningham, F.H.; Fiebelkorn, S.; Johnson, M.; Meredith, C. A novel application of the Margin of Exposure approach: Segregation of tobacco smoke toxicants. *Food Chem. Toxicol.* **2011**, *49*, 2921–2933. [CrossRef] [PubMed]
28. Soeteman-Hernández, L.G.; Bos, P.M.; Talhout, R. Tobacco smoke-related health effects induced by 1,3-butadiene and strategies for risk reduction. *Toxicol. Sci.* **2013**, *136*, 566–580. [CrossRef]
29. Safe, S.H. Polychlorinated biphenyls (PCBs): Environmental impact, biochemical and toxic responses, and implications for risk assessment. *Crit. Rev. Toxicol.* **1994**, *24*, 87–149. [CrossRef] [PubMed]
30. Reeves, W.R.; Barhoumi, R.; Burghardt, R.C.; Lemke, S.L.; Mayura, K.; McDonald, T.J.; Phillips, T.D.; Donnelly, K.C. Evaluation of methods for predicting the toxicity of polycyclic aromatic hydrocarbon mixtures. *Environ. Sci. Technol.* **2001**, *35*, 1630–1636. [CrossRef] [PubMed]
31. Boon, P.E.; Van der Voet, H.; Van Raaij, M.T.; Van Klaveren, J.D. Cumulative risk assessment of the exposure to organophosphorus and carbamate insecticides in the Dutch diet. *Food Chem. Toxicol.* **2008**, *46*, 3090–3098. [CrossRef]
32. Bil, W.; Zeilmaker, M.; Fragki, S.; Lijzen, J.; Verbruggen, E.; Bokkers, B. Risk Assessment of Per- and Polyfluoroalkyl Substance Mixtures: A Relative Potency Factor Approach. *Environ. Toxicol. Chem.* **2021**, *40*, 859–870. [CrossRef]
33. Stephens, W.E. Comparing the cancer potencies of emissions from vapourised nicotine products including e-cigarettes with those of tobacco smoke. *Tob. Control* **2017**, *27*, 10–17. [CrossRef]
34. Staal, Y.C.M.; Bil, W.; Bokkers, B.; Soeteman-Hernández, L.G.; Stephens, W.E.; Talhout, R. Challenges in predicting the change in the cumulative exposure of new tobacco and related products based on emissions and toxicity dose-response data. **2022**, accepted for publication in International Journal of Environmental Research and Public Health.
35. Owusu, D.; Huang, J.; Weaver, S.R.; Pechacek, T.F.; Ashley, D.L.; Nayak, P.; Eriksen, M.P. Patterns and trends of dual use of e-cigarettes and cigarettes among U.S. adults, 2015–2018. *Prev. Med. Rep.* **2019**, *16*, 101009. [CrossRef]
36. Havermans, A.; Krüsemann, E.J.Z.; Pennings, J.; de Graaf, K.; Boesveldt, S.; Talhout, R. Nearly 20,000 e-liquids and 250 unique flavour descriptions: An overview of the Dutch market based on information from manufacturers. *Tob. Control* **2021**, *30*, 57–62. [CrossRef]
37. Di Consiglio, E.; Pistollato, F.; Mendoza-De Gyves, E.; Bal-Price, A.; Testai, E. Integrating biokinetics and in vitro studies to evaluate developmental neurotoxicity induced by chlorpyrifos in human iPSC-derived neural stem cells undergoing differentiation towards neuronal and glial cells. *Reprod. Toxicol.* **2020**, *98*, 174–188. [CrossRef] [PubMed]
38. Meldrum, K.; Evans, S.J.; Vogel, U.; Tran, L.; Doak, S.H.; Clift, M.J.D. The influence of exposure approaches to in vitro lung epithelial barrier models to assess engineered nanomaterial hazard. *Nanotoxicology* **2022**, *16*, 114–134. [CrossRef] [PubMed]
39. Hayashi, Y. Designing in vitro assay systems for hazard characterization. basic strategies and related technical issues. *Exp. Toxicol. Pathol.* **2005**, *57* (Suppl. S1), 227–232. [CrossRef] [PubMed]
40. Lauterstein, D.; Savidge, M.; Chen, Y.; Weil, R.; Yeager, R.P. Nonanimal toxicology testing approaches for traditional and deemed tobacco products in a complex regulatory environment: Limitations, possibilities, and future directions. *Toxicol. Vitr.* **2020**, *62*, 104684. [CrossRef] [PubMed]
41. Mallock, N.; Pieper, E.; Hutzler, C.; Henkler-Stephani, F.; Luch, A. Heated Tobacco Products: A Review of Current Knowledge and Initial Assessments. *Front. Public Health* **2019**, *7*, 287. [CrossRef]
42. Bopp, S.K.; Barouki, R.; Brack, W.; Dalla Costa, S.; Dorne, J.C.M.; Drakvik, P.E.; Faust, M.; Karjalainen, T.K.; Kephalopoulos, S.; van Klaveren, J.; et al. Current EU research activities on combined exposure to multiple chemicals. *Environ. Int.* **2018**, *120*, 544–562. [CrossRef]
43. EFSA Scientific Committee. Guidance on harmonised methodologies for human health, animal health and ecotoxicological risk assessment of combined exposure to multiple chemicals. *EFSA J.* **2019**, *17*, 5634. [CrossRef]

44. Thompson, C.M.; Bhat, V.S.; Brorby, G.P.; Haws, L.C. Development of updated RfD and RfC values for medium carbon range aromatic and aliphatic total petroleum hydrocarbon fractions. *J. Air Waste Manag. Assoc.* **2021**, *71*, 1555–1567. [CrossRef]
45. Zavala, J.; Freedman, A.N.; Szilagyi, J.T.; Jaspers, I.; Wambaugh, J.F.; Higuchi, M.; Rager, J.E. New Approach Methods to Evaluate Health Risks of Air Pollutants: Critical Design Considerations for In Vitro Exposure Testing. *Int. J. Environ. Res. Public Health* **2020**, *17*, 2124. [CrossRef]
46. Kane, D.B.; Asgharian, B.; Price, O.T.; Rostami, A.; Oldham, M.J. Effect of smoking parameters on the particle size distribution and predicted airway deposition of mainstream cigarette smoke. *Inhal. Toxicol.* **2010**, *22*, 199–209. [CrossRef]
47. Sosnowski, T.R.; Kramek-Romanowska, K. Predicted Deposition of E-Cigarette Aerosol in the Human Lungs. *J. Aerosol Med. Pulm. Drug Deliv.* **2016**, *29*, 299–309. [CrossRef] [PubMed]
48. Apelberg, B.J.; Feirman, S.P.; Salazar, E.; Corey, C.G.; Ambrose, B.K.; Paredes, A.; Richman, E.; Verzi, S.J.; Vugrin, E.D.; Brodsky, N.S.; et al. Potential Public Health Effects of Reducing Nicotine Levels in Cigarettes in the United States. *N. Engl. J. Med.* **2018**, *378*, 1725–1733. [CrossRef] [PubMed]
49. Meek, M.E.; Boobis, A.R.; Crofton, K.M.; Heinemeyer, G.; Raaij, M.V.; Vickers, C. Risk assessment of combined exposure to multiple chemicals: A WHO/IPCS framework. *Regul. Toxicol. Pharmacol.* **2011**, *60* (Suppl. S1), S1–S14. [CrossRef]

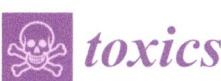

Article

Nose-Only Exposure to Cherry- and Tobacco-Flavored E-Cigarettes Induced Lung Inflammation in Mice in a Sex-Dependent Manner

Thomas Lamb, Thivanka Muthumalage, Jiries Meehan-Atrash and Irfan Rahman *

Department of Environmental Medicine, School of Medicine & Dentistry, University of Rochester Medical Center, Rochester, NY 14620, USA
* Correspondence: irfan_rahman@urmc.rochester.edu

Abstract: Flavoring chemicals in electronic nicotine delivery systems have been shown to cause cellular inflammation; meanwhile, the effects of fruit and tobacco flavors on lung inflammation by nose-only exposures to mice are relatively unknown. We hypothesized that exposure to flavored e-cigarettes would cause lung inflammation in C57BL/6 J mice. The mice were exposed to air, propylene glycol/vegetable glycerin, and flavored e-liquids: Apple, Cherry, Strawberry, Wintergreen, and Smooth & Mild Tobacco, one hour per day for three days. Quantification of flavoring chemicals by proton nuclear magnetic resonance spectroscopy (^{1}H NMR), differential cell counts by flow cytometry, pro-inflammatory cytokines/chemokines by ELISA, and matrix metalloproteinase levels by western blot were performed. Exposure to PG/VG increased neutrophil cell count in lung bronchoalveolar lavage fluid (BALF). KC and IL6 levels were increased by PG/VG exposure and female mice exposed to Cherry flavored e-cigarettes, in lung homogenate. Mice exposed to PG/VG, Apple, Cherry, and Wintergreen increased MMP2 levels. Our results revealed flavor- and sex-based e-cigarette effects in female mice exposed to cherry-flavored e-liquids and male mice exposed to tobacco-flavored e-liquids, namely, increased lung inflammation.

Keywords: e-cigarettes; ENDS; flavors; tobacco; mint; lung; inflammation

Citation: Lamb, T.; Muthumalage, T.; Meehan-Atrash, J.; Rahman, I. Nose-Only Exposure to Cherry- and Tobacco-Flavored E-Cigarettes Induced Lung Inflammation in Mice in a Sex-Dependent Manner. *Toxics* **2022**, *10*, 471. https://doi.org/10.3390/toxics10080471

Academic Editors: Andrzej Sobczak and Leon Kośmider

Received: 13 July 2022
Accepted: 8 August 2022
Published: 13 August 2022

Publisher's Note: MDPI stays neutral with regard to jurisdictional claims in published maps and institutional affiliations.

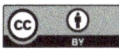

Copyright: © 2022 by the authors. Licensee MDPI, Basel, Switzerland. This article is an open access article distributed under the terms and conditions of the Creative Commons Attribution (CC BY) license (https://creativecommons.org/licenses/by/4.0/).

1. Introduction

Electronic nicotine delivery systems (ENDS), also referred to as electronic cigarettes (e-cigarettes), are devices that utilize an atomizer to aerosolize a liquid typically composed of propylene glycol/vegetable glycerin (PG/VG), nicotine, and flavoring chemicals at various concentrations [1]. In 2018, the United States had more than 8000 flavors and 250 e-cigarette brands available on the market [2]. In 2018, an estimated 8 million US adults (3.2%) were active e-cigarette users, with a high prevalence in young adults, with active e-cigarette users increasing to 4.5% in 2019 [3,4].

A majority of e-cigarette users list available flavor choices as their reason for initiation [5]. The Population Assessment of Tobacco and Health Study found age-dependent flavor preferences: adolescents have a higher affinity for fruit flavors than adults (52.8% vs. 30.8%), but a decreased preference for both menthol/mint (10.8% vs. 17.9%) and tobacco (5.1% vs. 24.5%) [6]. The 2021 National Youth Tobacco Survey also found fruit to be the preferred flavor among middle and high school students (71.6%), with mint and menthol trailing at 30.2% and 28.8%, respectively [7].

In the United States, current e-cigarette users believe that e-cigarettes are less harmful than traditional cigarettes [8,9]. Despite the fact that many flavoring chemicals are generally recognized as safe for ingestion (GRAS), emerging literature indicates that these chemicals may pose health risks to e-cigarette users [2]. A recent study demonstrated that ethyl maltol, maltol, ethyl vanillin, and furaneol exhibit cytotoxicity towards lung epithelial cells and mouse neuronal stem cells at concentrations found in e-liquids [10].

Monocytes treated with maltol, o-vanillin, and coumarin, and lung epithelial cells treated with maltol, o-vanillin, and diacetyl released significantly elevated levels of IL-8 [2,11,12]. Flavoring chemicals such as maltol and o-vanillin have been found in both fruit- and tobacco-flavored e-liquids [13]. Additionally, treatments with cinnamaldehyde-containing e-liquids decreased the phagocytotic activity of macrophages and neutrophils with concomitant increases in pro-inflammatory cytokine/chemokine secretion in the latter [14]. Recent studies also indicate that e-cigarette use is also beginning to be associated with lung remodeling and fibrosis-like events along with an increased risk for the development of respiratory diseases [15–18].

Given the high preference of flavored e-cigarette use in current users and in vitro data showing the induction of an inflammatory response by flavoring chemicals used in e-cigarettes, we hypothesize that nose-only exposure of mice to flavored e-cigarettes would result in lung inflammation. To conduct this study, we exposed mice to five different e-cigarette flavors to several puffs daily, a similar number to the daily puffs of e-cigarette users, by utilizing a puffing profile that mimicked the puffing topography of current e-cigarette users and measured pro-inflammatory cytokine levels, BALF cell counts, and lung protease levels to determine lung inflammation [19].

2. Materials and Methods

2.1. Ethics Statement

Experiments were performed following the standards established by the United States Animal Welfare Act. The Animal Research Committee of the University of Rochester (UCAR) approved the animal experimental protocol.

2.2. Animals

Six-week-old male and female C57 BL/6 J mice were ordered from Jackson Laboratory. Mice were housed at the University of Rochester for 1 week to acclimatize prior to nose-only tower training. All mice, regardless of exposure group, were trained by placing each mouse in the restraints of the Scireq nose-only tower one week prior to e-cigarette exposure. Mice were trained for fifteen minutes on the first day, thirty minutes on the second day, forty-five minutes on the third day, and one hour on the fourth and fifth days.

2.3. E-Cigarette Device and Liquids

A Joytech eVIC mini device (SCIREQ, Montreal) with KangerTech 0.15 Ω atomizers/coils (SCIREQ, Montreal) and the Scireq nose-only tower (SCIREQ, Montreal) were utilized for all e-cigarette exposures. E-liquids (0 mg nicotine), PG, and VG were purchased from the same company through local vendors/online vendors with e-liquids purchased under the following flavor categories, fruit (Apple, Cherry, and Strawberry), mint/menthol (Wintergreen), and tobacco (Smooth & Mild Tobacco). A 1:1 PG/VG mixture was used for all experiments.

2.4. E-Cigarette Exposure

E-cigarette nose-only exposure was performed utilizing the Scireq InExpose system using the Joytech eVIC mini device controlled by the Scireq Flexiware software. The puffing profile utilized to expose mice was set at two puffs per minute at an inter-puff interval of thirty seconds, with a three-second puff duration and a puff volume of 51 mL. Mice were split into six exposure groups (PG/VG, Apple, Cherry, Strawberry, Wintergreen, Smooth & Mild Tobacco) of equal numbers of males (3) and females (3) and exposed using the puffing profile (120 puffs daily) for a total of one hour per day for a three-day exposure. Air mice were exposed to room air following the same exposure methodology.

2.5. BALF Collection and Cell Counts

Mice were sacrificed 24 h after the last e-cigarette exposure and were euthanized by administering a mixture of ketamine and xylazine. Lungs were lavaged via tracheal catheterization three times each with 0.6 mL of 0.05% fetal bovine serum in 0.9% NaCl. The combined lavage fluids were centrifuged at 2000 rpm for 10 min at 4 °C. The supernatant was recovered and stored at −80 °C, while the cell pellet was resuspended in 1 mL of 1 × phosphate buffer saline (PBS). Total cell counts were measured by staining cells with acridine orange and propidium iodide (AO/PI) and counted using the Nexcelom Cellometer Auto 2000 cell viability counter. Differential cell counts were determined by flow cytometry using a Guava easyCyte flow cytometer with a minimum of 100,000 cells per sample. Cells from BALF were stained with CD16/32 (Tonbo biosciences 70-0161-u500, 1:10) to block nonspecific binding and then cells were stained using a master mix of CD45.1 (Biolegend Cat# 110728, 1:1000, San Diego, CA, USA), F4/80 (Biolegend Cat# 123110, 1:500, San Diego, CA, USA), Ly6 B.2 (Novus Biological Cat# NBP2-13077, 1:250, Littleton, CO, USA), CD4 (Invitrogen Cat# 25-0041-82, 1:500, Carlsbad, CA, USA), and CD8 (Invitrogen Cat# 17-0081-82, 1:500, Carlsbad, CA, USA).

2.6. Protein Extraction

Mouse lung lobes were collected and washed in 1 × PBS, dry blotted using a filter pad, and stored at −80 °C. Approximately 30 mg of lung tissue were mechanically homogenized in 350 µL of radioimmunoprecipitation assay buffer containing protease inhibitor and EDTA. After mechanical homogenization, samples were placed on ice for forty-five minutes before centrifugation at 14,000 rpm for thirty minutes at 4 °C. The supernatant was collected and stored at −80 °C in 50 µL aliquots for ELISA and Western blot. To determine the total protein concentration in each sample, the Pierce BCA Protein Assay kit (ThermoFisher Scientific, Cat# 23225, Waltham, MA, USA) was used and bovine serum albumin was utilized as the protein standard.

2.7. Pro-Inflammatory Cytokines/Chemokines

Pro-inflammatory cytokine/chemokine keratinocytes-derived chemokine (KC) (R&D DuoSet DY453), interleukin-6 (IL-6) (R&D Duoset DY406), and monocyte chemoattractant protein-1 (MCP-1) (R&D DuoSet DY479) levels were measured using ELISA following manufacturer protocol in BALF and lung homogenate. A dilution of 1:10 was utilized for lung homogenate samples and no dilution was utilized for BALF samples.

2.8. Immunoblot Assay

Equal concentration of lung homogenate samples, 10 µg of samples, were loaded per well of a 26 well 4–15% Criterion Precast Protein Gel (BioRad Cat# 5671085, GmbH, Feldkirchen, Germany) and proteins were ran at 200 V through the gel before being transferred to a nitrocellulose membrane. Nonspecific binding was blocked by incubating membranes in 5% non-fat milk in 1 × tris-buffer saline with 0.1% tween 20 (TBST) for one hour with rocking at room temperature. Membranes were then probed to determine protein levels using the following antibodies diluted in 5% non-fat milk in 1 × TBST: matrix metalloproteinase 9 (MMP9) (Abcam ab38898, 1:1000, Cambridge, MA, USA) and MMP2 (Abcam ab92536, 1:1000, Cambridge, MA, USA) and left rocking overnight at 4 °C. After overnight incubation, membranes were washed three times with 1 × TBST for ten minutes per wash and then incubated, with a secondary goat anti-rabbit antibody (BioRad Cat# 1706515, 1:10,000, GmbH, Feldkirchen, Germany) for one hour with rocking at room temperature. Membranes were then washed three times with 1 × TBST for ten minutes per wash and signals were measured using an ultra-sensitive enhanced chemiluminescent (Thermofisher Cat# 34096, Waltham, MA, USA) following the manufacturer's protocol. Images of the membrane were collected utilizing the Bio-Rad ChemiDoc MP Imaging system (Bio-Rad Laboratories, GmbH, Feldkirchen, Germany). Membranes were then stripped utilizing restore western stripping buffer (Thermofisher Cat# 21063, Waltham, MA, USA) and re-probed for the other MMP and finally for β-actin (cell signaling 12620 s, 1:2000). Band intensity was determined using densitometry analysis using image lab software and normalized to the levels of β-actin. Fold changes in protein levels were relative to the protein levels of air-exposed mice.

2.9. Proton Nuclear Magnetic Resonance Spectroscopy Chemical Assay

In total, 120 µL e-liquids, 600 µL of DMSO-d6 containing 0.3% tetramethylsilane (Cambridge Isotope Laboratories Inc., Cat#DLM-10 TC-25, Andover, MA, USA), and 10 µL of a 306 mM solution of 1,2,4,5-tetrachloro-3-nitrobenzene in DMSO-d6 were combined, after which 500 µL of this mixture was introduced into 5 mm Wilmad 528-PP-7 thin wall precision NMR tubes for analysis. ^{1}H NMR spectra were acquired on a Bruker Avance 500 MHz NMR spectrometer with 128 scans with a 4.7 s repetition rate, a 30° flip angle, with 64 k data points. Spectra were processed using Mestrenova with 0.3 Hz line-broadening factor to a final data size of 64 k real data points, manually phase-corrected, and baseline corrected using the Bernstein polynomial fit. Flavoring chemical concentrations were determined by comparing the peak integrations of the internal standard to flavoring chemicals, and the PG/VG ratio was determined by direct integration of their resonances. All samples were run in triplicates.

2.10. Statistical Analysis

Analysis was performed using GraphPad Prisma version 8.1.1 (San Diego, CA, USA) utilizing a one-way ANOVA with Dunnett's multiple comparisons test with data shown as mean ± standard error of the mean (SEM).

3. Results

3.1. NMR Analysis of Flavored E-liquids for Flavoring Chemicals

The chemical composition of all e-liquids was assessed by NMR to determine the ratio of PG to VG and quantify key flavoring chemicals in flavored e-liquids. In the Apple e-liquid, the concentration of hexyl acetate was determined to be 0.43 ± 0.04 mg/mL, and ethyl maltol was determined to be 0.30 ± 0.05 mg/mL with a 46:54 PG/VG ratio (Table 1). In the Cherry e-liquid, the concentration of benzaldehyde was determined to be 0.12 ± 0.01 mg/mL with a 51:49 PG/VG ratio (Table 1). In the Strawberry e-liquid, the concentration of ethyl maltol was determined to be 0.32 ± 0.05 mg/mL and maltol was determined to be 0.24 ± 0.04 mg/mL with a 50:50 PG/VG ratio (Table 1). In the Wintergreen e-liquid, the concentration of methyl salicylate was determined to be 9.70 ± 0.50 mg/mL with a 49:51 PG/VG ratio (Table 1). Finally, in the Smooth & Mild Tobacco e-liquid, the concentration of maltol was determined to be 1.13 ± 0.02 mg/mL with a 49:51 PG/VG ratio (Table 1).

Table 1. Flavoring chemical and propylene glycol and vegetable glycerin quantification in e-liquids. E-liquids were analyzed by ^{1}H NMR using a Bruker Advance 500 MHz NMR spectrometer with 128 scans with a 4.7 s repetition rate and a 30° flip angle, with 64 k data points. Flavoring chemical concentrations and propylene glycol and vegetable glycerin quantification were representatives of the average of the three samples ± SEM.

E-liquids	Flavoring Chemicals	Concentration	PG:VG
Apple	Hexyl Acetate	0.43 ± 0.04 mg/mL	46:54
	Ethyl Maltol	0.30 ± 0.05 mg/mL	
Cherry	Benzaldehyde	0.12 ± 0.01 mg/mL	51:49
Strawberry	Ethyl Maltol	0.32 ± 0.05 mg/mL	50:50
	Maltol	0.24 ± 0.04 mg/mL	
Wintergreen	Methyl Salicylate	9.70 ± 0.50 mg/mL	49:51
Smooth & Mild Tobacco	Maltol	1.13 ± 0.02 mg/mL	49:51

3.2. Alterations in Inflammatory Cell Influx in Lung by E-cigarette Flavors

To determine the effect of flavored e-cigarettes on the influx of inflammatory cells, differential cell counts were measured in BALF cells. In all mouse e-cigarette exposure groups, there were no significant alterations in total cell counts or macrophage cell counts compared to air controls (Figure 1A,B). In combined data, mice exposed to Smooth & Mild Tobacco resulted in a significant increase in the neutrophil cell count compared to air controls (Figure 1C). In male mice, exposure to Smooth & Mild Tobacco resulted in a significant increase in neutrophil cell counts, and in female mice, exposure to PG/VG and Apple resulted in a significant increase in neutrophil cell count compared to air controls (Figure 1C). Mice exposed to PG/VG resulted in a significant increase in the CD4 T-cell count compared to air controls (Figure 1D). In all mouse e-cigarette exposure groups, there were no significant alterations in CD8 T-cell count compared to air controls (Figure 1E).

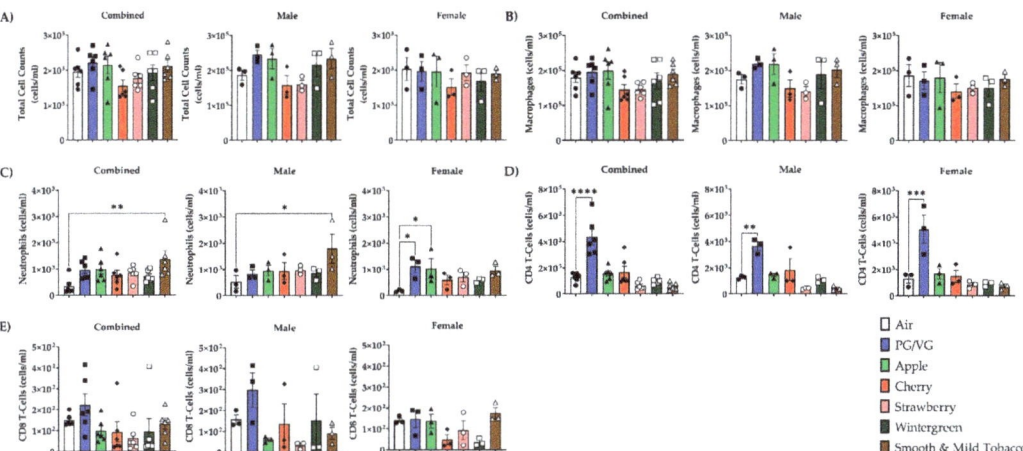

Figure 1. Sex-dependent effects of flavored e-cigarette exposure on inflammatory cell count in bronchoalveolar lavage fluid. Mice were exposed to air, PG/VG, and e-liquid flavors "Apple", "Cherry", "Strawberry", "Wintergreen", and "Smooth & Mild Tobacco" for 3 days for 1 h per day. Mice were sacrificed twenty-four hours after the final exposure. (**A**) Total cell counts were obtained by staining cells with AO/PI and counting with a cellometer. Differential cells were measured using flow cytometry: (**B**) F4/80+ macrophages, (**C**) Ly6 B.2+ neutrophils, (**D**) CD4+ T-cells, and (**E**) CD8+ T-cells. Data are shown as mean ± SEM with individual data points represented by the following symbols: Air (black circles), PG/VG (black squares), Apple (black triangles), Cherry (black diamonds), Strawberry (white circles), Wintergreen (white squares), Smooth & Mild Tobacco (white triangles), with * indicating $p < 0.05$, ** $p < 0.01$, *** $p < 0.001$, and **** $p < 0.0001$ vs. air controls. $n = 6$ for combined groups and $n = 3$ for male- and female-only groups.

3.3. Alteration of Pro-Inflammatory Cytokines/Chemokines Levels in Lungs by E-cigarette Flavors

To determine the potential for flavored e-cigarette to elicit an inflammatory response, pro-inflammatory cytokines/chemokines were measured in BALF and lung homogenate. In BALF, KC levels in combined data were significantly increased in Strawberry-exposed mice compared to air controls (Figure 2A). In lung homogenate, KC levels in combined data were significantly increased in Cherry and Smooth & Mild Tobacco exposed mice compared to air controls (Figure 3A). In lung homogenate, there was no significant change in any exposed groups in male mice, but in female mice, there was a significant increase in KC levels when exposed to PG/VG and Cherry compared to air controls (Figure 3A). In BALF, IL-6 levels in all exposed mice were not significantly changed compared to air controls (Figure 2B). In lung homogenate, IL-6 levels in combined data were significantly increased in PG/VG and Cherry exposed mice compared to air controls (Figure 3B). In lung homogenate, there was a significant increase in IL-6 levels in male mice exposed to PG/VG as compared to air controls, and female mice exposed to PG/VG and Cherry showed significant increases in IL-6 levels compared to air controls (Figure 3B). In BALF, MCP-1 levels were unchanged in all exposed mice compared to air controls (Figure 2C). In lung homogenate, MCP-1 levels in combined data were significantly decreased in Apple, Strawberry, Wintergreen, and Smooth & Mild Tobacco exposed mice compared to air controls (Figure 3C). In all male mice exposure groups, a significant decrease in MCP-1 levels compared to air controls in lung homogenate was observed, whereas for female mice, MCP-1 levels were not impacted by the exposures (Figure 3C).

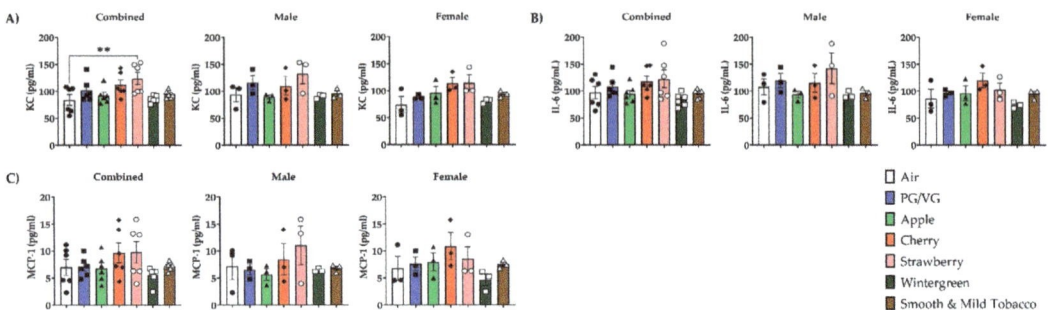

Figure 2. Sex-dependent effects of flavored e-cigarette exposure on pro-inflammatory cytokines/chemokine release in bronchoalveolar lavage fluid. Mice were exposed to air, PG/VG, and e-liquid flavors "Apple", "Cherry", "Strawberry", "Wintergreen", and "Smooth & Mild Tobacco" for 3 days for 1 h per day. Mice were sacrificed twenty-four hours after the final exposure. Pro-inflammatory cytokines/chemokines were measured in BALF. (**A**) KC levels, (**B**) IL-6 levels, (**C**) MCP-1 levels. Data are shown as mean ± SEM with individual data points represented by the following symbols: Air (black circles), PG/VG (black squares), Apple (black triangles), Cherry (black diamonds), Strawberry (white circles), Wintergreen (white squares), Smooth & Mild Tobacco (white triangles), with ** $p < 0.01$ vs. air controls. $n = 6$ for combined groups and $n = 3$ for male- and female-only groups.

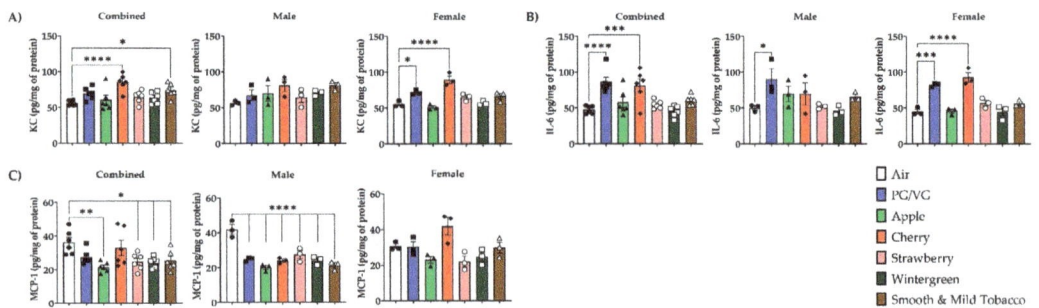

Figure 3. Sex-dependent effects of acute flavored e-cigarette exposure on pro-inflammatory cytokines/chemokine release in lung homogenate. Mice were exposed to air, PG/VG, and e-liquid flavors "Apple", "Cherry", "Strawberry", "Wintergreen", and "Smooth & Mild Tobacco" for 3 days for 1 h per day. Mice were sacrificed twenty-four hours after the final exposure. Pro-inflammatory cytokines/chemokines were measured in lung homogenate. (**A**) KC levels, (**B**) IL-6 levels, (**C**) MCP-1 levels. Data are shown as mean ± SEM with individual data points represented by the following symbols: Air (black circles), PG/VG (black squares), Apple (black triangles), Cherry (black diamonds), Strawberry (white circles), Wintergreen (white squares), Smooth & Mild Tobacco (white triangles), with * $p < 0.05$, ** $p < 0.01$, *** $p < 0.001$, and **** $p < 0.0001$ vs. air controls. $n = 6$ for combined groups and $n = 3$ for male- and female-only groups.

3.4. Alterations in Matrix Metalloproteinase Levels in Lungs by E-cigarette Flavors

To determine the effect of flavored e-cigarettes on extracellular remodeling proteins, MMP protein levels were measured in lung homogenate. In all female mice exposure groups, there was no significant change in the relative fold change of MMP9 protein levels compared to air controls (Figures 4B and S1–S3). Exposure to PG/VG, Apple, Cherry, and Wintergreen resulted in a significant increase in the relative fold change of MMP2 protein levels in female mice compared to air controls (Figures 4B and S1–S3). Male mice exposed to Apple displayed a significant decrease in the relative fold change of MMP9 protein levels compared to air controls (Figures 4B and S1–S3). In male mice exposed to PG/VG, Apple, Cherry, and Wintergreen resulted in a significant increase in the relative fold change of MMP2 protein levels compared to air controls (Figures 4B and S1–S3).

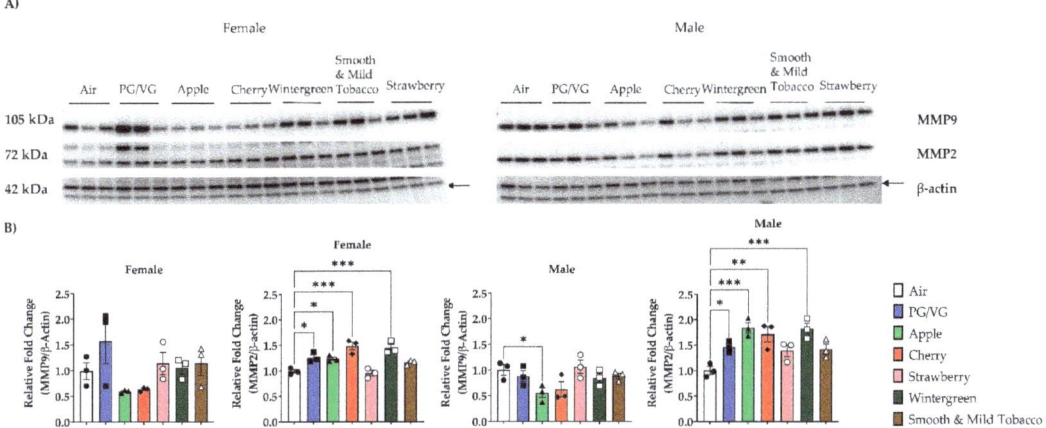

Figure 4. Effects of acute flavored e-cigarette exposure on matrix metalloprotease protein levels in lung homogenate. Mice were exposed to air, PG/VG, and e-liquid flavors "Apple", "Cherry", "Strawberry", "Wintergreen", and "Smooth & Mild Tobacco" for 3 days for 1 h per day. Mice were sacrificed twenty-four hours after the final exposure. Protein levels for matrix metalloproteinases were measured in lung homogenate using Western blot. (**A**) MMP2 and MMP9 protein abundance in mouse lung homogenate from male and female exposed mice. (**B**) Band intensity was measured using densitometry and data are shown as fold change compared to air control mice. Data are shown as mean ± SEM with individual data points represented by the following symbols: Air (black circles), PG/VG (black squares), Apple (black triangles), Cherry (black diamonds), Strawberry (white circles), Wintergreen (white squares), Smooth & Mild Tobacco (white triangles), with * $p < 0.05$, ** $p < 0.01$, and *** $p < 0.001$ vs. air controls. $n = 3$ for male- and female-only groups.

4. Discussion

In this study, we investigated the immune-inflammatory effects of exposure to flavored e-cigarettes. To determine the potential inhalation effects of flavoring chemicals added into e-liquids, we determined the concentration of five distinct flavoring chemicals (maltol, ethyl maltol, benzaldehyde, methyl salicylate, and hexyl acetate), but the presence of other flavorants are still under investigation. Prior literature also indicates that these compounds have an abundant and widespread presence in market-available e-liquids [13,20,21]. While quantification of flavorants are important, a recently published study showed the inherent variability in lung deposition of flavoring chemicals as a function of inhalation modality: in "lung inhalers" nearly 100% retention of flavorants was observed, but lower retention was observed for "mouth inhalers" [22].

The chemicals found in these e-liquids (maltol, ethyl maltol, benzaldehyde, hexyl acetate, methyl salicylate, and hexyl acetate) are GRAS for ingestion, but the inhalation and respiratory effects of these chemicals are relatively understudied. Diacetyl, which has been used commercially as flavor additives in food for butter flavoring, is a flavoring chemical that has been found in e-liquids, but despite being GRAS for ingestion, the inhalation of this chemical has been found to result in the respiratory disease bronchiolitis obliterans, which showed the potential risk of inhaling these chemicals [23]. Although there are limited studies, one study has previously been conducted on the inhalation effects of benzaldehyde in Sprague-Dawley rats and found that exposure to 500, 750, and 1000 ppm benzaldehyde displayed dose-dependent increases in nasal irritation [24]. Previous preliminary data from our lab exposing C57 BL/6 J mice (n = 2–3) to PG/VG and benzaldehyde, following the same methodology described in thisstudy, has shown a potential trend of an increase in pro-inflammatory cytokine production in BALF, although the small sample size does not allow for the determination of significant changes (Figure S4).

Few studies have focused solely on the effect of flavors/flavoring chemicals in e-cigarette exposure, with most studies focusing on the effects of nicotine or the effects of the base components of e-liquids. One study that has investigated the respiratory effects of the flavoring chemical vanillin exposed C57 BL/6 J mice to 70:30 VG:PG with or without vanillin for 6 weeks. This study found similar results to the results herein, with no significant change in macrophages count and CD8 T cells from VG/PG with or without vanillin, while also finding a significant increase in CD4 T cells in mice exposed to VG/PG but also found an increase in VG/PG with vanillin contrary to the flavor exposure results herein [25]. Another study conducted on flavored e-cigarettes, in which C57 BL/6 J mice were exposed for two weeks to a menthol-flavored e-cigarette with 1.8% nicotine. Contrary to the results herein, macrophage cells were significantly increased in e-cigarette-exposed mice; meanwhile, no significant changes were found in neutrophil and lymphocyte cell counts such as the results herein [26]. One study conducted on the base component of e-liquids exposed female BALB/c to PG and VG alone. Similar to the results of our female mice exposed to PG/VG, PG and VG alone resulted in no significant change in total cell count and macrophage cell count compared to air controls, while contrary to the results herein, PG and VG alone did not result in a significant increase in neutrophil count [27]. In another study looking at the base component of e-liquids, female C57 BL/6 J mice were exposed to 60:40 PG:VG for four months. Comparable to the results herein, there was no significant change in macrophage cell counts in PG/VG; meanwhile, unlike the results herein, there was no significant change in neutrophil or lymphocyte cell counts in PG/VG exposures [28]. In another study conducted on exposure to PG for a three-day exposure, contrary to the results herein, exposure to PG resulted in a significant decrease in total cell counts and macrophage cell count, along with no significant change in neutrophil and CD4 T-cells [15]. A study conducted on the effects of PG for 1 month, similar to the results herein, found no significant change in total cell count, macrophage cell counts, or CD8 T-cells compared to air controls, while, differing from the results herein, there was no significant change in CD4 T-cells [29].

In line with the increase in IL-6 levels by PG/VG and Cherry exposures in lung homogenate, exposure of C57 BL/6 J mice to e-cigarette with 18 mg/mL nicotine found a significant increase in IL-6 RNA levels in the lung tissue [30]. However, exposure to 60:40 PG:VG in C57 BL/6 J female mice found no change in IL-6 levels in lung homogenate [28]. In line with the results from the Wintergreen flavor exposure, menthol-flavored C57 BL/6 J mouse exposure had no change in MCP-1 levels, although this exposure resulted in a significant decrease in IL-6 levels in BALF [26]. In contrast to results herein, another C57 BL/6 J e-cigarette exposure found that PG/VG did not alter IL-6 levels, but tobacco flavored exposure significantly increased IL-6 levels in lung homogenate [31]. In alternative mice strains, ENDS exposure in βENaC resulted in a significant increase in cytokines associated with lung fibrosis [32]. While exposure to PG/VG with nicotine in A/J mice resulted in a significant increase in RNA levels of cytokines associated with chronic obstructive pulmonary disease (COPD) [33].

The results of this study are one of the first evidence to show the sex-specific effects of nose-only exposure to e-cigarette flavors. The results herein found that male mice exposed to Smooth & Mild tobacco resulted in a significant increase in neutrophil count in BALF, while all e-cigarette exposures resulted in a significant decrease in MCP-1 levels in lung homogenate. In female mice exposed to Cherry, there was a significant increase in levels of KC and IL-6 in lung homogenate, while in female mice exposed to Apple, there was a significant increase in neutrophil count in BALF. In PG/VG-exposed female mice, there was a significant increase in neutrophils in BALF and a significant increase in KC levels in lung homogenate. There are limited current studies that have investigated the sex-specific effects of e-cigarette exposure. One study investigating the effects of PG and PG with nicotine on C57 BL/6 J mice in a sex-specific manner found that female mice exposed to PG with nicotine had a significant increase in neutrophil and CD8 T-cell counts, while male mice exposed to PG with nicotine were found to have a significant increase in lung inflammatory cytokines [15]. A study conducted on cigarette smoke exposure on spontaneously hypertensive rats found that male mice had significant increases in macrophage cell counts and tumor necrosis factor-alpha levels showing a male-specific increase in inflammation contrary to the results herein but similar to the results of Wang et al. [34].

Alterations in MMP2 and MMP9 levels due to e-cigarette exposures are important, since both MMP2 and MMP9 gelatinolytic activity have been found to be increased in the sputum in both asthmatic and COPD patients [35]. Comparable to the results herein, exposure of C57 BL/6 J mice to PG found that there was no change in MMP9 levels in exposed mice [15]. However, e-cigarette exposures to PG/VG with nicotine resulted in an increase in MMP9 and other lung protease levels [33]. Cell studies have found that alveolar macrophages and neutrophils treated with e-cigarette condensate significantly increased MMP9 [36,37]. MMP9 levels have also been found to be elevated in the plasma and bronchoalveolar lavage in e-cigarette users [38,39]. Consistent with our MMP2 results, increased MMP2 levels have also been found in mice exposed to PG and increased MMP2 levels in the bronchoalveolar lavage of chronic e-cigarette users [15,29,39]. Although the effects of e-cigarette exposures on cytokine/chemokine levels, MMP levels, and BALF cell counts have different effects in this and other studies, these differences may come down to the methodology for e-cigarette exposures. Each study utilizes different devices and puffing profiles for mouse exposures, along with different e-liquids with differences in nicotine concentration, flavors, and the ratio of PG and VG. These differences between studies demonstrate the need for a standardized methodology for mouse exposures to reduce potential differences between studies and allow for greater comparisons between studies.

5. Conclusions

Based on the results in this study, flavored e-cigarettes showed both increases in lung inflammation and resolution. Mice exposed to PG/VG, Cherry, and Smooth & Mild Tobacco resulted in an increase in lung inflammation due to the increases in KC and IL-6 levels in lung homogenate along with infiltration of neutrophils in BALF. These exposures may also have sex-specific alterations, with Smooth & Mild Tobacco exposure only resulting in a significant increase in neutrophil cell counts in male mice. Meanwhile, in Cherry exposure, KC and IL-6 levels were increased in lung homogenate only in female mice. In PG/VG exposures, only female mice had a significant increase in neutrophil cell count and a significant increase in KC levels in lung homogenate. Despite the increases in inflammatory cytokines in Cherry and PG/VG, the increases in MMP2 levels potentially indicate that these exposures have begun to shift away from inflammation and towards tissue repair and resolution. In contrast, other exposures, such as Wintergreen flavor, resulted in a decrease in lung inflammation, with a decrease in MCP-1 levels and increases in MMP2 levels. Further studies are in progress to determine the chronic exposures to flavored e-cigarettes on long-term pulmonary effects and the potential sex-specific effects. This study revealed that flavor-based e-cigarette exposure elicited sex-specific alterations in lung inflammation, with cherry flavors/benzaldehyde eliciting female-specific and tobacco flavor resulting in male-specific increases in lung inflammation. This highlights the toxicity of flavored chemicals and the further need for the regulation of flavoring chemicals.

Supplementary Materials: The following supporting information can be downloaded at: https://www.mdpi.com/article/10.3390/toxics10080471/s1, Figure S1: Full image of MMP2 for male and female exposed mice; Figure S2: Full image of MMP9 for male and female exposed mice; Figure S3: Full image of β-actin for male and female exposed mice; Figure S4: Alterations in pro-inflammatory cytokines/chemokine release in bronchoalveolar lavage fluids due to acute exposure to PG/VG and PG/VG with benzaldehyde.

Author Contributions: T.L., T.M., J.M.-A. and I.R. conceived and designed the experiments; T.L. conducted the experiments; T.L. and J.M.-A. analyzed the data; T.L., T.M., J.M.-A. and I.R. wrote and edited the manuscript. All authors have read and agreed to the published version of the manuscript.

Funding: WNY Center for Research on Flavored Tobacco Products (CRoFT) # U54 CA228110 and Toxicology Training Program grant T32 ES007026.

Institutional Review Board Statement: The animal study protocol was approved by the Animal Research Committee of the University of Rochester (UCAR) of the University of Rochester (2007–070).

Data Availability Statement: Not applicable.

Conflicts of Interest: The authors declare no conflict of interest.

References

1. Cao, Y.; Wu, D.; Ma, Y.; Ma, X.; Wang, S.; Li, F.; Li, M.; Zhang, T. Toxicity of electronic cigarettes: A general review of the origins, health hazards, and toxicity mechanisms. *Sci. Total Environ.* **2021**, *772*, 145475. [CrossRef] [PubMed]
2. Kaur, G.; Muthumalage, T.; Rahman, I. Mechanisms of toxicity and biomarkers of flavoring and flavor enhancing chemicals in emerging tobacco and non-tobacco products. *Toxicol. Lett.* **2018**, *288*, 143–155. [CrossRef] [PubMed]
3. Cornelius, M.E.; Wang, T.W.; Jamal, A.; Loretan, C.G.; Neff, L.J. Tobacco Product Use Among Adults—United States, 2019. *MMWR Morb. Mortal. Wkly. Rep.* **2020**, *69*, 1736–1742. [CrossRef] [PubMed]
4. Villarroel, M.A.; Cha, A.E.; Vahratian, A. Electronic Cigarette Use among US Adults, 2018. *NCHS Data Brief.* **2020**, *365*, 1–8.
5. Soneji, S.S.; Knutzen, K.E.; Villanti, A.C. Use of Flavored E-Cigarettes Among Adolescents, Young Adults, and Older Adults: Findings From the Population Assessment for Tobacco and Health Study. *Public Health Rep.* **2019**, *134*, 282–292. [CrossRef]
6. Schneller, L.M.; Bansal-Travers, M.; Goniewicz, M.L.; McIntosh, S.; Ossip, D.; O'Connor, R.J. Use of Flavored E-Cigarettes and the Type of E-Cigarette Devices Used among Adults and Youth in the US-Results from Wave 3 of the Population Assessment of Tobacco and Health Study (2015–2016). *Int. J. Environ. Res. Public Health* **2019**, *16*, 2991. [CrossRef] [PubMed]
7. Park-Lee, E.; Ren, C.; Sawdey, M.D.; Gentzke, A.S.; Cornelius, M.; Jamal, A.; Cullen, K.A. Notes from the Field: E-Cigarette Use Among Middle and High School Students—National Youth Tobacco Survey, United States, 2021. *MMWR Morb. Mortal. Wkly. Rep.* **2021**, *70*, 1387–1389. [CrossRef] [PubMed]
8. Amrock, S.M.; Zakhar, J.; Zhou, S.; Weitzman, M. Perception of e-cigarette harm and its correlation with use among US adolescents. *Nicotine Tob. Res.* **2015**, *17*, 330–336. [CrossRef] [PubMed]
9. Huang, J.; Feng, B.; Weaver, S.R.; Pechacek, T.F.; Slovic, P.; Eriksen, M.P. Changing Perceptions of Harm of e-Cigarette vs. Cigarette Use Among Adults in 2 US National Surveys From 2012 to 2017. *JAMA Netw. Open* **2019**, *2*, e191047. [CrossRef]
10. Hua, M.; Omaiye, E.E.; Luo, W.; McWhirter, K.J.; Pankow, J.F.; Talbot, P. Identification of Cytotoxic Flavor Chemicals in Top-Selling Electronic Cigarette Refill Fluids. *Sci. Rep.* **2019**, *9*, 2782. [CrossRef]
11. Gerloff, J.; Sundar, I.K.; Freter, R.; Sekera, E.R.; Friedman, A.E.; Robinson, R.; Pagano, T.; Rahman, I. Inflammatory Response and Barrier Dysfunction by Different e-Cigarette Flavoring Chemicals Identified by Gas Chromatography-Mass Spectrometry in e-Liquids and e-Vapors on Human Lung Epithelial Cells and Fibroblasts. *Appl. Vitro Toxicol.* **2017**, *3*, 28–40. [CrossRef]
12. Muthumalage, T.; Prinz, M.; Ansah, K.O.; Gerloff, J.; Sundar, I.K.; Rahman, I. Inflammatory and Oxidative Responses Induced by Exposure to Commonly Used e-Cigarette Flavoring Chemicals and Flavored e-Liquids without Nicotine. *Front. Physiol.* **2017**, *8*, 1130. [CrossRef] [PubMed]
13. Tierney, P.A.; Karpinski, C.D.; Brown, J.E.; Luo, W.; Pankow, J.F. Flavour chemicals in electronic cigarette fluids. *Tob. Control* **2016**, *25*, e10–e15. [CrossRef] [PubMed]
14. Clapp, P.W.; Lavrich, K.S.; van Heusden, C.A.; Lazarowski, E.R.; Carson, J.L.; Jaspers, I. Cinnamaldehyde in flavored e-cigarette liquids temporarily suppresses bronchial epithelial cell ciliary motility by dysregulation of mitochondrial function. *Am. J. Physiol. Lung Cell. Mol. Physiol.* **2019**, *316*, L470–L486. [CrossRef] [PubMed]
15. Wang, Q.; Khan, N.A.; Muthumalage, T.; Lawyer, G.R.; McDonough, S.R.; Chuang, T.D.; Gong, M.; Sundar, I.K.; Rehan, V.K.; Rahman, I. Dysregulated repair and inflammatory responses by e-cigarette-derived inhaled nicotine and humectant propylene glycol in a sex-dependent manner in mouse lung. *FASEB Bioadv.* **2019**, *1*, 609–623. [CrossRef] [PubMed]
16. Hariri, L.P.; Flashner, B.M.; Kanarek, D.J.; O'Donnell, W.J.; Soskis, A.; Ziehr, D.R.; Frank, A.; Nandy, S.; Berigei, S.R.; Sharma, A.; et al. E-Cigarette Use, Small Airway Fibrosis, and Constrictive Bronchiolitis. *NEJM Evid.* **2022**, *1*, EVIDoa2100051. [CrossRef]

17. Osei, A.D.; Mirbolouk, M.; Orimoloye, O.A.; Dzaye, O.; Uddin, S.M.I.; Benjamin, E.J.; Hall, M.E.; DeFilippis, A.P.; Bhatnagar, A.; Biswal, S.S.; et al. Association Between E-Cigarette Use and Chronic Obstructive Pulmonary Disease by Smoking Status: Behavioral Risk Factor Surveillance System 2016 and 2017. *Am. J. Prev. Med.* **2020**, *58*, 336–342. [CrossRef]
18. Bhatta, D.N.; Glantz, S.A. Association of E-Cigarette Use with Respiratory Disease among Adults: A Longitudinal Analysis. *Am. J. Prev. Med.* **2020**, *58*, 182–190. [CrossRef] [PubMed]
19. Dautzenberg, B.; Bricard, D. Real-Time Characterization of E-Cigarettes Use: The 1 Million Puffs Study. *J. Addict. Res. Ther.* **2015**, *6*, 4172. [CrossRef]
20. Eshraghian, E.A.; Al-Delaimy, W.K. A review of constituents identified in e-cigarette liquids and aerosols. *Tob. Prev. Cessat.* **2021**, *7*, 10. [CrossRef] [PubMed]
21. Krusemann, E.J.Z.; Pennings, J.L.A.; Cremers, J.; Bakker, F.; Boesveldt, S.; Talhout, R. GC-MS analysis of e-cigarette refill solutions: A comparison of flavoring composition between flavor categories. *J. Pharm. Biomed. Anal.* **2020**, *188*, 113364. [CrossRef] [PubMed]
22. Khachatoorian, C.; McWhirter, K.J.; Luo, W.; Pankow, J.F.; Talbot, P. Tracing the movement of electronic cigarette flavor chemicals and nicotine from refill fluids to aerosol, lungs, exhale, and the environment. *Chemosphere* **2022**, *286*, 131494. [CrossRef]
23. Allen, J.G.; Flanigan, S.S.; LeBlanc, M.; Vallarino, J.; MacNaughton, P.; Stewart, J.H.; Christiani, D.C. Flavoring Chemicals in E-Cigarettes: Diacetyl, 2,3-Pentanedione, and Acetoin in a Sample of 51 Products, Including fruit-, Candy-, and Cocktail-Flavored E-Cigarettes. *Environ. Health Perspect.* **2016**, *124*, 733–739. [CrossRef] [PubMed]
24. Andersen, A. Final report on the safety assessment of benzaldehyde. *Int. J. Toxicol.* **2006**, *25* (Suppl. S1), 11–27. [CrossRef]
25. Szafran, B.N.; Pinkston, R.; Perveen, Z.; Ross, M.K.; Morgan, T.; Paulsen, D.B.; Penn, A.L.; Kaplan, B.L.F.; Noel, A. Electronic-Cigarette Vehicles and Flavoring Affect Lung Function and Immune Responses in a Murine Model. *Int. J. Mol. Sci.* **2020**, *21*, 6022. [CrossRef]
26. Sussan, T.E.; Gajghate, S.; Thimmulappa, R.K.; Ma, J.; Kim, J.H.; Sudini, K.; Consolini, N.; Cormier, S.A.; Lomnicki, S.; Hasan, F.; et al. xposure to electronic cigarettes impairs pulmonary anti-bacterial and anti-viral defenses in a mouse model. *PLoS ONE* **2015**, *10*, e0116861. [CrossRef] [PubMed]
27. Larcombe, A.N.; Janka, M.A.; Mullins, B.J.; Berry, L.J.; Bredin, A.; Franklin, P.J. The effects of electronic cigarette aerosol exposure on inflammation and lung function in mice. *Am. J. Physiol. Lung Cell. Mol. Physiol.* **2017**, *313*, L67–L79. [CrossRef] [PubMed]
28. Madison, M.C.; Landers, C.T.; Gu, B.H.; Chang, C.Y.; Tung, H.Y.; You, R.; Hong, M.J.; Baghaei, N.; Song, L.Z.; Porter, P.; et al. Electronic cigarettes disrupt lung lipid homeostasis and innate immunity independent of nicotine. *J. Clin. Investig.* **2019**, *129*, 4290–4304. [CrossRef] [PubMed]
29. Wang, Q.; Sundar, I.; Li, D.; Lucas, J.; Muthumalage, T.; McDonough, S.; Rahman, I. E-cigarette-Induced Pulmonary Inflammation and Dysregulated Repair are Mediated by nAChR alpha7 Receptor: Role of nAChR alpha7 in ACE2 Covid-19 receptor regulation. *Respir. Res.* **2020**, *21*, 154. [CrossRef] [PubMed]
30. Husari, A.; Shihadeh, A.; Talih, S.; Hashem, Y.; El Sabban, M.; Zaatari, G. Acute Exposure to Electronic and Combustible Cigarette Aerosols: Effects in an Animal Model and in Human Alveolar Cells. *Nicotine Tob. Res.* **2016**, *18*, 613–619. [CrossRef] [PubMed]
31. Glynos, C.; Bibli, S.I.; Katsaounou, P.; Pavlidou, A.; Magkou, C.; Karavana, V.; Topouzis, S.; Kalomenidis, I.; Zakynthinos, S.; Papapetropoulos, A. Comparison of the effects of e-cigarette vapor with cigarette smoke on lung function and inflammation in mice. *Am. J. Physiol. Lung Cell. Mol. Physiol.* **2018**, *315*, L662–L672. [CrossRef] [PubMed]
32. Han, H.; Peng, G.; Meister, M.; Yao, H.; Yang, J.J.; Zou, M.H.; Liu, Z.R.; Ji, X. Electronic Cigarette Exposure Enhances Lung Inflammatory and Fibrotic Responses in COPD Mice. *Front. Pharmacol.* **2021**, *12*, 726586. [CrossRef]
33. Garcia-Arcos, I.; Geraghty, P.; Baumlin, N.; Campos, M.; Dabo, A.J.; Jundi, B.; Cummins, N.; Eden, E.; Grosche, A.; Salathe, M.; et al. Chronic electronic cigarette exposure in mice induces features of COPD in a nicotine-dependent manner. *Thorax* **2016**, *71*, 1119–1129. [CrossRef] [PubMed]
34. Shen, Y.H.; Pham, A.K.; Davis, B.; Smiley-Jewell, S.; Wang, L.; Kodavanti, U.P.; Takeuchi, M.; Tancredi, D.J.; Pinkerton, K.E. Sex and strain-based inflammatory response to repeated tobacco smoke exposure in spontaneously hypertensive and Wistar Kyoto rats. *Inhal. Toxicol.* **2016**, *28*, 677–685. [CrossRef] [PubMed]
35. Demedts, I.K.; Brusselle, G.G.; Bracke, K.R.; Vermaelen, K.Y.; Pauwels, R.A. Matrix metalloproteinases in asthma and COPD. *Curr. Opin. Pharmacol.* **2005**, *5*, 257–263. [CrossRef] [PubMed]
36. Higham, A.; Rattray, N.J.; Dewhurst, J.A.; Trivedi, D.K.; Fowler, S.J.; Goodacre, R.; Singh, D. Electronic cigarette exposure triggers neutrophil inflammatory responses. *Respir. Res.* **2016**, *17*, 56. [CrossRef]
37. Scott, A.; Lugg, S.T.; Aldridge, K.; Lewis, K.E.; Bowden, A.; Mahida, R.Y.; Grudzinska, F.S.; Dosanjh, D.; Parekh, D.; Foronjy, R.; et al. Pro-inflammatory effects of e-cigarette vapour condensate on human alveolar macrophages. *Thorax* **2018**, *73*, 1161–1169. [CrossRef]
38. Singh, K.P.; Lawyer, G.; Muthumalage, T.; Maremanda, K.P.; Khan, N.A.; McDonough, S.R.; Ye, D.; McIntosh, S.; Rahman, I. Systemic biomarkers in electronic cigarette users: Implications for noninvasive assessment of vaping-associated pulmonary injuries. *ERJ Open Res.* **2019**, *5*, 00182–2019. [CrossRef]
39. Ghosh, A.; Coakley, R.D.; Ghio, A.J.; Muhlebach, M.S.; Esther, C.R., Jr.; Alexis, N.E.; Tarran, R. Chronic E-Cigarette Use Increases Neutrophil Elastase and Matrix Metalloprotease Levels in the Lung. *Am. J. Respir. Crit. Care Med.* **2019**, *200*, 1392–1401. [CrossRef]

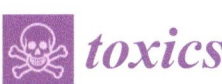

Article

Differences in Acellular Reactive Oxygen Species (ROS) Generation by E-Cigarettes Containing Synthetic Nicotine and Tobacco-Derived Nicotine

Shaiesh Yogeswaran and Irfan Rahman *

Department of Environmental Medicine, University of Rochester Medical Center, Box 850, 601 Elmwood Avenue, Rochester, NY 14642, USA; shaiesh_yogeswaran@urmc.rochester.edu
* Correspondence: irfan_rahman@urmc.rochester.edu; Tel.: +1-(585)-275-6911

Abstract: Electronic nicotine delivery systems (ENDS) containing synthetic nicotine have yet to be classified as tobacco products; consequently, there is ambiguity over whether Food and Drug Administration (FDA) regulatory authority can be extended to include tobacco-free nicotine (TFN) e-cigarettes. In recent years, a more significant number of e-cigarette companies have been manufacturing TFN-containing e-cigarettes and e-liquids to circumvent FDA regulations. While studies have shown that aerosols generated from tobacco-derived nicotine-containing e-cigarettes contain significant reactive oxygen species (ROS) levels, no comparison studies have been conducted using TFN e-cigarettes. This study uses a single puff aerosol generator to aerosolize TFN and tobacco-derived nicotine-containing vape products and subsequently involves semi-quantifying the ROS generated by these vape products in H_2O_2 equivalents. We found that the differences between ROS levels generated from TFN and tobacco-derived nicotine-containing vape products vary by flavor. TFN tobacco flavored and fruit flavored products are more toxic in terms of ROS generation than menthol/ice and drink/beverage flavored products using TFN. Our study provides further insight into understanding how flavoring agents used in vape products impact ROS generation from e-cigarettes differently in TFN e-cigarettes than e-cigarettes using tobacco-derived nicotine.

Keywords: tobacco-free nicotine (TFN); synthetic nicotine; tobacco-derived nicotine; vape-bar; electronic nicotine delivery systems; reactive oxygen species (ROS)

Citation: Yogeswaran, S.; Rahman, I. Differences in Acellular Reactive Oxygen Species (ROS) Generation by E-Cigarettes Containing Synthetic Nicotine and Tobacco-Derived Nicotine. *Toxics* **2022**, *10*, 134. https://doi.org/10.3390/toxics10030134

Academic Editors: Andrzej Sobczak and Leon Kośmider

Received: 7 February 2022
Accepted: 8 March 2022
Published: 11 March 2022

Publisher's Note: MDPI stays neutral with regard to jurisdictional claims in published maps and institutional affiliations.

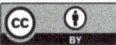

Copyright: © 2022 by the authors. Licensee MDPI, Basel, Switzerland. This article is an open access article distributed under the terms and conditions of the Creative Commons Attribution (CC BY) license (https://creativecommons.org/licenses/by/4.0/).

1. Introduction

Based on data from the 2021 National Youth Tobacco Survey (NYTS), a report published in the Morbidity and Mortality Weekly Report estimated 11.3% (1.72 million) of high school students and an estimated 2.8% (320,000) of middle school students currently use e-cigarettes [1]. E-cigarette aerosols contain numerous toxic chemicals, including acrolein, formaldehyde, and acetaldehyde; the latter two are known to cause lung disease and cardiovascular disease [2,3]. Previous studies have shown that aerosols generated from e-cigarette vapor contain exogenous reactive oxygen species (ROS) [4–6]. Additionally, studies have shown that exogenous ROS found in cigarette smoke and air pollutants can induce oxidative stress in the lungs and are the main factor in the development of chronic obstructive pulmonary disease (COPD) [7].

The 2021 NYTS found that out of all youth e-cigarette users surveyed, 85% used flavored e-cigarettes [1]. Additionally, one study has shown that ROS levels within e-cigarette aerosols vary amongst different flavored e-cigarettes and e-cigarettes of differing nicotine concentrations [4]. Regarding analyses of e-cigarette sales trends, a study conducted by the Office on Smoking and Health, a part of the Center for Disease Control and Prevention (CDC), found that 98.7% of flavored e-cigarettes sold in the United States in 2015 contain nicotine [8]. Ongoing efforts to reduce youth usage of e-cigarettes include the Food and Drug Administration (FDA) extending its tobacco regulatory authority to cover electronic nicotine delivery systems (ENDS), like e-cigarettes, in 2016 [9]. In May 2016, the FDA issued the Deeming Tobacco Products to be Subject to the Federal Food, Drug, and Cosmetic Act, commonly known as the "Deeming Rule" [9]. Under the "deeming rule," the FDA can regulate the sales of any product that contains tobacco or uses components derived from tobacco, like tobacco-derived nicotine; this includes e-cigarettes [9]. Moreover, since May 2016, the FDA has required all e-cigarette manufacturers and retailers to file premarket tobacco market applications (PMTAs) to gain permission from the agency to market their products [9]. The Center for Tobacco Products (CTP) oversees all products containing tobacco-derived nicotine; however, the FDA has not decided how to regulate synthetic nicotine-containing vape products; these products continue to remain unregulated [2,10,11]. In recent years, a more significant number of e-cigarette manufacturers have been using synthetic nicotine instead of tobacco-derived nicotine when producing e-cigarettes and e-liquids, all to bypass/evade FDA regulations [10]. Synthetic nicotine is chemically identical to nicotine from tobacco plants, with the former being made within a lab without the need of a tobacco plant [12]. In February 2021, Puff Bar, a prominent e-cigarette manufactured in the U.S., reintroduced their disposable vape-bar products, claiming them to contain synthetic nicotine and not containing tobacco or anything derived from tobacco [13]. Since Puff Bar's synthetic nicotine-containing vape bars entered the market in April 2021, Puff Bar has become the most popular company from which disposable e-cigarettes are purchased in the U.S., the company holding 51.3% of the national disposable e-cigarette market share [13]. No studies to date have been conducted involving comparative analyses in exogenous ROS levels between aerosols generated by synthetic-nicotine-containing e-cigarettes and those by e-cigarettes containing tobacco-derived nicotine. With the substantial rise in youth usage of e-cigarettes and a more significant number of e-cigarette manufacturers producing TFN e-cigarettes, more studies examining differences in ROS levels between aerosols generated by tobacco-based nicotine and synthetic nicotine-containing e-cigarettes are needed [11]. Unlike previous studies which have analyzed the ROS concentration levels within aerosols generated by tobacco-derived nicotine-containing e-cigarettes, our study includes analyses of the acellular ROS levels generated by TFN e-cigarettes [4–6]. Adding to the novelty of this study, we seek to understand the role the type of salt nicotine used in e-flavored e-cigarettes (synthetic or tobacco-derived) has in altering acellular ROS levels within generated aerosols. In this study, we quantify ROS levels generated by synthetic nicotine-containing ENDS products and compare them to ROS levels generated from their flavor-specific tobacco-derived nicotine-containing counterparts.

2. Materials and Methods

2.1. Procurement of Vape-Bars and E-Liquids

Three different TFN vape-bars and three different TFN e-liquids were analyzed in this study (Table 1). In addition to the six TFN vape-products analyzed, six different tobacco-derived nicotine-containing vape-bars were analyzed in this study. All vape-products (vape-bars and e-liquids) used in this study were either purchased from online vendors or local stores in the Rochester, NY area. All vape-bars and e-liquids used in this study have a salt nicotine concentration of 50 mg/mL or 5.0% nicotine by volume.

Table 1. Tobacco-derived and tobacco-free nicotine ENDS used in this study.

Company	Flavor	Nicotine Concentration (mg/mL)	Nicotine Salt-Type
Air Factory	Pink Punch (Pink Punch Lemonade)	50.0	TFN
Bad Drip	Rawberry Melon	50.0	TFN
Flair Plus	Pink Lemonade	50.0	Tobacco-Derived
Glas (BASIX Series)	Blue Razz	50.0	TFN
Hyppe	Blue Raz	50.0	Tobacco-Derived
Hyde	Spearmint	50.0	Tobacco-Derived
JUUL	Virginia Tobacco	50.0	Tobacco-Derived
Lit	Strawmelon	50.0	Tobacco-Derived
Pachamama	Banana Ice	50.0	TFN
Puff Bar	Banana Ice	50.0	Tobacco-Derived
Salty Man	Creamy Tobacco	50.0	TFN
Salty Man	Spearmint	50.0	TFN

2.2. Acellular ROS Quantification within Generated Aerosols

ROS levels within aerosols generated from all twelve vape-products were quantified via spectrofluorometry and in H_2O_2 equivalents. Aerosols from each individual TFN vape-product used in the study were generated using a Buxco Individual Cigarette Puff Generator (Data Sciences International (DSI), St. Paul, MN, USA) (Cat#601-2055-001) (Figure 1). Upon inserting the e-cigarette device into the central orifice apart of the adapter on the front side of the Puff Generator, the aerosol is generated and puffed by the mechanical part of the Puff Generator. Via tubing, the generated aerosols are then exposed to 10 mL of fluorogenic dye for a single puffing regimen at 1.5 L/min (Figure 1). One puffing regimen lasted for 10 min; 2 puffs/min, with each puff having a volume of 55.0 mL to simulate vaping topography parameters like puff volume, puff length, and puff duration This specific puffing regimen is identical to the puffing regimen used in our previous study analyzing acellular ROS levels with different flavored tobacco-derived nicotine-containing vape-bars and similar to the one used in another one of our previous studies examining acellular ROS levels generated by JUUL pods [4,14]. The fluorogenic dye used in the study was made from 0.01 N NaOH, $2'7'$ dichlorofluorescein diacetate (H_2DCF-DA) (EMD Biosciences, San Diego, CA, USA) (Cat#287810), phosphate (PO_4) buffer, and horseradish peroxidase (Thermo Fisher Scientific, Waltham, MA, USA (Cat#31491). Each TFN e-liquid was aerosolized using a new, empty refillable JUUL Pod (OVNStech, Shenzhen, China) (Model: WO1 JUUL Pods) inserted into a JUUL device (JUUL Labs Inc., Washington, DC, USA) (Model: Rechargeable JUUL Device w/USB charger). Subsequently, this JUUL device was inserted into the Individual Cigarette Puff Generator.

Each vape-bar and JUUL Pod containing TFN e-liquid had undergone three separate puffing regimens to prepare three individual samples of 10 mL dye solution exposed to e-cigarette aerosols. For our negative control, filtered air was passed through fluorogenic dye using the previously mentioned puffing regimen and inserting a filter into the Individual Puff Generator instead of an e-cigarette. For our positive control, the smoke generated from a conventional cigarette (Kentucky Tobacco Research & Development Center in the University of Kentucky, Lexington, KY, USA) (Model Reference: 3R4F) was exposed to fluorogenic dye under the previously mentioned puffing regimen. To avoid cross-contamination, once a specific e-cigarette had undergone a single puffing regimen, the tubing connecting the Puff Generator to the 50 mL conical tube containing dye was rinsed with 70% ethanol and then double-distilled water (ddH_2O). The tubing was also rinsed with 70% ethanol and ddH_2O prior to generating puffs from a different e-cigarette model.

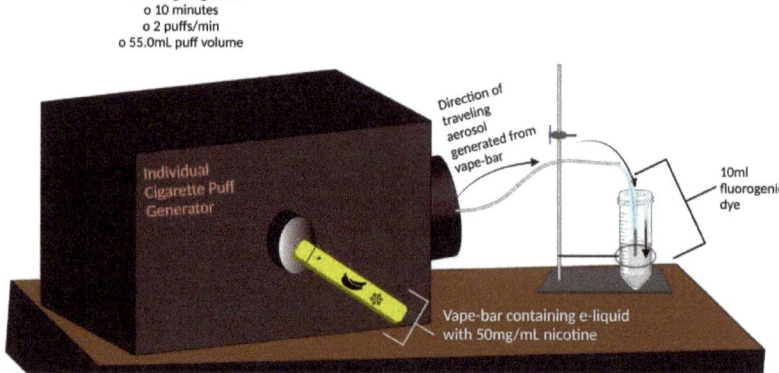

Figure 1. E-cigarette puff generator apparatus. The schematic shows the apparatus used to aerosolize each vape-bar and e-liquid included in this study. Once inserted into the Individual Cigarette Puff Generator, the component e-liquid within each vape bar was aerosolized for one individual puffing regimen; the generated aerosol was then exposed to 10 mL of fluorogenic dye during those ten minutes. One puffing regimen consisted of a vape-bar being aerosolized for 10 min and generating 20 total puffs, each puff lasting 3.0 s and having a volume of 55.0 mL. The entirety of the aerosolization process and the subsequent exposure of the generated aerosols to fluorogenic dye was done within a chemical fume hood. The pictogram was made using Adobe Illustrator and BioRender.

Subsequently, 0 µM, 10 µM, 15 µM, 20 µM, 30 µM, 40 µM, and 50 µM H_2O_2 standards were prepared using 30% H_2O_2 (Thermo Fischer Scientific, Waltham, MA, USA) (Cat#H323-500) and ddH_2O. After aerosolizing each vape product and exposing its generated aerosols to three separate 10 mL samples of fluorogenic dye, each resulting fluorogenic dye sample and standard was placed in a 37 °C degree water bath (VWR International, Radnor, PA) (Model: 1228 Digital Water Bath) for fifteen minutes. After placing each sample and standard into the water bath, the resulting solutions were analyzed via fluorescence spectroscopy (Ex = 475 nm and Em = 535 nm). Readings were taken on a spectrofluorometer (Thermo Fischer Scientific, Waltham, MA, USA) (Model: FM109535) in fluorescence intensity units (FIU) and measured as H_2O_2 equivalents.

2.3. Statistical Analyses

One-way ANOVA and Tukey's post-hoc test for multiple pairwise comparisons via GraphPad Prism Software version 8.1.1 was used to conduct statistical analyses of significance. Samples were run in triplicates. The results are shown as mean ± SEM with triplicate analyses. Data were considered to be statistically significant for p values < 0.05.

3. Results

Differences in ROS Levels within Aerosols Generated by TFN Vape-Products and Tobacco-Derived Nicotine-Containing Vape-Products Vary with Flavor

For the blueberry-raspberry-flavored vape-products analyzed, the level of ROS generated from the Hyppe: Blue Raz (5.0% tobacco-derived nicotine) bar (4.92–6.61 µM) did not significantly differ from that generated from the GLAS Basix Blue Razz (5.0% synthetic nicotine) e-liquid (4.97–7.44 µM) (Figure 2a). Among the strawberry watermelon flavored vape-bars analyzed, the difference in acellular ROS levels in aerosols generated by the Bad Drip: Rawberry Melon (5.0% synthetic nicotine) vape-bar (3.82–7.48 µM) and Lit: Strawmelon (5.0% tobacco-derived nicotine) vape-bar (4.10–4.77 µM) was not significant (Figure 2b).

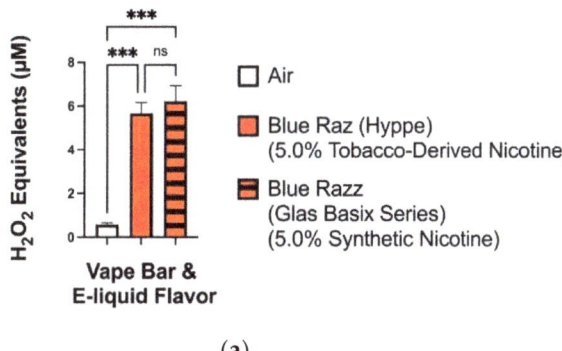

(a)

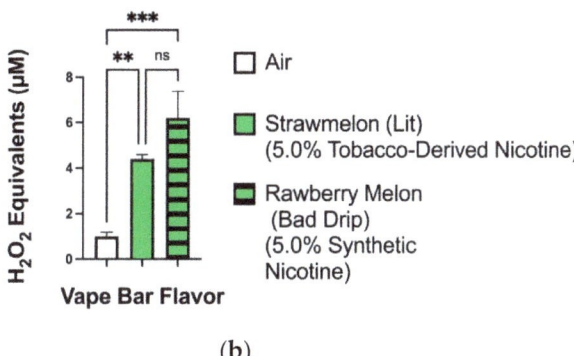

(b)

Figure 2. ROS levels within aerosols generated from blueberry-raspberry (**a**) and strawberry-melon (**b**) flavored tobacco-derived nicotine-containing and TFN vape-products. ROS levels within the generated aerosols from each individual TFN vape-product and tobacco-derived nicotine-containing vape-product was measured via spectrofluorometry and quantified as H_2O_2 equivalents. During analysis, the level of ROS generated from each individual vape-product was compared to the ROS generated from the filtered air control. Data are represented as mean ± SEM, and significance was determined by one-way ANOVA. ** $p < 0.01$ and *** $p < 0.001$ versus air controls. ns is abbreviated for "Non-Significant" versus air-controls ($p > 0.05$). Sample size (N) = 3–4.

Regarding minty/iced (cooled) flavored vape products, there appear to be significant differences in ROS levels generated between TFN vape products and their corresponding flavor-specific tobacco-derived nicotine counterparts (Figure 3). The level of ROS generated from the Pachamama: Banana Ice (5.0% synthetic nicotine) vape-bar (7.19–8.40 µM) differed significantly from that generated from the Puff Bar: Banana Ice (5.0% tobacco-derived nicotine) bar (9.69–15.87 µM) (Figure 3a). Similarly, the level of ROS generated from aerosolized Salty Mann: Spearmint (5.0% synthetic nicotine) e-liquid (1.33–2.11 µM) differed significantly from that generated from the Hyde: Spearmint (5.0% tobacco-derived nicotine) bar (3.28–4.50 µM) (Figure 3b).

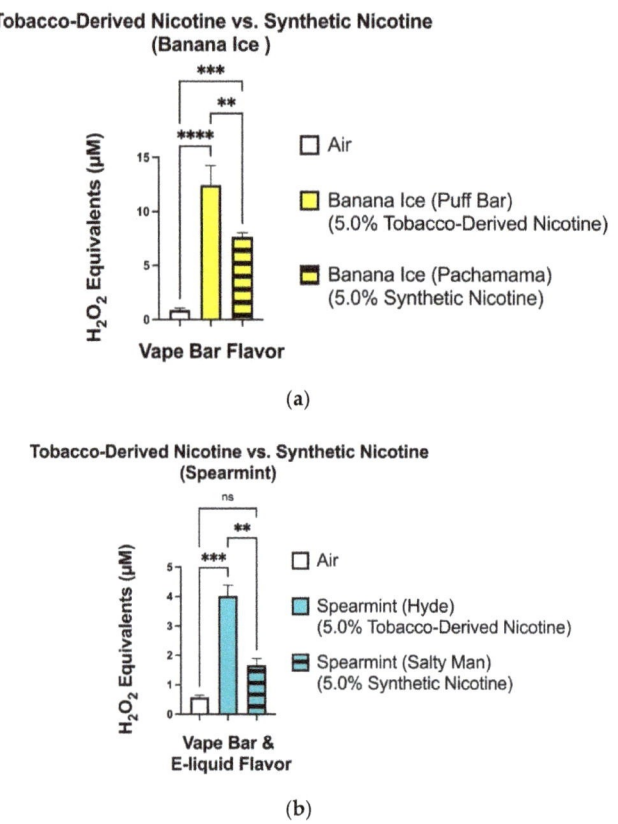

Figure 3. ROS generation among aerosols generated from banana ice (**a**) and spearmint (**b**) flavored TFN and tobacco-derived nicotine-containing vape-products. ROS levels within the generated aerosols from each individual minty/iced (cooled) flavored TFN and tobacco-derived nicotine-containing vape-product was measured via spectrofluorometry and quantified as H_2O_2 equivalents. During analysis, the level of ROS generated from each individual vape-bar was compared to the ROS generated from the filtered air control. Data are represented as mean ± SEM, and significance was determined by one-way ANOVA. ** $p < 0.01$, *** $p < 0.001$, and **** $p < 0.0001$ versus air controls. ns is abbreviated for "Non-Significant" versus air-controls ($p > 0.05$). Sample size (N) = 3–4.

When comparing tobacco-flavored vape products, the level of ROS generated from the aerosolized Salty Man: Creamy Tobacco (5.0% synthetic nicotine) e-liquid (2.32–3.96 µM) did not significantly differ from that generated from the JUUL: Virginia Tobacco (5.0% tobacco-derived nicotine) bar (1.26–5.14 µM) (Figure 4a). However, regarding drink-flavored ENDS, the level of ROS generated from the Flair Plus: Pink Lemonade (5.0% tobacco-derived nicotine) bar (1.84–2.47 µM) was significantly different from that generated from the aerosolized Air Factory: Pink Punch (5.0% synthetic nicotine) e-liquid (0.61–0.92 µM) (Figure 4b). Regarding comparisons of the differences in ROS production between all flavors that had tobacco-derived nicotine and all flavors that had synthetic nicotine, we found particular flavored e-cigarettes containing Tobacco-derived nicotine generated significantly higher levels of ROS compared to the air control (0.21–1.59 µM) than their TFN-containing counterpart (Figure 5). More specifically, the difference in ROS levels generated by the Blue Razz, Strawberry Melon, and Tobacco-flavored vape-products containing tobacco-derived nicotine and the air control was higher than that between the corresponding flavored TFN vape-products and the air control (Figure 5).

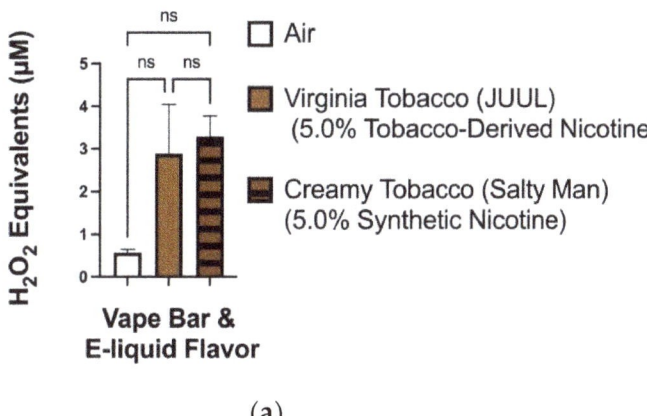

(a)

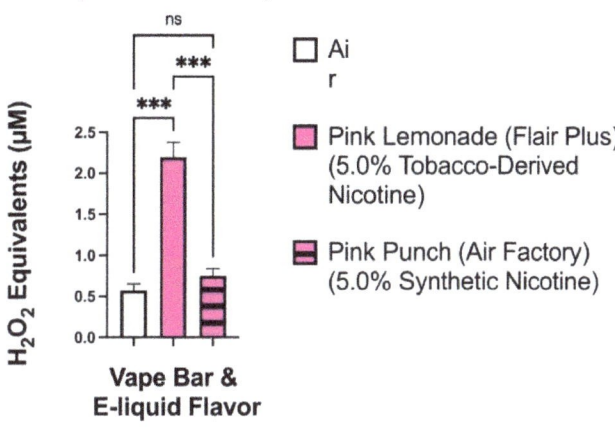

(b)

Figure 4. ROS generation among aerosols generated from tobacco (**a**) and drink flavored (**b**) TFN and tobacco-derived nicotine-containing vape-products. ROS levels within the generated aerosols from each individual tobacco and drink-flavored TFN e-liquid and tobacco-derived nicotine-containing vape-bar was measured via spectrofluorometry and quantified as H_2O_2 equivalents. During analysis, the level of ROS generated from each individual vape-bar was compared to the ROS generated from the filtered air control. Data are represented as mean ± SEM, and significance was determined by one-way ANOVA. *** $p < 0.001$ versus air controls. ns is abbreviated for "Non-Significant" versus air-controls ($p > 0.05$). Sample size (N) = 3–4.

Tobacco-derived Nicotine-containing Vape Products

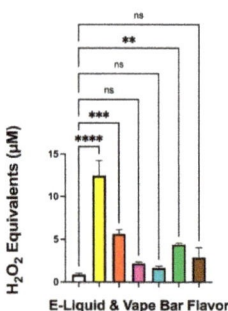

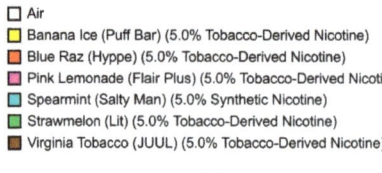

(a)

Synthetic Nicotine-containing Vape Products

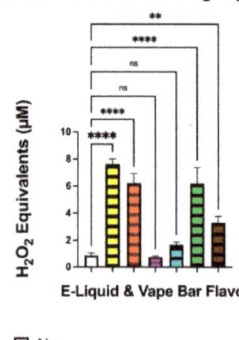

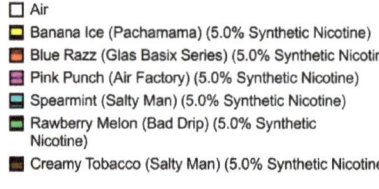

(b)

Figure 5. ROS generation among aerosols generated from tobacco-derived nicotine-containing (a) and TFN (b) vape-products ROS levels within the generated aerosols from each individual flavored TFN e-liquid and tobacco-derived nicotine-containing vape products were measured via spectrofluorometry and quantified as H_2O_2 equivalents. During analysis, the level of ROS generated from each individual vape-bar and e-liquid was compared to the ROS generated from the filtered air control. Data are represented as mean ± SEM, and significance was determined by one-way ANOVA. ** $p < 0.01$, *** $p < 0.001$, and **** $p < 0.0001$ versus air controls. ns is abbreviated for "Non-Significant" versus air-controls ($p > 0.05$). Sample size (N) = 3–4.

4. Discussion

Our data suggest that the type of nicotine salt used in e-liquids and vape-bars, tobacco-derived or synthetic, plays a role in modulating ROS generation upon component e-liquid aerosolization. To further explain, significant differences in ROS generation were observed between TFN and tobacco-derived nicotine-containing vape-products containing drink and minty/iced flavoring. However, non-significant differences in ROS generation were observed between TFN and tobacco-derived nicotine-containing vape-products with fruity and tobacco flavoring. Our data suggest that flavoring agents used in e-cigarettes containing synthetic nicotine play a role in modulating ROS levels within generated aerosols. Our data also indicate that flavoring agents used in e-liquids affect acellular ROS generation from synthetic-nicotine-containing e-cigarettes and tobacco-derived nicotine-containing e-cigarettes of comparable flavors differently.

Similarly, the results of our study seem to concur with our previous study, the data of which suggested that flavoring agents used in tobacco-derived nicotine-containing vape-bars play a role in modulating ROS generation upon component e-liquid aerosolization [4]. Regarding the effects of nicotine content on ROS generation and oxidative stress, one study had found that nicotine increases oxidative stress in rat mesencephalic cells in a dose-dependent manner [15]. Another study found that aerosols from flavored e-cigarettes and e-liquids promoted oxidative stress in H292 lung epithelial cells as well as in the lungs of mice [16]. Additionally, one study found that ROS generated from e-cigarettes was highly dependent on the flavor of e-liquid used (fruity and tobacco) [5]. However, studies examining the differences in ROS generation within cellular and acellular systems due to the usage of tobacco-derived nicotine-containing and TFN vape-products are lacking. While previous studies have shown that voltage, flavoring, and nicotine concentration have a role in modulating e-cigarette generated ROS levels, the results of our study show that the type of nicotine salt used (synthetic or tobacco-derived) does as well [4–6].

Interestingly, we noticed that amongst the minty/cooled flavored vape-products analyzed (Spearmint and Banana Ice), the level of ROS generated by the synthetic-nicotine vape-product was significantly less than that generated by its flavor specific tobacco-derived nicotine-containing counterpart. Additionally, amongst the drink/beverage-flavored vape-products analyzed, the synthetic nicotine-containing vape product generated significantly less ROS than its tobacco-derived nicotine-containing counterpart. Synthetic nicotine lacks the impurities contained within tobacco-derived nicotine [11,17]. Vape products using synthetic nicotine lack tobacco specific nitrosamines (TSNAs), a carcinogen found in tobacco and tobacco-derived nicotine [11,17,18]. In our study, the differences in exogenous ROS between aerosols generated by TFN and tobacco-derived nicotine-containing vape-products with Pink Lemonade, Spearmint, and Banana-Ice flavoring may be due to the differences in impurities within each type of nicotine salt (tobacco-derived or synthetic) used. However, to determine whether the results observed for the Pink Punch Lemonade, Spearmint, and Banana Ice flavored ENDS are due to differences in the level of impurities within the salt nicotine used, e-cigarette screening via inductively coupled plasma mass spectrometry (ICP-MS) is needed.

Regarding the limitations of this study, due to there being very few companies that manufacture both TFN and tobacco-derived nicotine-containing vape-products, we could not control for the e-cigarette brand in our pairwise comparisons between TFN products and their flavor specific tobacco-derived nicotine-containing counterparts, as well as differences between enantiomers or stereoisomers (R-nicotine vs. S-nicotine) of nicotine in both the products. Many vendors which utilize synthetic nicotine in their vape products either never sold e-cigarettes using tobacco-derived nicotine or stopped selling them entirely due to the cost-burden associated with submitting PMTAs and lack of public interests, and confirming the validity of synthetic vs. natural nicotine. One study has shown that even amongst e-cigarettes of the same flavor, ROS levels within generated aerosols vary by brand [4]. Future studies examining the differences in ROS levels generated by TFN vape products and their flavor-specific tobacco-derived nicotine-containing counterparts of the same company are needed, as well as cellular studies.

5. Conclusions

Our data suggest that TFN tobacco flavors and fruit flavors are more toxic in terms of ROS generation than menthol/ice and drink/beverage flavored products using TFN. In other words, beverage flavor and minty/iced (cool) flavored TFN products generate significantly less ROS than their corresponding flavor-specific tobacco-derived nicotine-containing counterparts. Our study provides insight into how interactions between flavoring agents and salt-nicotine used in e-cigarettes impact ROS levels generated by TFN e-cigarettes differently than e-cigarettes using tobacco-derived nicotine.

Author Contributions: Conceptualization, I.R.; methodology, I.R. and S.Y.; software, S.Y.; validation, S.Y. and I.R.; formal analysis, S.Y.; investigation, S.Y.; resources, I.R.; data curation, S.Y.; writing—original draft preparation, S.Y.; writing—review and editing, I.R.; editing, S.Y. and I.R.; visualization, S.Y.; supervision, I.R.; project administration, I.R.; funding acquisition, I.R. All authors have read and agreed to the published version of the manuscript.

Funding: This research was supported by our TCORS Grant: CRoFT 1 U54 CA228110-01.

Institutional Review Board Statement: All assays and experiments performed in this study were approved and in accordance with the University of Rochester Institutional Biosafety Committee. Additionally all protocols, procedures, and data analysis in this study followed the NIH guidelines and standards of reproducibility and scientific rigor by an unbiased approach. (Biosafety Study approval #Rahman/102054/09-167/07-186; identification code: 07-186; date of approval: 1 May 2019). No animals or human subjects were used.

Informed Consent Statement: Not applicable as study did not involve humans.

Data Availability Statement: We declare that we have provided all the data in figures.

Acknowledgments: Graphical Abstract and Figure 1 were made using BioRender and Adobe Illustrator. Figures 2–5 were made using GraphPadprism.

Conflicts of Interest: The authors declare that they have no conflict of interest.

References

1. Park-Lee, E.; Ren, C.; Sawdey, M.D.; Gentzke, A.S.; Cornelius, M.; Jamal, A.; Cullen, K.A. Notes from the Field: E-Cigarette Use among Middle and High School Students—National Youth Tobacco Survey, United States, 2021. *MMWR. Morb. Mortal. Wkly. Rep.* **2021**, *70*, 1387–1389. [CrossRef] [PubMed]
2. Bein, K.; Leikauf, G.D. Acrolein—A pulmonary hazard. *Mol. Nutr. Food Res.* **2011**, *55*, 1342–1360. [CrossRef] [PubMed]
3. Ogunwale, M.A.; Li, M.; Raju, M.V.R.; Chen, Y.; Nantz, M.H.; Conklin, D.J.; Fu, X.-A. Aldehyde Detection in Electronic Cigarette Aerosols. *ACS Omega* **2017**, *2*, 1207–1214. [CrossRef] [PubMed]
4. Yogeswaran, S.; Muthumalage, T.; Rahman, I. Comparative Reactive Oxygen Species (ROS) Content among Various Flavored Disposable Vape Bars, including Cool (Iced) Flavored Bars. *Toxics* **2021**, *9*, 235. [CrossRef] [PubMed]
5. Zhao, J.; Zhang, Y.; Sisler, J.D.; Shaffer, J.; Leonard, S.S.; Morris, A.M.; Qian, Y.; Bello, D.; Demokritou, P. Assessment of reactive oxygen species generated by electronic cigarettes using acellular and cellular approaches. *J. Hazard. Mater.* **2018**, *344*, 549–557. [CrossRef] [PubMed]
6. Haddad, C.; Salman, R.; El-Hellani, A.; Talih, S.; Shihadeh, A.; Saliba, N.A. Reactive Oxygen Species Emissions from Supra- and Sub-Ohm Electronic Cigarettes. *J. Anal. Toxicol.* **2018**, *43*, 45–50. [CrossRef] [PubMed]
7. Rahman, I.; MacNee, W. Role of oxidants/antioxidants in smoking-induced lung diseases. *Free Radic. Biol. Med.* **1996**, *21*, 669–681. [CrossRef]
8. Marynak, K.L.; Gammon, D.; Rogers, T.; Coats, E.M.; Singh, T.; King, B.A. Sales of Nicotine-Containing Electronic Cigarette Products: United States, 2015. *Am. J. Public Health* **2017**, *107*, 702–705. [CrossRef] [PubMed]
9. Food and Drug Administration. Deeming Tobacco Products To Be Subject to the Federal Food, Drug, and Cosmetic Act, as Amended by the Family Smoking Prevention and Tobacco Control Act; Restrictions on the Sale and Distribution of Tobacco Products and Required Warning Statements for Tobacco Products. Final Rule. *Fed. Regist.* **2016**, *81*, 28973–29106.
10. Cwalina, S.N.; McConnell, R.; Benowitz, N.L.; Barrington-Trimis, J.L. Tobacco-free Nicotine—New Name, Same Scheme? *N. Engl. J. Med.* **2021**, *385*, 2406–2408. [CrossRef] [PubMed]
11. Jordt, S.-E. Synthetic nicotine has arrived. *Tob. Control* **2021**. PMID:34493630. Available online: https://tobaccocontrol.bmj.com/content/tobaccocontrol/early/2021/09/07/tobaccocontrol-2021-056626.full.pdf (accessed on 6 February 2022).

12. Zettler, P.J.; Hemmerich, N.; Berman, M.L. Closing the Regulatory Gap for Synthetic Nicotine Products. *Boston Coll. Law Rev.* **2018**, *59*, 1933–1982. [PubMed]
13. Chen-Sankey, J.; Ganz, O.; Seidenberg, A.; Choi, K. Effect of a 'tobacco-free nicotine' claim on intentions and perceptions of Puff Bar e-cigarette use among non-tobacco-using young adults. *Tob. Control* **2021**. [CrossRef] [PubMed]
14. Muthumalage, T.; Lamb, T.; Friedman, M.R.; Rahman, I. E-cigarette flavored pods induce inflammation, epithelial barrier dysfunction, and DNA damage in lung epithelial cells and monocytes. *Sci. Rep.* **2019**, *9*, 19035. [CrossRef] [PubMed]
15. Barr, J.; Sharma, C.S.; Sarkar, S.; Wise, K.; Dong, L.; Periyakaruppan, A.; Ramesh, G.T. Nicotine induces oxidative stress and activates nuclear transcription factor kappa B in rat mesencephalic cells. *Mol. Cell. Biochem.* **2006**, *297*, 93–99. [CrossRef] [PubMed]
16. Lerner, C.A.; Sundar, I.K.; Yao, H.; Gerloff, J.; Ossip, D.J.; McIntosh, S.; Robinson, R.; Rahman, I. Vapors Produced by Electronic Cigarettes and E-Juices with Flavorings Induce Toxicity, Oxidative Stress, and Inflammatory Response in Lung Epithelial Cells and in Mouse Lung. *PLoS ONE* **2015**, *10*, e0116732. [CrossRef] [PubMed]
17. Hellinghausen, G.; Lee, J.T.; Weatherly, C.A.; Lopez, D.A.; Armstrong, D.W. Evaluation of nicotine in tobacco-free-nicotine commercial products. *Drug Test. Anal.* **2017**, *9*, 944–948. [CrossRef] [PubMed]
18. Yalcin, E.; de la Monte, S. Tobacco nitrosamines as culprits in disease: Mechanisms reviewed. *J. Physiol. Biochem.* **2016**, *72*, 107–120. [CrossRef] [PubMed]

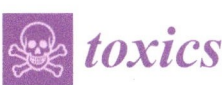

Article

The Impact of the Storage Conditions and Type of Clearomizers on the Increase of Heavy Metal Levels in Electronic Cigarette Liquids Retailed in Romania

Alexandra Jităreanu [1], Irina Gabriela Cara [2,*], Alexandru Sava [3], Ioana Mârțu [4], Ioana-Cezara Caba [1] and Luminița Agoroaei [1]

1. Department of Toxicology, Faculty of Pharmacy, University of Medicine and Pharmacy "Grigore T. Popa", 700115 Iași, Romania; jitareanu.alexandra@umfiasi.ro (A.J.); ioana-cezara.caba@umfiasi.ro (I.-C.C.); luminita.agoroaei@umfiasi.ro (L.A.)
2. Research Institute for Agriculture and Environment, "Ion Ionescu de la Brad" University of Life Sciences, 700115 Iasi, Romania
3. Department of Analytical Chemistry, Faculty of Pharmacy, University of Medicine and Pharmacy "Grigore T. Popa", 700115 Iași, Romania; alexandru-i-sava@d.umfiasi.ro
4. Department of Dental Technology, Faculty of Dental Medicine, University of Medicine and Pharmacy "Grigore T. Popa", 700115 Iași, Romania; ioana.martu@umfiasi.ro
* Correspondence: carairina@uaiasi.ro

Abstract: The growing popularity of electronic cigarettes has raised several public health concerns, including the risks associated with heavy metals exposure via e-liquids and vapors. The purpose of this study was to determine, using atomic absorption spectrometry, the concentrations of Pb, Ni, Zn, and Co in some commercially available e-liquid samples from Romania immediately after purchase and after storage in clearomizers. Lead and zinc were found in all investigated samples before storage. The initial concentrations of Pb ranged from 0.13 to 0.26 mg L^{-1}, while Zn concentrations were between 0.04 and 0.07 mg L^{-1}. Traces of nickel appeared in all investigated e-liquids before storage but in very small amounts (0.01–0.02 mg L^{-1}). Co was below the detection limits. We investigated the influence of the storage period (1, 3, and 5 days), storage temperature (22 °C and 40 °C), and type of clearomizer. In most cases, the temperature rise and storage period increase were associated with higher concentrations of heavy metals. This confirms that storage conditions can affect metal transfer and suggests that the temperature of storage is another parameter that can influence this phenomenon.

Keywords: e-liquids; heavy metals; storage

1. Introduction

Over the past decade, electronic nicotine-delivery systems, assigned as e-cigarettes, have been viewed as a substitute with fewer health risks compared to conventional tobacco cigarettes [1,2].

The progress of these products' technology generated a diverse range of e-cigarettes types available on the market worldwide. The generation of e-cigarettes design consists of closed- and open-system devices as described by Chen et al. [3]. Open-system devices have three fundamental items: a battery, a clearomizer, and a refillable tank where users can mix different e-liquids [3]. Typically, e-cigarettes transform a liquid solution consisting of propylene glycol, vegetable glycerol, as well as nicotine, and flavors into aerosols, which are inhaled [4–7].

The composition of e-liquids and e-cigarettes aerosol is crucial in determining potential health implications. The analysis can be challenging due to the great variety of

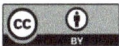

e-liquids present on the market. Several studies identified toxicants, such as tobacco-specific nitrosamines and other nicotine decomposition products, metals, and carbonyl compounds [4,5,8].

Toxic metals, such as nickel (Ni), zinc (Zn), and lead (Pb), may be present in electronic cigarettes as well as in the aerosols formed, exposing users and those in immediate proximity (passive vaping). These metals can originate from e-liquids but mostly from the metal coils included in the clearomizer of the e-cigarette device. The Scanning Electron Microscopy Energy–Dispersive X-Ray (Sem-EDX) analysis of e-cigarette coils revealed the presence of metals, such as chromium (Cr), nickel (Ni), lead (Pb), zinc (Zn), and copper (Cu), and consequently, the transfer to the e-liquids and aerosols is possible [9–12].

Several metals, including cadmium (Cd), chromium (Cr), lead (Pb), nickel (Ni), zinc (Zn), copper (Cu), iron (Fe), and arsenic (As), have been found in e-cigarette samples and further detected in human biological samples collected from e-cigarette users. Inductively Coupled Plasma Mass Spectrometry (ICP-MS), Atomic Absorption Spectrometry (AAS), Total Reflection X-ray Fluorescence (TRXF), and Molecular Fluorescence are common techniques used to analyze heavy metals in e-cigarettes [13–15]. Therefore, with the exception of Cd, similar metals' concentrations were found in the biological samples collected from e-cigarette users compared with conventional tobacco cigarette smokers [16]. Although cobalt (Co) is not a common element found in the environment or in the composition of alloys used in the construction of e-cigarettes or other ENDS (electronic nicotine delivery systems), small amounts of this metal were identified in the components of clearomizers from all generations [17].

The longer-term effects of e-cigarettes exposure are still inconclusive, but the existing literature reports revealed their inflammatory, irritant, and cytotoxic potential [18]. The major route of metal exposure is through direct or secondary inhalation of e-liquids, which is associated with serious health threats, such as carcinogenic and neurotoxic risks [19]. The risks are augmented by the size of the particles. E-cigarette aerosols contain nanoparticles (11–25 nm median diameter) and submicron particles (96–175 nm median diameter) [20]. The size of the inhaled particles is important for the depth of airway penetration, and the toxic potential can be enhanced by the high penetration of small-sized particles in tissues and organs [21,22]. Re et al. found a connection between chronic e-cigarette aerosol exposure and endogen metal dyshomeostasis, which has been linked to the onset of neurodegenerative diseases, such as Alzheimer's and Parkinson's [19]. The risk of neurotoxicity is significantly higher for young people's developing brains. They proved that neurotoxic levels of metals accumulated in the striatum, the frontal cortex, and the ventral midbrain of rodents after exposure to e-cigarette aerosols, increasing the risks of developing neurological disorders and neurodegenerative diseases [19]. Metal accumulation in the nervous system in the case of e-cigarette use is enhanced by the alteration of the blood–brain barrier integrity [23].

Long-term Pb exposure could be related to a variety of neurological and peripheral structure illnesses, cardiovascular issues, and muscle system abnormalities in humans [24]. Chronic inhalation of lead nanoparticles is associated with cardiovascular, respiratory, and central nervous system alterations. The results of the studies concerning lead exposure for e-cigarette users are still contradictory. Wiener and Bhandari found similar blood lead levels in subjects who used or did not use e-cigarettes, while Goniewicz et al. showed that the urinary level of lead was lower in never-users than in e-cigarette smokers [25,26]. In a study performed on 100 participants, Olmedo et al. evaluated exposure to metals through e-cigarettes by assessing the metal levels in non-invasive biological samples (urine, hair, and exhaled breath condensate) [27]. Metals such as Cr, Cu, Pb, and Sn were found in higher quantities in the urine of e-cigarette users, but the study could not correlate the metal levels in the biological samples with the concentrations determined in e-vapors. It could not confirm that vaping was the main source of metal exposure [27].

Ni is a toxic metal, and its adverse health effects are linked to changes in heart rate, oxidative stress, and the consequent lung, nasal, and paranasal cancers [9,28,29]. The possible toxic effects of e-cigarette are also related to respiratory system damage. Ni is classified as inhalation carcinogens, and the lung represents the most sensitive target of Ni toxicity [16,30]. The results of Fowles et al. estimated the toxicity of heavy metals (especially chromium and nickel) in e-liquids and aerosols and related to major health issues, such as cancer [24]. The prolonged exposure of Ni in the human body can significantly increase the risk of cancer [24].

Another metal of concern is Co. Cobalt exposure can cause hematopoietic effects, cardiomyopathy, hypothyroidism, and thyroid hyperplasia, and it also has irritant effects on the respiratory tract [31]. A recent study investigated the association between cobalt exposure (cobalt lung) and e-cigarette users who developed giant cell interstitial pneumonia and hard metal pneumoconiosis [32], but several inconsistencies were identified in this report (cobalt was not determined in the original method cited by the authors, and Co was not found in the lung samples collected from the patient) [33].

In accordance with its function to human growth and development, Zn is one of the more fundamental elements and a cofactor for the activity of many enzymes, but inhaling large amounts of Zn and Zn-derivative nanoparticles can cause airway inflammation [16,34]. Increased Zn concentrations have been associated with copper deficiencies in the liver and heart along with metalloenzymes function interference and iron storage, resulting in anemia [35]

Several parameters were investigated to see their influence on metal concentrations in both e-liquids and aerosols. Zhao et al. determined the concentrations in e-cigarette aerosols produced in open- and closed-systems devices and concluded that the device type influenced metal release to aerosols; aerosols generated in open-system devices presented higher concentrations of metals [1]. Furthermore, metal concentrations increased with power setting, and a higher voltage is associated with an increased coil temperature and a higher probability of degradation and metal emissions. Differences in coil composition can also affect metal levels in aerosols [1].

In some cases, the e-liquids can remain in clearomizers for several days, stored at different environmental temperatures, and it is important to identify the factors that influence metal emissions of the components of the clearomizers. Na et al. investigated the metal release phenomenon during storage and use [11]. They concluded that metal transfer is influenced by the duration of storage in the e-cigarette device and that the concentrations of heavy metals found in e-liquids were significantly higher after e-cigarette use [11].

Starting from these findings, the present study aimed to determine the concentration of some important heavy metals (Pb, Ni, Zn, and Co) in some e-liquids found on the Romanian market. Samples from five (5) different e-cigarette brands were obtained from national retail markets. The heavy metal content after purchasing (from e-liquid bottles) and storage period (1, 3, and 5 days) at different temperatures (22 °C and 40 °C) were analyzed, and their concentrations were linked to World Health Organization (WHO) and Food and Agriculture Organization (FAO) recommended limits.

2. Materials and Methods

2.1. Sample Preparation

The types of electronic cigarette samples (ECS) were purchased from the national market outlets (from VapePoint and Etigareta shops, Iasi, Romania). A total of five commercially available e-liquid samples of various nicotine concentrations and different flavoring agents were selected for this study (Table 1). The samples were selected randomly, but the variable nicotine concentration and the different flavor and propylene glycol:vegetable glycerin ratio were taken into consideration for the selection. The packaging of the liquids consisted of 10 mL plastic dropper bottles (the dropper lids were also made from plastic). The samples coded from A to E were kept at room temperature (22 °C) until analysis. The basic composition description of the EC liquids (according to the manufacturer) consists predominantly of propylene glycol (PG) and vegetable glycerin (VG).

Table 1. Basic composition of EC liquids selected in this study.

Sample	Nicotine (mg/mL)	PG:VG Ratio (w/w)	Flavor
A	0	50:50	Dark tobacco
B	6	70:30	Cherry
C	12	50:50	Apple
D	18	70:30	Tobacco
E	18	50:50	Cuban cigar

Data presented were available on the labels of the products.

For each sample, their heavy metal content was analyzed under three variables/conditions:

- I: The initial phase: the EC liquids were directly taken from EC liquid bottles as purchased from retail;
- II: EC liquid analyzed for storage period and clearomizer effect: the samples were stored for 1, 3, and 5 days in 2 different types of EC clearomizers purchased from specialized shops (VapePoint and Etigareta shops, Iasi, Romania). The clearomizers were selected based on their popularity. According to the employees from the vape shops, at the time of the purchase, these models were requested most frequently by the customers. Both clearomizers were "tank-style" electronic cigarettes and belonged to the second generation of electronic cigarettes [36,37]; clearomizer 1 was a CE4 type, while clearomizer 2 was a T3S type. The clearomizers (Figure 1) presented different tank capacities (1.6 mL and, respectively, 3.0 mL) and were made from dark plastic material (clearomizer 1) and clear, resistant plastic (clearomizer 2). Inside the tank, an atomizing unit with metallic coil and wick material were visible. The prices for the two clearomizers were also different (rating as "low"—clearomizer 1 and "high"—clearomizer 2);
- III: EC liquid analyzed for storage period and temperature effect: EC liquids were stored in the two clearomizers mentioned above at two different temperatures: 22 °C (room temperature) and 40 °C. In this step, the samples were maintained in room with controlled temperature (22 °C), in the absence of direct sunlight, and in a programmable furnace (Model Nobertherm, Germany) at 40 °C for 1, 3, and 5 days in order to investigate the concentration of heavy metals that can be released through their storage under improper/inadequate conditions. For each clearomizer and both the variables (storage period and temperature), three replicates of each sample were performed. The clearomizers were filled and sealed with the e-liquid, from which an aliquot of 1 mL was separated and analyzed.

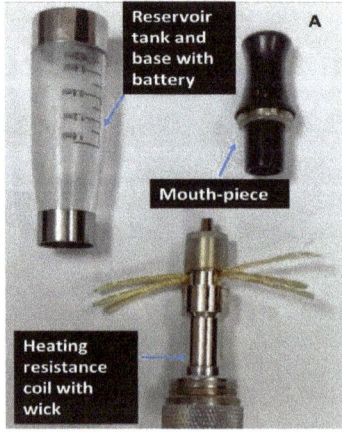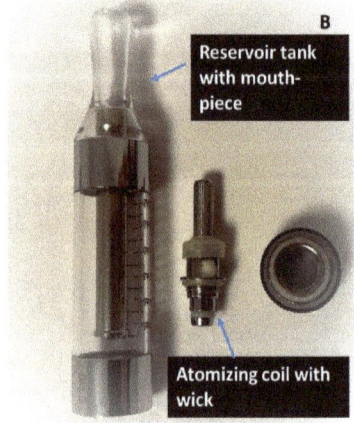

Figure 1. Anatomy of the clearomizers used in the experiment ((**A**) clearomizer 1; (**B**) clearomizer 2).

The storage period and temperature were chosen in order to mimic real-life scenarios. Electronic cigarette users do not keep e-liquids inside the clearomizers for more than a few days before using them, and that is why we chose a five-day limit for the storage period. The room temperature is usually around 22 °C, but it can reach 40 °C during very hot summer days; we have chosen these two temperature values to evaluate the storage temperature's influence on metal transfer.

For heavy metal analysis, 1 mL of each e liquid sample was performed by diluting with 10 mL of 5% HNO_3 solution. This mixture was sonicated for 30 min (Elma S180, Elmasonic sonicator), and then, the solution were analyzed by AAS [11]. A blank e-liquid sample was prepared by mixing PG and VG at the same ratio (1:1, w/w) and analyzed according to real sample method.

2.2. Reagents and Standards

All reagents and chemicals used in this study were of analytical grade. Nitric acid (HNO_3 Suprapur 65%, Merck, Darmstadt, Germany) and mono-element containing stock standard solutions of Ni, Pb, Zn, and Co (1000 mg L^{-1}, Merck, Darmstadt, Germany) were used to obtain the standard solution for the calibration curve.

Calibration standards were prepared by diluting the primary standard with 5% HNO_3 at five different concentration levels (0.05, 0.1, 0.2, 0.25, and 0.5 mg L^{-1}). All dilutions were performed using high-purity deionized water obtained from a Milli-Q water purification system (Millipore, Bedford, MA, USA).

The samples were prepared in 25 mL glass flasks (class A), which were previously immersed in 1% HNO_3 warm aqueous solution for at least 6 h and then rinsed with ultrapure water.

2.3. Instrument

An atomic absorption spectrometer-AAS (ContrAA 700, Analytikjena, Jena, Germany) was conducted to assess the metals concentrations. The parameters that were used to determine the concentration of heavy metal by AAS were a high-resolution continuum source, equipped with a xenon short lamp with UV arc in hot spot mode and a high-resolution echelle grating monochromator. The flame was generated using an air-acetylene mixture with 99.95% purity.

Accuracy, linearity, precision, limit of detection (LOD), and limit of quantification (LOQ) are some of the analytical criteria used to validate the optimized method.

The correlation coefficient (R^2) of the calibration curves was used to calculate the linearity. As part of the instrument's performance and method accuracy, the recovery of standard spiked samples was assessed using 5% HNO_3 method [11]. It was performed at each stage by spiking the e-liquid samples with two different concentrations (1.0 and 5.0 mg L^{-1}) of a mono-element standard. A blank sequence and spiked blanks were performed at each stage to ensure the results and cancel the matrix interferences.

The relative standard deviation (RSD) of the triplicate measurements of each e-liquid sample was used to compute the precision value. As a result, the values of this procedure are reported as an average RSD of triplicate measurements.

The limit of detection (LOD) was the lowest amount of metal that can be detected and was estimated by dividing the SD of three measurements of the PG/VG mixture with the slope of the calibration curve. The limit of quantification (LOQ) was defined as the smallest amount that can be quantitatively identified at a specified precision and accuracy.

2.4. Data Analysis

Three replicates were taken for each sample, and the average value was calculated. The mean values were statistically analyzed using the *t*-test with a 95% confidence level.

3. Results

3.1. Calibration and Detection Limit

Table 2 presents the calibration results for the determination of heavy metals Pb, Zn, Ni, and Co by AAS technique. The correlation coefficient was used to confirm the linearity of each trace element (R^2). The concentration ranged between 0.05–0.50 mg L^{-1} was established among absorbance and metal concentration; all calibration curves showed good linearity ($R^2 > 0.997$). The obtained LOD values ranging between 0.001–0.04 mg L^{-1} highlights the sensitivity of the method, as the analytical parameters are low compared with other analytical techniques [38].

Table 2. Calibration results for the determination of heavy metals in e-cigarettes.

Metal	Wavelength (nm)	Linear Range (mg L^{-1})	Detection Limit (mg L^{-1})	Correlation Coefficient (R^2)	RSD (%)
Pb	217.00	0.1–0.5	0.04	0.998	1.9
Zn	213.85	0.05–0.5	0.001	0.999	2.1
Ni	232.00	0.05–0.5	0.01	0.999	1.7
Co	240.72	0.05–0.5	0.005	0.997	3.4

The measurements were done in triplicate; RSD, Relative Standard Deviation of the triplicate measurements.

PG/VG mixture and e-liquids' samples spiked with concentration of 1.0 and 5.0 mg L^{-1} using mono-element standard registered 94.8 to 101% and 94.1 to 107.3% of the recoveries, with RSD less than 20% at all spiked quantities (Table 3). The method's accuracy was found to be appropriate and was confirmed for each heavy metal through real and spiked values measured in comparison.

Table 3. The average recovery (%) and RSD (%) of spiked samples.

Metal	E-Liquid Sample				PG/VG Mixture			
	1.0 mg L^{-1}		5.0 mg L^{-1}		1.0 mg L^{-1}		5.0 mg L^{-1}	
	Recovery (%)	RSD (%)	Recovery (%)	RSD (%)	Recovery (%)	RSD (%)	Recovery (%)	RSD (%)
Pb	94.1	2.5	96.2	1.9	95.7	7.8	95.9	4.1
Zn	98.3	4.5	107.3	2.1	94.8	4.6	95.5	6.9
Ni	95.4	1.7	95.7	2.3	98.1	3.9	101.3	4.8
Co	96.4	5.5	104.2	3.4	95.7	4.2	98.1	2.4

RSD, Relative Standard Deviation of the triplicate measurements; PG, propylene glycol; V, vegetable glycerin.

The recoveries for the reliability assessment of our experimental method based on spiked samples ranged between 94–107% with relative standard deviation ranged between 1.7–7.8%. According to these findings, the method presents good performance characteristics.

3.2. Heavy Metals Concentration in E-Cigarettes

The results of the heavy metal analysis using AAS for e-cigarette items being sold in Romania markets are presented. Consequently, the five e-cigarette brands were discovered to contain quantifiable levels of heavy metals (Table 4).

Table 4. Heavy metals (Pb, Ni, Zn) concentrations in EC liquids under different conditions.

Sample	Initial Conc. (mg L^{-1})	Clearomizer 1		Clearomizer 2	
		22 °C (mg L^{-1})	40 °C (mg L^{-1})	22 °C (mg L^{-1})	40 °C (mg L^{-1})
		Pb			
A(1)		0.28 ± 0.01	0.53 ± 0.01	0.37 ± 0.02	0.81 ± 0.01
A(3)	0.17 ± 0.02	0.58 ± 0.03	0.84 ± 0.02	0.74 ± 0.05	0.88 ± 0.09
A(5)		0.98 ± 0.04	1.84 ± 0.04	1.84 ± 0.07	1.94 ± 0.07
B(1)		0.47 ± 0.01	0.67 ± 0.03	0.50 ± 0.06	0.86 ± 0.02
B(3)	0.15 ± 0.03	0.78 ± 0.02	1.15 ± 0.11	0.78 ± 0.03	1.30 ± 0.06
B(5)		2.99 ± 0.15	3.22 ± 0.21	1.97 ± 0.7	1.98 ± 0.8
C(1)		0.58 ± 0.11	1.02 ± 0.16	0.49 ± 0.08	1.12 ± 0.21
C(3)	0.26 ± 0.06	0.78 ± 0.16	1.45 ± 0.18	0.85 ± 0.10	1.73 ± 0.36
C(5)		0.98 ± 0.20	1.86 ± 0.11	1.89 ± 0.08	2.38 ± 0.31
D(1)		0.20 ± 0.01	0.29 ± 0.04	0.76 ± 0.14	6.63 ± 1.32
D(3)	0.13 ± 0.01	0.42 ± 0.03	0.90 ± 0.07	0.94 ± 0.19	8.56 ± 1.78
D(5)		0.74 ± 0.04	1.77 ± 0.11	1.85 ± 0.21	10.48 ± 1.91
E(1)		1.20 ± 0.19	4.72 ± 0.83	1.98 ± 0.73	4.48 ± 1.03
E(3)	0.19 ± 0.01	2.56 ± 0.53	5.36 ± 0.38	3.69 ± 1.03	7.88 ± 2.11
E(5)		2.95 ± 0.74	7.27 ± 0.95	5.16 ± 1.38	9.23 ± 2.18
		Ni			
A(1)		0.11 ± 0.02	0.22 ± 0.08	0.15 ± 0.01	0.25 ± 0.02
A(3)	0.01 ± 0.01	0.18 ± 0.01	0.31 ± 0.05	0.23 ± 0.05	0.31 ± 0.06
A(5)		0.33 ± 0.05	0.46 ± 0.11	0.58 ± 0.09	2.30 ± 0.29
B(1)		0.09 ± 0.01	0.25 ± 0.05	1.10 ± 0.11	1.02 ± 0.11
B(3)	0.02 ± 0.01	0.60 ± 0.09	0.89 ± 0.07	1.73 ± 0.21	1.95 ± 0.18
B(5)		1.19 ± 0.12	1.59 ± 0.22	2.08 ± 0.26	2.83 ± 0.13
C(1)		0.03 ± 0.01	0.27 ± 0.09	0.19 ± 0.03	0.15 ± 0.04
C(3)	0.02 ± 0.01	0.05 ± 0.01	1.02 ± 0.26	0.89 ± 0.11	0.83 ± 0.09
C(5)		0.16 ± 0.03	1.61 ± 0.28	0.78 ± 0.08	0.87 ± 0.17
D(1)		0.18 ± 0.07	0.57 ± 0.11	0.15 ± 0.06	2.56 ± 0.42
D(3)	0.01 ± 0.01	0.33 ± 0.1	0.66 ± 0.18	0.63 ± 0.07	3.59 ± 0.38
D(5)		0.51 ± 0.11	0.87 ± 0.12	1.06 ± 0.11	4.04 ± 0.96
E(1)		0.18 ± 0.06	1.62 ± 0.53	1.28 ± 0.52	3.60 ± 0.84
E(3)	0.02 ± 0.01	0.32 ± 0.09	2.45 ± 0.78	2.63 ± 0.31	4.56 ± 0.91
E(5)		0.56 ± 0.15	3.96 ± 0.82	5.01 ± 0.79	8.19 ± 0.78
		Zn			
A(1)		0.17 ± 0.02	0.62 ± 0.12	0.17 ± 0.01	0.31 ± 0.08
A(3)	0.04 ± 0.01	0.30 ± 0.09	0.79 ± 0.19	0.19 ± 0.01	0.37 ± 0.11
A(5)		0.31 ± 0.07	0.85 ± 0.39	0.25 ± 0.03	0.45 ± 0.18
B(1)		1.36 ± 0.25	1.93 ± 0.43	0.91 ± 0.09	0.51 ± 0.17
B(3)	0.07 ± 0.01	4.02 ± 0.72	4.95 ± 0.61	3.50 ± 0.72	2.41 ± 0.77
B(5)		5.52 ± 0.73	6.98 ± 0.95	4.03 ± 0.90	3.78 ± 0.85
C(1)		0.78 ± 0.01	5.59 ± 0.67	0.16 ± 0.08	0.20 ± 0.02
C(3)	0.05 ± 0.01	1.25 ± 0.82	7.14 ± 0.85	0.88 ± 0.81	0.79 ± 0.14
C(5)		4.59 ± 0.91	7.84 ± 0.73	1.46 ± 0.93	1.84 ± 0.20
D(1)		0.69 ± 0.09	0.93 ± 0.15	1.01 ± 0.12	1.54 ± 0.84
D(3)	0.07 ± 0.01	2.60 ± 0.55	4.33 ± 0.83	1.12 ± 0.05	4.89 ± 0.66
D(5)		3.45 ± 0.86	4.56 ± 0.79	1.72 ± 0.09	5.89 ± 0.90
E(1)		3.35 ± 0.94	3.65 ± 0.25	2.40 ± 0.38	2.53 ± 0.62
E(3)	0.06 ± 0.01	7.45 ± 0.92	7.52 ± 0.89	3.12 ± 0.67	5.35 ± 0.88
E(5)		8.45 ± 0.85	8.20 ± 0.96	7.38 ± 0.73	8.75 ± 0.97

Data are presented as mean ± SD (standard deviation). Sample code: Sample number (number of storage days in the clearomizer).

3.2.1. Lead Concentration

In the present study, lead was found in all investigated samples before storage. The initial mean values of this metal ranged from 0.13 to 0.26 mg L^{-1}. The highest concentration of Pb was exhibited by sample C.

In Figure 2 are shown the Pb concentrations obtained for the five samples and their variation under different experimental conditions.

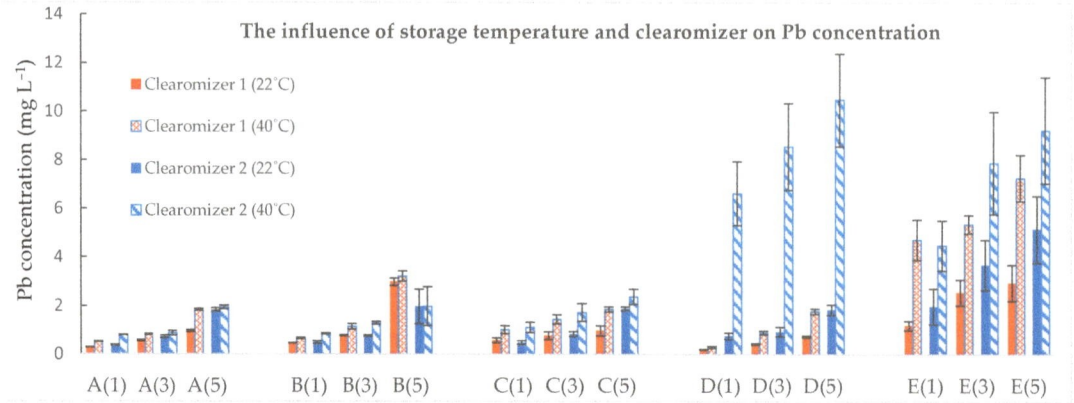

Figure 2. The influence of storage temperature and of the clearomizer on Pb concentration. Sample code: Sample number (number of storage days in the clearomizer).

As the storage period increased (from 1 to 5 days), the reported values in the five E-liquid samples for Pb also tended to increase. This pattern of Pb concentration was found in both types of clearomizers after storage, which showed that there are significantly higher differences after storage than the initial ones at the 0.05 level (p-value < 0.05) (Table 5).

Table 5. The influence of the duration of storage on Pb concentration; p-value for the paired t-test (t-test: Paired Two Sample for Means).

Storage Conditions	I vs. 1 D	I vs. 3 D	I vs. 5 D	1 D vs. 3 D	1 D vs. 5 D	3 D vs. 5 D
Clearomizer 1 (22 °C)	0.048	0.048	**0.019**	0.048	**0.022**	0.068
Clearomizer 1 (40 °C)	0.099	0.054	**0.023**	**0.0006**	**0.003**	**0.008**
Clearomizer 2 (22 °C)	0.048	0.049	**0.011**	0.055	**0.004**	**0.0001**
Clearomizer 2 (40 °C)	**0.045**	**0.042**	**0.029**	**0.049**	**0.018**	**0.0043**

I, initial; 1 D, storing for 1 day; 3 D, storing for 3 days; 5 D, storing for 5 days. Bold numbers denote the cases in which differences are statistically significant at 95% confidence level. Clearomizer 1, CE4-type clearomizer; Clearomizer 2, T3S-type clearomizer.

In addition, the current study investigated the influence of temperature on Pb transfer after storage in the two types of clearomizers (Figure 1). After increasing the storage temperature from 22 °C to 40 °C, higher Pb concentrations in the e-cigarette samples were obtained. The Pb content found in e-liquids sample E (after storage in both clearomizers) and sample D (after storage in clearomizer 2) showed the greatest increase, which suggests the release and transfer of heavy elements from the metal substrates of different components of clearomizers. The statistical analysis regarding the influence of temperature on Pb transfer was performed using the t-test. For clearomizer 1, the results of the analysis showed a significant difference at the 0.05 level only for samples B, C, and E, while for clearomizer 2, the results were significantly different at the 0.05 level for samples C, D, and E.

The research also included a comparison of the clearomizer type on Pb transfer when stored at temperatures of 22 °C and 40 °C. The results obtained were heterogeneous; for e-liquid samples A, C, D, and E, the average transfer of Pb was higher after storage in clearomizer 2, while for sample B, the transfer was higher for clearomizer 1.

The statistical analysis regarding the influence of the clearomizer on Pb transfer was performed using the *t*-test. At 22 °C, the results showed a significant difference at the 0.05 level only for samples D and E, while after storage at 40 °C, there was a significant difference only for sample D.

3.2.2. Nickel Concentration

The present study recorded small concentrations of Ni (0.01–0.02 mg L^{-1}) in each investigated EC liquid sample before storage. The related values for Ni content in the EC liquids are presented in Table 4.

As a general trend, storage at a higher temperature (40 °C in comparison to 22 °C) increased Ni transfer. The ascending trend of Ni levels in e-liquids in relation to the storage period and temperature is visible in Figure 3.

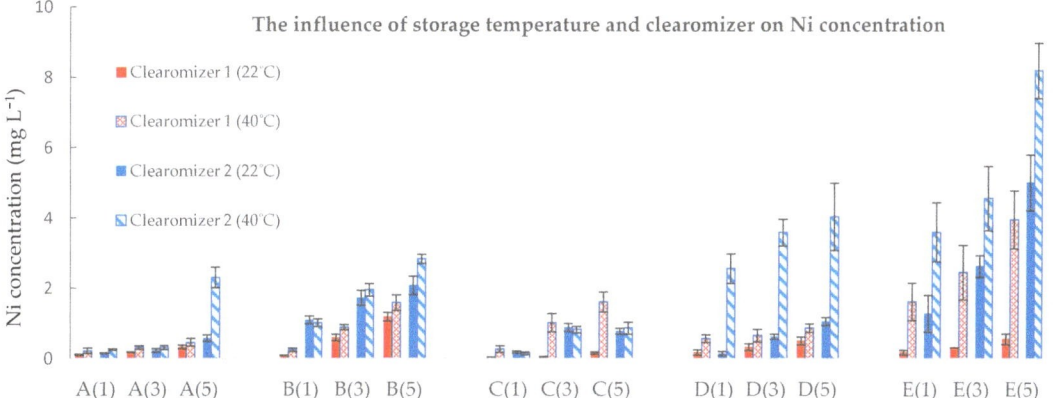

Figure 3. The influence of storage temperature and of the clearomizer on Ni concentration. Sample code: Sample number (number of storage days in the clearomizer).

According to our results, the concentrations of Ni were higher after the storage period, sustaining the possible metal transfer from the metallic parts of the clearomizer to the solutions. It is likely that Ni concentrations increased after storage in both clearomizers, with values significantly greater than the initial ones at the 0.05 level (Table 6).

Table 6. The influence of the duration of storage on Ni concentration; *p*-value for the paired *t*-test (*t*-test: Paired Two Sample for Means).

Storage Conditions	I vs. 1 D	I vs. 3 D	I vs. 5 D	1 D vs. 3 D	1 D vs. 5 D	3 D vs. 5 D
Clearomizer 1 (22 °C)	**0.013**	**0.018**	**0.018**	0.054	**0.033**	**0.021**
Clearomizer 1 (40 °C)	**0.049**	**0.022**	**0.024**	**0.020**	**0.023**	**0.030**
Clearomizer 2 (22 °C)	**0.045**	**0.023**	**0.041**	**0.017**	**0.047**	0.096
Clearomizer 2 (40 °C)	**0.045**	**0.025**	**0.021**	**0.007**	**0.015**	**0.048**

I, initial; 1 D, storing for 1 day; 3 D, storing for 3 days; 5 D, storing for 5 days. Bold numbers denote the cases in which differences are statistically significant at 95% confidence level. Clearomizer 1, CE4-type clearomizer; Clearomizer 2, T3S-type clearomizer.

The statistical analysis regarding the influence of temperature on the metal transfer was performed using the *t*-test. For clearomizer 1, the results of the analysis showed a significant difference at the 0.05 level for all samples, while for clearomizer 2, the results were significantly different at the 0.05 level only for samples D and E.

When analyzing the influence of the clearomizer (Figure 2), the data suggested that Ni transfer was more pronounced in the case of the EC liquids stored in clearomizer 2. The statistical analysis was performed using the *t*-test. At 22 °C, the results of the analysis showed a significant difference at the 0.05 level for samples B, C, and E, while at 40 °C, the results were significantly different at the 0.05 level for samples B, D, and E ($p < 0.05$).

3.2.3. Zinc Concentration

The concentrations of Zn in EC-liquid samples established during the present study are indicated in Table 4.

Concentrations of Zn were identified in EC liquid samples before storage. Zn initial concentrations were lower than the determined concentration of lead and ranged between 0.04–0.07 mg L^{-1}.

The concentrations of Zn increased significantly according to the storage period (from 1 to 5 days), and also, high levels of Zn were associated with storage at 40 °C temperature (Figure 4).

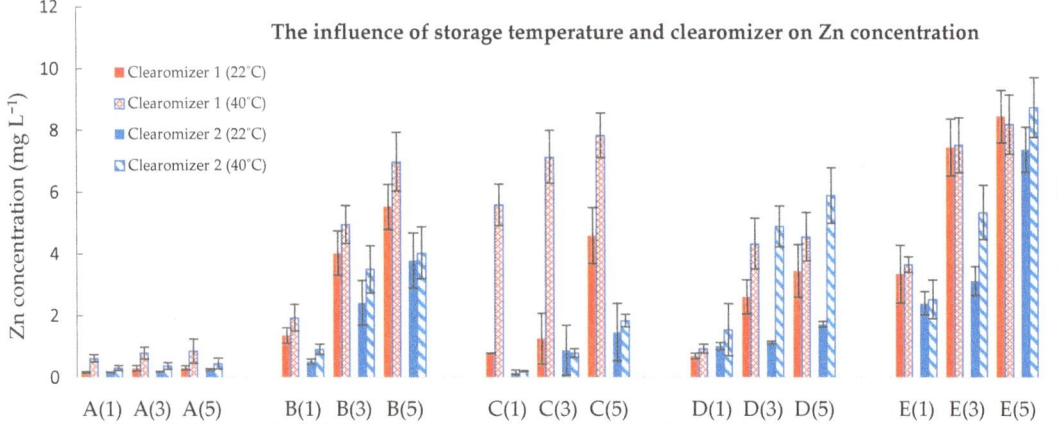

Figure 4. The influence of storage temperature and of the clearomizer on Zn concentration. Sample code: Sample number (number of storage days in the clearomizer).

In several samples, the amount of Zn as a result of the storage period in both types of clearomizers was more than 100 times higher, with statistically significant differences at the 0.05 level (Table 7). Moreover, our findings were very comparable to those of other studies all supporting the claim that heavy metals can be transported to the liquids via EC devices [11,39].

The *t*-test analysis was performed for the influence of temperature on zinc transfer. For clearomizer 1, the results of the analysis showed a significant difference at the 0.05 level for samples A, B, and C, while for clearomizer 2, the results were significantly different at the 0.05 level only for sample A. Moreover, we found that the two types of clearomizers released different amounts of metals when the same temperature (40 °C) was used; while the concentrations of Ni released was more powerful after storage in clearomizer 2, Zn concentration tended to be higher after storage in clearomizer 1 (Figure 3). In addition, the *t*-test analysis showed at 22 °C no significant difference, while at 40 °C, a significant difference at the 0.05 level was found for samples A, B, C, and D.

Table 7. The influence of the duration of storage on Zn concentration; *p*-value for the paired *t*-test (*t*-test: Paired Two Sample for Means).

Storage Conditions	I vs. 1 D	I vs. 3 D	I vs. 5 D	1 D vs. 3 D	1 D vs. 5 D	3 D vs. 5 D
Clearomizer 1 (22 °C)	**0.046**	**0.041**	**0.017**	**0.041**	**0.012**	**0.036**
Clearomizer 1 (40 °C)	**0.027**	**0.009**	**0.008**	**0.015**	**0.013**	**0.049**
Clearomizer 2 (22 °C)	0.064	**0.024**	**0.041**	0.053	**0.041**	0.070
Clearomizer 2 (40 °C)	**0.035**	**0.023**	**0.023**	**0.025**	**0.021**	0.051

I, initial; 1 D, storing for 1 day; 3 D, storing for 3 days; 5 D, storing for 5 days. Bold numbers denote the cases in which differences are statistically significant at 95% confidence level. Clearomizer 1, CE4-type clearomizer; Clearomizer 2, T3S-type clearomizer.

3.2.4. Cobalt Concentrations

Cobalt levels were in most cases below the LOD even as the period of storage and temperature increased. More data are needed to evaluate the significance of e-liquids as exposure sources for Co.

4. Discussion

The systemic toxicity of heavy metals has become a subject of great interest in the last few years. Several research groups investigated this phenomenon and the factors that influence the levels of heavy metals in e-liquids and aerosols produced during vaping. The e-liquids are able to heighten the heavy metal content depending on the manufacturing material and design of the used devices but also in relation to their composition (the ratio of propylene glycol to glycerol, nicotine, pH modifiers, and different flavors) [10,40]. The quality of the constituents (propylene glycol, glycerol, nicotine, and flavors) can be important because they can be a source of heavy metals. A study conducted by Kamilari et al. found high levels of Cd and Ni in the nicotine and two flavoring agents used for the production of e-liquids [15].

Another key element is the electronic device itself. Palazzolo et al. also found higher concentrations of metals (e.g., Ni and Zn) in the aerosols produced during vaping than in the e-liquids, pointing to the electronic cigarette device as the source of the metals [14]. They indicated the source for Ni to be, most likely, the core tip, the resistance coil, and the wiring and welding within the core assembly [14]. The analysis performed on the elemental composition of clearomizers revealed that the materials used included metals, such as chromium, nickel, tin, zinc, and copper, and that the components in these devices were very similar regardless of the brand and generation [41]. As Olmedo et al. pointed out, the spike of metal levels (like nickel) in e-liquid samples after they were exposed to the heating element suggests that heating coils are a potential source of the metals [39,42]. When electrical power is applied, the heating coils can produce metallic nanoparticles, which can condense and coagulate into nanoparticle clusters. Wilson et al. analyzed the characteristics of metallic nanoparticles generated by the heating of an electronic cigarette coil in the absence of a nicotine solution [43]. According to their results, using a low-resistance coil can reduce metal exposure [43]. Modifying the electronic devices' designs and using materials of suitable quality are ways for lowering the concentration of potentially dangerous metals in e-liquids and e-vapors [42,44].

A research subject imminently related to the assessment of the levels of heavy metals in e-liquids (and the understanding of the various factors that can influence these concentrations) is to evaluate to what extent heavy metals are transferred from e-liquids to aerosols. Previous studies revealed that the transfer of heavy metals to aerosols is not uniform; it depends on the different topographies for aerosol production (puffing protocol), but the results obtained are especially sensitive to the efficiencies of the methods of aerosol collection [36]. Thus far, several methods were reported for e-cigarette aerosol collection in the literature [36,45,46], but the absence of a standardized procedure makes it difficult to evaluate the real quantity of metals delivered through e-cigarette aerosols and to estimate potential health effects.

Our study investigated the concentrations of some heavy metals (Pb, Ni, Zn, and Co) in e-liquid samples, but we focused more on evaluating the impact of the storage conditions and type of clearomizer on the increase of heavy metals content in e-liquids.

In the case of lead, the initial concentrations (determined in e-liquids prior to the contact with the clearomizers) varied between 0.13 and 0.26 mg L^{-1}. In their review, Zhao et al. pointed out that different studies reported metal levels in different ways, and for easy comparison, they recommended the conversion to the weight/weight basis using a value of 1:16 g/mL for the density of e-liquids [16]. If this algorithm of conversion would be used for our results, the values obtained would be in the range 0.11 to 0.22 mg kg^{-1}. No regulations regarding heavy metals content were established until now, but JECFA (Joint FAO/WHO Expert Committee on Food Additives) adopted a general limit of 2 mg kg^{-1} for lead and a limit of 1 mg kg^{-1} or lower in case of high consumption [47]. Similar studies about the transfer characteristics of heavy metals in EC liquids reported average values of Pb between 0.12–0.25 mg kg^{-1} for the e-liquid samples analyzed before placement in the electronic cigarette device [11], while a study from Canada and the United States conducted by Dunbar et al. evaluated the heavy metals levels in e-liquids samples bottled in individual containers and in e-liquids that were extracted from inside disposable electronic devices [48]. They reported that the Pb concentrations in bottled e-liquids were not detectable above the limit of quantitation of 0.0091 mg L^{-1} (9.1 ppb) [48]. Furthermore, Olmedo et al. determined the concentrations of metals from both the e-liquids directly from the refilling dispenser (without contact with the coil) and from the tanks after the device was used [39]. They determined a value of 0.476 µg kg^{-1} (0.000476 mg kg^{-1}) for the median concentration of Pb in 56 e-liquid samples in the absence of the previous contact with the electronic device [39].

Our results showed a direct link between the storage period in clearomizers and the Pb levels. These results are in agreement with the reported results of a study conducted by Na et al. [11]. They also found that the average concentration of Pb significantly increases after storage in the clearomizer [11].

In the case of nickel, the initial concentrations found in e-liquids were very low. At present, there are no maximum contaminant levels for heavy metals in e-liquids, but the European Food Safety Authority (EFSA) analyzed the risks to public health related to the presence of nickel in food and drinking water and reported the limit values established for Ni by different international organisms [49]. A value of 20 µg/L (0.02 mg L^{-1}) for nickel was set in Council Directive 98/83/EC, while the WHO established a limit value 70 µg nickel/L and a tolerable daily intake (TDI) of 11 µg nickel/kg b.w. [49–51]. All our results did not exceed those limits.

Some of the previous studies have also reported traces of concentrations of Ni in EC liquids. Na et al. reported values of Ni in the investigated samples (represented by EC liquid bottles directly analyzed as purchased from retail) below the detection limit, 0.04 mg kg^{-1} [11]. Kamilari et al. used Total Reflection X-ray Fluorescence Spectrometry for the quantification, and the Ni concentrations found in the 22 analyzed samples varied between 0.002 and 0.017 µg g^{-1} (mg kg^{-1}) [15]. For easy comparison between our results and the finding from other studies, a conversion to mg kg^{-1} could be performed using the formula of the density and considering the value of 1.16 g/mL for the density of e-liquids as recommended by Zhao et al. [16].

E-cigarette devices have a metallic coil, which heats the e-liquid generating the aerosol; these metallic coils are manufactured with nickel (Ni) and chromium (Cr) alloys, which can be released to the e-liquids during the storage and heating process [9,29]. Other data support that the nichrome from the heating elements is resistant to oxidation (even at high temperatures) and suggest other alloys as possible sources of chromium, iron, and nickel oxide. However, the authors cannot exclude a limited degree of degradation of nichrome heating elements caused by extensive use periods [21].

The Ni levels increased after storage in the clearomizers. The results of the current study are in accordance with the findings of Na et al. [11]. This means that the clearomizer composition and conditions influenced the concentration of heavy metals. Thus, even without the heating procedure, the majority of the metallic components in the liquids are enhanced just by being stored in the clearomizer. Olmedo et al. determined a value of 2.03 µg/kg (0.0023 mg kg^{-1}) for the median concentration of Ni in e-liquids sampled directly from the refilling dispenser (without contact with the coil), while in the liquids after puffing the e-cigarettes, the Ni median concentration was 100 times higher [39].

In the case of zinc, the Joint FAO/WHO Expert Committee on Food Additives established a provisional maximum tolerable daily intake (PMTDI) of 1.0 mg/kg of body weight [52]. The Zn levels determined in the e-liquids after purchase ranged from 0.04–0.07 mg L^{-1}. If we applied the conversion algorithm mentioned by Zhao et al., our results would range between 0.03–0.06 mg kg^{-1}. We can state that the results of the current research are in accordance with previously published results of Na et al., which determined the heavy metals concentrations in e-liquids directly taken from bottles as purchased from retail [11]. They reported Zn concentrations between 0.05–0.63 mg kg^{-1} [11]. In the samples they analyzed, Olmedo et al. obtained a median concentration of 13.1 µg/kg (0.0131 mg kg^{-1}) without previous contact with the device [39]. Another study conducted by Gray et al. reported a connection between the higher Zn concentration in samples from devices with brass electrical connectors [10].

In the case of cobalt, a limit value of 0.1 mg kg^{-1} (per day) was identified to be the reliable dose of the substance for non-toxic level (NOAEL), while for chronic exposure via inhalation, a MRL of 1×10^{-4} mg m^{-3} was set by ATSDR (The Agency for Toxic Substances and Disease Registry) [53,54]. In our samples, the cobalt levels were below the detection limit (0.005 mg L^{-1}).

In our study, sample 5 had the highest concentration of nicotine (18 mg/mL) and a ratio of propylene glycol:glycerol of 50:50, and it presented the highest values for Pb, Ni, and Zn after storage in both clearomizers. A study conducted by Zervas et al. concluded that the transfer of Fe, Ni, Cu, Zn, and Pb increased with nicotine concentration and that glycerol also facilitated metal transfer in comparison to propylene glycol [55]. However, in our case, the investigation of more samples is needed to fully support this statement.

Looking at the behavior of the five e-liquids in the two clearomizers, we observed that lead and nickel transfer were more pronounced after storage in clearomizer 2, while zinc levels increased more after the storage of the e-liquids in clearomizer 1. The most likely explanation is the differences in the design and the materials used for the electronic devices, but we can only support this statement using the results of other research [29,36,44].

This study is the first to determine the concentrations of heavy metals in e-liquids marketed in Romania, but its major limitation is the low number of samples analyzed. From these preliminary results, there is no indication of low-quality counterfeit products sold in Romania, but more extensive research is needed in the future to conclusively evaluate the safety of these products for Romanian consumers. The findings in the present paper also emphasized and confirmed that the levels of heavy metals are greatly influenced by simply storing the e-liquids clearomizers and that storage conditions can also influence this transfer process. The storage temperature (investigated for the first time, to our knowledge) is another parameter that can influence metal transfer from the components of the clearomizer to the e-liquid inside.

5. Conclusions

The concentrations of four heavy metals (Pb, Ni, Zn, and Co) with potentially serious implications for human health were estimated in five e-liquid samples purchased from the Romanian market. The initial concentrations were reduced in the analyzed e-liquids and increased after their storage in clearomizers at different temperatures for various periods.

Co was found to be non-detectable in all the stages of the study. These findings support and consolidate the idea that heavy metals are transferred to e-liquids through the direct contact between the e-liquids and the metallic components of the devices. Heavy metals transfer depends on the characteristics of the electronic device and the composition of the e-liquids (as revealed by previous studies) but also on the storage conditions. Longer periods of storage inside the clearomizer were associated with higher levels of metals in e-liquids. Besides the period of storage, we also pointed out that storage temperature (22 °C vs. 40 °C) can also affect metal transfer from the parts of the clearomizers. This is an important aspect that needs to be taken into consideration by the manufacturers and regulatory agencies, which can introduce new recommendations that could reduce metal release during storage. Furthermore, an interesting subject for future research would be the investigation of the combined influence of certain chemical composition parameters of e-liquids and different storage conditions.

Author Contributions: Conceptualization, A.J., I.G.C., and L.A.; methodology, I.G.C.; validation, I.G.C.; formal analysis, I.-C.C., I.M.; investigation, A.J., I.G.C., and A.S.; resources, I.-C.C.; data curation, I.G.C. and I.-C.C.; writing—original draft preparation, A.J., I.G.C., and L.A.; writing—review and editing, A.J., I.G.C., and L.A.; supervision, L.A.; project administration, A.J., L.A., and I.M.; funding acquisition, A.J. All authors have read and agreed to the published version of the manuscript.

Funding: This research was funded by "Grigore T. Popa" University of Medicine and Pharmacy Iași, Romania, grant number. 4717/25.02.2021.

Institutional Review Board Statement: Not applicable.

Informed Consent Statement: Not applicable.

Data Availability Statement: Not applicable.

Conflicts of Interest: The authors declare no conflict of interest.

References

1. Zhao, D.; Navas-Acien, A.; Ilievski, V.; Slavkovich, V.; Olmedo, P.; Adria-Mora, B.; Domingo-Relloso, A.; Aherrera, A.; Kleiman, N.; Rule, A.M.; et al. Metal concentrations in electronic cigarette aerosol: Effect of open-system and closed-system devices and power settings. *Environ. Res.* **2019**, *174*, 125–134. [CrossRef]
2. Short, M.; Cole, A.G. Factors Associated with E-Cigarette Escalation among High School Students: A Review of the Literature. *Int. J. Environ. Res. Public Health* **2021**, *18*, 10067. [CrossRef] [PubMed]
3. Chen, C.; Zhuang, Y.-L.; Zhu, S.-H. E-Cigarette Design Preference and Smoking Cessation: A U.S. Population Study. *Am. J. Prev. Med.* **2016**, *51*, 356–363. [CrossRef] [PubMed]
4. Margham, J.; McAdam, K.; Forster, M.; Liu, C.; Wright, C.; Mariner, D.; Proctor, C. Chemical Composition of Aerosol from an E-Cigarette: A Quantitative Comparison with Cigarette Smoke. *Chem. Res. Toxicol.* **2016**, *29*, 1662–1678. [CrossRef] [PubMed]
5. Cheng, T. Chemical evaluation of electronic cigarettes. *Tob. Control* **2014**, *23* (Suppl. 2), ii11–ii17. [CrossRef]
6. Callahan-Lyon, P. Electronic cigarettes: Human health effects. *Tob. Control* **2014**, *23* (Suppl. 2), ii36–ii40. [CrossRef]
7. Do, E.K.; O'Connor, K.; Perks, S.N.; Soule, E.K.; Eissenberg, T.; Amato, M.S.; Graham, A.L.; Martin, C.K.; Höchsmann, C.; Fuemmeler, B.F. E-cigarette device and liquid characteristics and E-cigarette dependence: A pilot study of pod-based and disposable E-cigarette users. *Addict. Behav.* **2021**, *124*, 107117. [CrossRef]
8. Cao, Y.; Wu, D.; Ma, Y.; Ma, X.; Wang, S.; Li, F.; Li, M.; Zhang, T. Toxicity of electronic cigarettes: A general review of the origins, health hazards, and toxicity mechanisms. *Sci. Total Environ.* **2021**, *772*, 145475. [CrossRef]
9. Hess, C.A.; Olmedo, P.; Navas-Acien, A.; Goessler, W.; Cohen, J.E.; Rule, A.M. E-cigarettes as a source of toxic and potentially carcinogenic metals. *Environ. Res.* **2017**, *152*, 221–225. [CrossRef]
10. Gray, N.; Halstead, M.; Gonzalez-Jimenez, N.; Valentin-Blasini, L.; Watson, C.; Pappas, R.S. Analysis of Toxic Metals in Liquid from Electronic Cigarettes. *Int. J. Environ. Res. Public Health* **2019**, *16*, 4450. [CrossRef]
11. Na, C.-J.; Jo, S.-H.; Kim, K.-H.; Sohn, J.-R.; Son, Y.-S. The transfer characteristics of heavy metals in electronic cigarette liquid. *Environ. Res.* **2019**, *174*, 152–159. [CrossRef] [PubMed]
12. McAlinden, K.D.; Lu, W.; Eapen, M.S.; Sohal, S.S. Electronic cigarettes: Modern instruments for toxic lung delivery and posing risk for the development of chronic disease. *Int. J. Biochem. Cell Biol.* **2021**, *137*, 106039. [CrossRef] [PubMed]
13. Bansal, V.; Kim, K.-H. Review on quantitation methods for hazardous pollutants released by e-cigarette (EC) smoking. *TrAC Trends Anal. Chem.* **2016**, *78*, 120–133. [CrossRef]

14. Palazzolo, D.L.; Crow, A.P.; Nelson, J.M.; Johnson, R.A. Trace Metals Derived from Electronic Cigarette (ECIG) Generated Aerosol: Potential Problem of ECIG Devices That Contain Nickel. *Front. Physiol.* **2017**, *7*, 663. [CrossRef] [PubMed]
15. Kamilari, E.; Farsalinos, K.; Poulas, K.; Kontoyannis, C.G.; Orkoula, M.G. Detection and quantitative determination of heavy metals in electronic cigarette refill liquids using Total Reflection X-ray Fluorescence Spectrometry. *Food Chem. Toxicol.* **2018**, *116 Pt B*, 233–237. [CrossRef]
16. Zhao, D.; Aravindakshan, A.; Hilpert, M.; Olmedo, P.; Rule, A.M.; Navas-Acien, A.; Aherrera, A. Metal/Metalloid Levels in Electronic Cigarette Liquids, Aerosols, and Human Biosamples: A Systematic Review. *Environ. Health Perspect.* **2020**, *128*, 36001. [CrossRef] [PubMed]
17. Omaiye, E.E.; Williams, M.; Bozhilov, K.N.; Talbot, P. Design features and elemental/metal analysis of the atomizers in pod-style electronic cigarettes. *PLoS ONE* **2021**, *16*, e0248127. [CrossRef]
18. Merecz-Sadowska, A.; Sitarek, P.; Zielinska-Blizniewska, H.; Malinowska, K.; Zajdel, K.; Zakonnik, L.; Zajdel, R. A Summary of In Vitro and In Vivo Studies Evaluating the Impact of E-Cigarette Exposure on Living Organisms and the Environment. *Int. J. Mol. Sci.* **2020**, *21*, 652. [CrossRef] [PubMed]
19. Re, D.B.; Hilpert, M.; Saglimbeni, B.; Strait, M.; Ilievski, V.; Coady, M.; Talayero, M.; Wilmsen, K.; Chesnais, H.; Balac, O.; et al. Exposure to e-cigarette aerosol over two months induces accumulation of neurotoxic metals and alteration of essential metals in mouse brain. *Environ. Res.* **2021**, *202*, 111557. [CrossRef]
20. Mikheev, V.B.; Brinkman, M.C.; Granville, C.A.; Gordon, S.M.; Clark, P.I. Real-Time Measurement of Electronic Cigarette Aerosol Size Distribution and Metals Content Analysis. *Nicotine Tob. Res.* **2016**, *18*, 1895–1902. [CrossRef]
21. Pappas, R.S.; Gray, N.; Halstead, M.; Valentin-Blasini, L.; Watson, C. Toxic Metal-Containing Particles in Aerosols from Pod-Type Electronic Cigarettes. *J. Anal. Toxicol.* **2021**, *45*, 337–347. [CrossRef]
22. Farsalinos, K.E.; Voudris, V.; Poulas, K. Are Metals Emitted from Electronic Cigarettes a Reason for Health Concern? A Risk-Assessment Analysis of Currently Available Literature. *Int. J. Environ. Res. Public Health* **2015**, *12*, 5215–5232. [CrossRef] [PubMed]
23. Heldt, N.A.; Seliga, A.; Winfield, M.; Gajghate, S.; Reichenbach, N.; Yu, X.; Rom, S.; Tenneti, A.; May, D.; Gregory, B.D.; et al. Electronic cigarette exposure disrupts blood-brain barrier integrity and promotes neuroinflammation. *Brain Behav. Immun.* **2020**, *88*, 363–380. [CrossRef] [PubMed]
24. Fowles, J.; Barreau, T.; Wu, N. Cancer and Non-Cancer Risk Concerns from Metals in Electronic Cigarette Liquids and Aerosols. *Int. J. Environ. Res. Public Health* **2020**, *17*, 2146. [CrossRef] [PubMed]
25. Wiener, R.C.; Bhandari, R. Association of electronic cigarette use with lead, cadmium, barium, and antimony body burden: NHANES 2015-2016. *J. Trace Elements Med. Biol.* **2020**, *62*, 126602. [CrossRef] [PubMed]
26. Goniewicz, M.L.; Smith, D.M.; Edwards, K.C.; Blount, B.C.; Caldwell, K.L.; Feng, J.; Wang, L.; Christensen, C.; Ambrose, B.; Borek, N.; et al. Comparison of Nicotine and Toxicant Exposure in Users of Electronic Cigarettes and Combustible Cigarettes. *JAMA Netw. Open* **2018**, *1*, e185937. [CrossRef]
27. Olmedo, P.; Rodrigo, L.; Grau-Pérez, M.; Hilpert, M.; Navas-Acién, A.; Téllez-Plaza, M.; Pla, A.; Gil, F. Metal exposure and biomarker levels among e-cigarette users in Spain. *Environ. Res.* **2021**, *202*, 111667. [CrossRef]
28. Gaur, S.; Agnihotri, R. Health Effects of Trace Metals in Electronic Cigarette Aerosols—A Systematic Review. *Biol. Trace Element Res.* **2019**, *188*, 295–315. [CrossRef]
29. Williams, M.; Bozhilov, K.; Ghai, S.; Talbot, P. Elements including metals in the atomizer and aerosol of disposable electronic cigarettes and electronic hookahs. *PLoS ONE* **2017**, *12*, e0175430. [CrossRef]
30. Agoroaei, L.; Bibire, N.; Apostu, M.; Strugaru, M.; Grigoriu, I.; Butnaru, E. Content of Heavy Metals in Tobacco of Commonly Smoked Cigarettes in Romania. *Rev. Chim.* **2014**, *65*, 1026–1028.
31. Bouktif, M.; Maatouk, I.; Leblanc, J.C.; Gharbi, N.; Landoulsi, A. Dietary Intake of Tunisian Adult Population Aged from 19 To 65 in Cobalt. *J. Food Nutr.* **2021**, *7*, 1–7.
32. Elliott, D.R.F.; Shah, R.; Hess, C.A.; Elicker, B.; Henry, T.S.; Rule, A.M.; Chen, R.; Golozar, M.; Jones, K.D. Giant cell interstitial pneumonia secondary to cobalt exposure from e-cigarette use. *Eur. Respir. J.* **2019**, *54*, 1901922. [CrossRef]
33. Gonzalez-Jimenez, N.; Gray, N.; Pappas, R.S.; Halstead, M.; Lewis, E.; Valentin-Blasini, L.; Watson, C.; Blount, B. Analysis of Toxic Metals in Aerosols from Devices Associated with Electronic Cigarette, or Vaping, Product Use Associated Lung Injury. *Toxics* **2021**, *9*, 240. [CrossRef] [PubMed]
34. Monsé, C.; Raulf, M.; Hagemeyer, O.; Van Kampen, V.; Kendzia, B.; Gering, V.; Marek, E.-M.; Jettkant, B.; Bünger, J.; Merget, R.; et al. Airway inflammation after inhalation of nano-sized zinc oxide particles in human volunteers. *BMC Pulm. Med.* **2019**, *19*, 266. [CrossRef] [PubMed]
35. Kalokalin, B.; Velimirovic, D. Potentiometric stripping analysis of zinc, cadmium and lead in tabacco leaves (*Nicotiana tabacum* L.) and soil samples. *Int. J. Electrochem. Sci.* **2012**, *7*, 313–323.
36. Williams, M.; Li, J.; Talbot, P. Effects of Model, Method of Collection, and Topography on Chemical Elements and Metals in the Aerosol of Tank-Style Electronic Cigarettes. *Sci. Rep.* **2019**, *9*, 13969. [CrossRef] [PubMed]
37. Williams, M.; Talbot, P. Design Features in Multiple Generations of Electronic Cigarette Atomizers. *Int. J. Environ. Res. Public Health* **2019**, *16*, 2904. [CrossRef]

38. Cheng, D.; Ni, Z.; Liu, M.; Shen, X.; Jia, Y. Determination of trace Cr, Ni, Hg, As, and Pb in the tipping paper and filters of cigarettes by monochromatic wavelength X-ray fluorescence spectrometry. *Nucl. Instrum. Methods Phys. Res. Sect. B Beam Interact. Mater. At.* **2021**, *502*, 59–65. [CrossRef]
39. Olmedo, P.; Goessler, W.; Tanda, S.; Grau-Perez, M.; Jarmul, S.; Aherrera, A.; Chen, R.; Hilpert, M.; Cohen, J.E.; Navas-Acien, A.; et al. Metal Concentrations in e-Cigarette Liquid and Aerosol Samples: The Contribution of Metallic Coils. *Environ. Health Perspect.* **2018**, *126*, 27010. [CrossRef]
40. Zhao, D.; Ilievski, V.; Slavkovich, V.; Olmedo, P.; Domingo-Relloso, A.; Rule, A.M.; Kleiman, N.J.; Navas-Acien, A.; Hilpert, M. Effects of e-liquid flavor, nicotine content, and puff duration on metal emissions from electronic cigarettes. *Environ. Res.* **2021**, *204 Pt C*, 112270. [CrossRef]
41. Williams, M.; Bozhilov, K.N.; Talbot, P. Analysis of the elements and metals in multiple generations of electronic cigarette atomizers. *Environ. Res.* **2019**, *175*, 156–166. [CrossRef] [PubMed]
42. Arnold, C. Between the Tank and the Coil: Assessing How Metals End Up in E-Cigarette Liquid and Vapor. *Environ. Health Perspect.* **2018**, *126*, 64002. [CrossRef] [PubMed]
43. Wilson, M.D.; Prasad, K.A.; Kim, J.S.; Park, J.H. Characteristics of metallic nanoparticles emitted from heated Kanthal e-cigarette coils. *J. Nanopart. Res.* **2019**, *21*, 156. [CrossRef]
44. Williams, M.; To, A.; Bozhilov, K.; Talbot, P. Strategies to Reduce Tin and Other Metals in Electronic Cigarette Aerosol. *PLoS ONE* **2015**, *10*, e0138933. [CrossRef] [PubMed]
45. Aszyk, J.; Kubica, P.; Namieśnik, J.; Kot-Wasik, A.; Wasik, A. New approach for e-cigarette aerosol collection by an original automatic aerosol generator utilizing melt-blown non-woven fabric. *Anal. Chim. Acta* **2018**, *1038*, 67–78. [CrossRef]
46. Olmedo, P.; Navas-Acien, A.; Hess, C.; Jarmul, S.; Rule, A. A direct method for e-cigarette aerosol sample collection. *Environ. Res.* **2016**, *149*, 151–156. [CrossRef]
47. *Limit Test for Heavy Metals in Food Additive Specifications—Explanatory Note*; Joint FAO/WHO Expert Committee on Food Additives (JECFA): Rome, Italy, 2002. Available online: https://www.fao.org/documents/card/en/c/f9d29932-9975-479c-8528-b8d3cc8ed34e/ (accessed on 18 February 2022).
48. Dunbar, Z.R.; Das, A.; O'Connor, R.J.; Goniewicz, M.L.; Wei, B.; Travers, M.J. Brief Report: Lead Levels in Selected Electronic Cigarettes from Canada and the United States. *Int. J. Environ. Res. Public Health* **2018**, *15*, 154. [CrossRef]
49. EFSA CONTAM Panel (EFSA Panel on Contaminants in the Food Chain). Scientific Opinion on the Risks to Public Health Related to the Presence of Nickel in Food and Drinking Water. *EFSA J.* **2015**, *13*, 4002. [CrossRef]
50. Council Directive 98/83/EC of 3 November 1998 on the Quality of Water Intended for Human Consumption. Available online: https://eur-lex.europa.eu/legal-content/EN/TXT/?uri=celex%3A31998L0083 (accessed on 18 February 2022).
51. Nickel in Drinking-Water. Available online: https://www.who.int/water_sanitation_health/gdwqrevision/nickel2005.pdf (accessed on 18 February 2022).
52. Summary of Evaluations Performed by the Joint FAO/WHO Expert Committee on Food Additives—Zinc. Available online: https://inchem.org/documents/jecfa/jeceval/jec_2411.htm (accessed on 18 February 2022).
53. Cobalt and Its Compounds Chemical Substances Control Law. Available online: https://www.env.go.jp/en/chemi/chemicals/profile_erac/profile11/pf1-09.pdf (accessed on 15 November 2021).
54. Provisional Peer Reviewed Toxicity Values for Cobalt. Available online: https://cfpub.epa.gov/ncea/pprtv/documents/Cobalt.pdf (accessed on 15 November 2021).
55. Zervas, E.; Matsouki, N.; Kyriakopoulos, G.; Poulopoulos, S.; Ioannides, T.; Katsaounou, P. Transfer of metals in the liquids of electronic cigarettes. *Inhal. Toxicol.* **2020**, *32*, 240–248. [CrossRef]

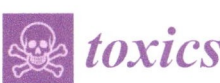

Article

E-Liquids from Seven European Countries–Warnings Analysis and Freebase Nicotine Content

Patryk Krystian Bębenek [1], Vinit Gholap [2], Matthew Halquist [2], Andrzej Sobczak [1] and Leon Kośmider [1,*]

[1] Department of General and Inorganic Chemistry, Faculty of Pharmaceutical Sciences in Sosnowiec, Medical University of Silesia in Katowice, Jagiellonska 4, 41-200 Sosnowiec, Poland; patryk.krystian.bebenek@gmail.com (P.K.B.); asobczak@sum.edu.pl (A.S.)
[2] Department of Pharmaceutics, School of Pharmacy, Virginia Commonwealth University, Richmond, VA 23298, USA; vinitgholap21@gmail.com (V.G.); halquistms@vcu.edu (M.H.)
* Correspondence: lkosmider@sum.edu.pl

Abstract: Electronic cigarettes are available in a variety of devices with e-liquids also available in many flavors, and nicotine concentrations, albeit less than 20 mg/mL in Europe. Given the dynamics of these products, it is important to evaluate product content, including labeling, nicotine content versus labeled claim, nicotine form, and other aspects that may help policy decisions and align with the Tobacco Product Directive (TPD). Herein, we performed a study on 86 e-liquids from seven European countries (Croatia, Czech Republic, France, Germany, Italy, Poland, and the United Kingdom) with 34 different liquid brands and 57 different flavors. Nicotine content versus labeled claim, labeling, volume, pH, and nicotine form (i.e., freebase nicotine) were evaluated. From all tested products, eight of them from Germany, Poland, and UK (from 3 to 18 mg/mL) met the ±2% criteria. The ±10% criteria was fulfilled by 50 (58.1%) liquids from all countries. Among 71 liquids which contained nicotine, (one e-liquid labeled as 6 mg/mL had no nicotine level quantified), the amount of freebase nicotine differed from 0 to 97.8%, with a mean value 56.5 ± 35.7. None of the tested liquids had nicotine salt listed in the ingredients. Therefore, a low level of freebase nicotine in some liquids was most likely achieved by added flavorings. All tested liquids presented in this study met the basic requirements of the TPD. There were differences in the scope of information about harmfulness, type of warnings on packaging, attaching leaflets, placing graphic symbols, and discrepancies between the declared and quantified nicotine concentrations.

Keywords: nicotine; nicotine form; e-liquids; European legislation

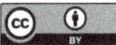

1. Introduction

Electronic-cigarette companies have sold their products as a cheaper, tobacco-free, or smoke-free alternative to cigarettes, cigars, and other tobacco goods [1]. Marketing campaigns are focused on the attractiveness of these products: a variety of flavors, different designs, and devices perfect for tobacco smokers or people trying this type of product for the first time [2]. Companies presenting e-cigarettes focus on the absence of real tobacco in their devices and what comes with it—the lack of a characteristic irritating smell and ash—as a new way of a more socially acceptable form of nicotine consumption [3]. Although nicotine is an addictive component of tobacco, negative health effects are induced by other components of tobacco smoke [4,5]. E-cigarettes can be used with a wide range of nicotine concentrations, including without nicotine; however unlike traditional cigarettes, e-cigarettes do not contain tobacco and emit smoke, because their use is not based on combustion, which leads to lower harmfulness of e-cigarette aerosol [6]. There is little evidence that e-cigarette emissions harm the health of bystanders [6]. Using e-cigarettes can increase the amount of particulate matter in the air; however, the composition is different from that caused by cigarette smoke and the concentration is much lower, and sometimes at the same level as in rooms without smoking or using e-cigarettes [7–11].

The WHO Tobacco-Free initiative commissioned a report to help countries around the world develop policies to regulate e-cigarettes. This report, published in 2013, contained detailed political suggestions for countries regarding the regulation of e-cigarettes. These include: (1) a ban on the use of e-cigarettes wherever the use of traditional cigarettes is prohibited, (2) a ban on the sale of e-cigarettes to anyone who cannot legally buy cigarettes or other places where the sale of traditional cigarettes is prohibited, (3) apply the same marketing restrictions for e-cigarettes that apply to traditional cigarettes, (4) prohibition of using branded cigarettes or e-cigarettes, which promotes dual use, (5) a ban on the use of distinctive flavors in e-cigarettes like candy and alcohol flavors, (6) forbidding companies to make claims regarding the cessation of tobacco use (until e-cigarette manufacturers and companies provide sufficient evidence of this, that Electronic Nicotine Delivery System (ENDS) products can be effectively used to quit smoking) and (7) prohibiting e-cigarette companies from making health claims about their products, unless made by independent regulatory agencies, and (8) calls for standards to regulate the ingredients and functioning of the product [12,13].

The "Europe against cancer" program started in 1985, resulting in the introduction of a number of tobacco control measures and one of these was the 2001 Tobacco Products Directive (2001/37/EC), which regulates the production, sale and presentation of tobacco products [14–16]. In 2009, the European Commission published a report of this directive in the light of new market and scientific developments and the WHO Framework Convention on Tobacco Control (FCTC) [17]. The European Union (EU) Tobacco Products Directive was passed in 2014 and implemented in 2016. Article 20 of the Directive has brought forward specific regulations regarding components reporting, emissions, production quality control and potential design parameters that could reduce risk. At the same time, all members of the European Union banned placing on the market cigarettes containing characteristic flavors, such as menthol, chocolate, or vanilla since May 2020. However, these regulations do not apply e-cigarettes, which can be found with many different types of flavors. Among adolescent, flavors are especially appealing and increase youth preferences for e-cigarettes [18]. Flavored e-cigarettes also effect receptivity to use, willingness to use and perception on associated risk. Some studies present results that e-cigarettes can become a gateway for future cigarette use among youths [19,20]. The agents used in e-cigarettes to impart different flavors are widely recognized as not harmful when consumed in most consumer products available in the market. However, the potentially harmful effects on health during single inhalation and repeated inhalation of many of these flavoring agents are still barely known and uncertain [21]. The results of in vitro and laboratory studies indicate that fruit flavors, one of the most popular types of flavors added to e-cigarettes, have been associated with exposure to higher concentrations of known irritants agents during inhalation, lower activity of bronchial epithelial cells, and increased release of pro-inflammatory cytokines [22–24]. Fruit flavors are also implicated with the possibility of increasing the delivery of nicotine compared to other e-cigarette flavors, which may affect to the addictive potential of these products [25,26].

One of the greatest challenges surrounding e-cigarettes is whether these devices are used like recreational drugs like cigarettes or for abuse treatment. It is likely that e-cigarettes constitute both, making it difficult for regulatory efforts. The United Kingdom has long focused on the potential of using e-cigarettes as tools for tobacco harm reduction and smoking cessation. In 2015, Public Health England (PHE) published a report including information that e-cigarettes were approximately 95% safer than traditional smoking [27]. Furthermore, in 2010, the PHE created a possibility confirmed by English law for e-cigarettes as a medicine, what would involve meeting medicinal standards and advertising conditions for these products [27]. Taking into consideration the high costs of the application to get the license for e-cigarettes as medicine and the difficulty of meeting the medicinal requirements, since this report, no e-cigarette manufacturer has attempted to obtain a license. The UK Medicines and Healthcare Products Regulatory Agency set new rules in May 2016, introducing safety and quality standards for e-cigarettes, including restrictions on the total content of nicotine for all e-cigarette consumers, according to the European Union 2014 Tobacco Products Directive [28].

European countries like Denmark [29], Norway [30], Switzerland [31], and Sweden [32] that have registered e-cigarettes only for therapeutic purposes in the past have changed their law to dual-track regulations that permit them to be sold either as a consumer product, or medicine for therapeutical treatment. Some countries (Singapore, Thailand and Western Australia) completely banned the sale, and in special circumstances, the possession and use of all vaping products, even including those devices that did not contain nicotine [33].

In most European countries, e-cigarette regulation focuses on their classification as tobacco, and preparation for medicinal purposes or consumer products. Governments of some of these countries (e.g., Austria, Czech Republic, Denmark, Croatia, Ireland, Finland, Poland) established two or more classifications for e-cigarettes, which results in several regulatory approaches for these products [34]. Commonly used rules for classic tobacco products, like restriction to sale and advertisement, were included for e-cigarettes. Other tobacco control laws were expanded to e-cigarettes also, like e-cigarette-free public places and banning purchase laws for adolescents. About a third of countries that regulate e-cigarettes only apply existing tobacco control regulations to these products and fail to perform separate policies for e-cigarettes [34]. Some rules that have been adopted for tobacco products, such as health warning labels (HWLs), are challenges for e-cigarette manufacturers and legislation, considering that we currently have many different devices and different types of packaging. Furthermore, governments from European countries still have not decided on exactly what health warnings should be included on e-cigarettes and their packages, which results in different warnings used in the European Union, despite the Tobacco Product Directive. Few countries around the world tax e-cigarettes or liquids, and there were no policies about regulating the concentration of liquid ingredients, excluding nicotine levels [34].

The ambiguity in the regulatory approach in various EU countries was noted in the report of the European Commission [35]. The report concludes that Member States have had good experience with the implementation of some e-cigarette legislation, with the possibility for improvement in other specific areas. Pursuant to Art. 20 paragraph 2, more can be done to provide higher quality information, particularly toxicological data and uniform doses of nicotine during product consumption, such as by standardizing assessment methods.

In this survey, the team focused on which regulatory domains due to the Tobacco Directive were being applied to liquids, mainly on the warnings and HWLs on the liquid packaging. It was important to identify which information and HWLs are on the package and what they depend on. To achieve this goal, the team gathered information placed by manufacturers from the liquid package and bottle. The next step was to verify obtained information from liquids, compare them with regulations given by the Tobacco Directive, and collate data from samples with each other, including comparing nicotine level, HWLs on the package and bottle label, and other warnings included on labels.

Due to the latest data, the information related to the concentration of nicotine is especially important. The practice of producers to date was associated with the information about its total concentration. Meanwhile, nicotine depending on the pH can be presented as a freebase (non-protonated), mono-protonated, or diprotonated form (Figure 1). The freebase and protonated nicotine yield of the e-cigarettes is found to have different effects on the plasma nicotine concentration-time profile in vapers [36–39]. As the possible reasons for such differences are being studied, it becomes necessary to determine the freebase or protonated nicotine yield of liquids and classify them based on this yield. Such classification would eventually help in better regulation of the liquid/e-cigarette market [37,40].

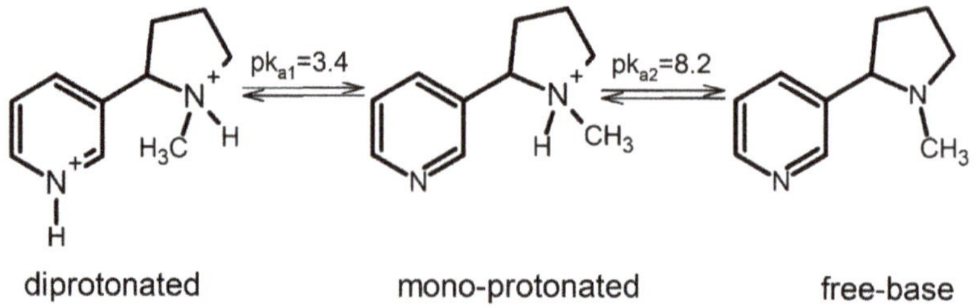

Figure 1. Nicotine forms.

2. Materials and Methods

In total, 86 liquids from seven European countries (Croatia, Czech Republic, France, Germany, Italy, Poland, and the United Kingdom) with 34 different liquid brands and 57 different flavors were used in this study. Randomly selected liquids were purchased at the turn of 2018 and 2019 in stationary stores (mainly kiosks, cigarette and tobacco stores or vape shops) in respective countries by researchers. The team obtained e-liquids with different nicotine concentrations; however, not every type of nicotine concentration was available in stationary stores. It is probably due to this fact that not every nicotine level is popular among users in respective countries. The nicotine level in individual liquids varies from 0 mg nicotine concentration to 18 mg per ml. The research group consisted of 14, 3, 23, 3, 15, 1, 14, 2 and 11 liquids with nicotine concentrations of 0 mg/mL, 1.5 mg/mL, 3 mg/mL, 4 mg/mL, 6 mg/mL, 9 mg/mL, 12 mg/mL, 16 mg/mL, and 18 mg/mL, respectively. All samples were stored in the refrigerator prior to analysis.

The e-liquids were grouped by country of purchase and type of flavor (fruity, sweet, menthol, tobacco groups). Flavor groups were assigned by two scientists based on labeling; in the case of one e-liquid where the results for classification differed, it was marked as "unassigned" (Energy Drink). Details of the e-liquid classification can be found in Supplementary Table S1.

The total nicotine in liquids was determined by a previously published method using the HPLC-PDA detection method [41]. All chromatographic conditions used were described previously [40]. A Waters Alliance 2695 quaternary pump HPLC equipped with a Waters 996 PDA Detector was used, along with a Hypersil Gold Phenyl column (150 mm × 4.6 mm, 3 µm, Thermo Scientific™, Greenville, NC, USA) and a Security Guard Cartridge Phenyl (4 mm × 2.0 mm, Phenomenex, Torrance, CA, USA). Waters Empower 2 software was used for processing data.

Similarly, freebase nicotine was calculated using a 10× dilution approach followed by the Henderson Hasselbalch method using a TruLab pH 1310P (YSI Incorporated, Xylem Inc, Yellow Springs, OH, USA) potentiometric pH meter with a TruLine 15 glass electrode selective to H+ ions and containing silver chloride reference electrodes [40]. Limit of detection was 0.007 mg/mL and limit of quantification 0.02 mg/mL for e-liquid analysis.

Seventy-two refill solutions containing nicotine (in accordance to labeling) were analyzed further. The difference between labeled nicotine content and the quantified nicotine content were calculated. Data were analyzed using Statistica 13.0 software. Differences between the mean freebase nicotine content of refill solutions/declare nicotine content (for e-liquids with nicotine and labeled concentrations as 1.5, 3, 6, 12 and 18 mg/mL) or flavor (for sweet, fruity, menthol and tobacco) were examined using ANOVA, and Scheffe's method was used for post hoc testing ($p < 0.05$).

3. Results

3.1. Health Warning Labels

On every tested liquid from countries that participated in this study which contained nicotine, manufacturers placed information about the nicotine concentration in mg/mL or in percentages. Twenty-seven (31.4%) of them had information about the total nicotine level per bottle and nicotine level per puff on their package. All information about nicotine concentration (nicotine level per ml, per bottle and per puff) had only 14 (16.3%) tested liquids. A total of 59 (68.6%) liquids also had carton packaging. A total of 28 (32.5%) tested liquids were bought without an additional box. All nicotine liquids had carton boxes (if it was included) with warnings about nicotine as a compound of the product. Forty-nine (57%) of them had warnings that it should not be used by children, adolescents, or those aged under 18. Eight (9.3%) tested liquids had warnings on their packaging in regard to pregnant women. General warnings like "attention" or "danger" were placed on 31 (36%) liquids. Information about toxicity properties of tested liquids were noticed on 15 (17.4%) samples. On 26 (30.2%), liquid producers placed more specific information about health risks linked with using this product, like "harmful if swallowed", "wash hands thoroughly after handling", "do not eat, drink or smoke when using this product", "toxic to the skin", "not allowed for people with cardiovascular diseases, high blood pressure and lung diseases", and "not suitable for non-smokers". Three (3.5%) liquids without nicotine had information about the presence of propylene glycol and its harmful effects on health. An acute toxicity symbol was on 30 (34.9%) of them. Danger or attention labels were placed on 35 (59.3%) boxes of tested liquids. Producers placed "not allowed under 18 HWLs on 25 (42.4%) samples; however, the "not allowed for pregnant" mark were set only on 14 (23.7%) of them. The "keep away from children" symbol was observed on 20 (33.9%) packages. In summary, from 59 liquids with an additional carton package, 47 (79.7%) of them had HWLs.

On four (4.6%) tested bottles, there were no warnings. Three (3.5%) of them contained nicotine and one did not. From 72 liquids with nicotine, only on 58 (80.5%) liquids, producers placed additional information about nicotine level or the presence of this alkaloid on the bottle label. On 65 (75.6%) of all tested samples, the team identified information about banning sale to or use by children, adolescents, or people under 18. Information like "not allowed for pregnant women" were placed only on 18 (20.9%) liquids. Warnings about danger or paying attention when using these products or about the general toxicity of these products were noticed on 33 (38.4%) samples. More specific information about toxic effects during the use of these products, like "toxic to the skin", "harmful if swallowed", "do not eat, drink or smoke when using this product", "toxic to the skin", "not allowed for people with cardiovascular diseases, high blood pressure and lung diseases" were set by manufacturers on 22 (25.6%) bottle labels. Only on two labels were there warnings about propylene glycol, and these liquids were without nicotine. In the case of other tested samples, information about the presence of propylene glycol in the ingredients section was observed, though without warnings directed to consumers. Nineteen (22.1%) liquids from the 86 tested in this study had no HWLs on the bottle labels. Only four (4.6%) of them were without nicotine. Sixteen (18.6%) liquids which contained nicotine with different levels of this alkaloid and no HWLs about toxicity or paying attention were noticed in this survey. On 58 (67.4) bottle labels, we identified HWLs like "attention", "danger", or "acute toxic". HWLs like "not allowed for children" or "not allowed under 18" were placed by producers on 45 (52.3%) labels on bottles. Information conducted with health effects for pregnant women were noticed on 19 (22.1%) liquid bottles.

Forty (46.5%) tested samples had additional information about the liquid's components, how it should be used, and even more descriptions of the side effects of these liquids. From 86 liquids, the basic components of 83 (96.5%) of them were glycerin and propylene glycol. In three (3.5%) liquids, the main components were propane-1,2,3-triol and propane-1,2-diol. In one (1.2%) liquid, the main component of the liquid base was propane-1,2-diol. Liquids with different flavors had additional substances, like geraniol, vanillin, methyl cinnamate, or d-limonene, that have a characteristic smell and taste when used. All nicotine-containing and non-nicotine containing refill containers in this study were child- and tamper-proof, with protection against breakage and leakage.

3.1.1. Germany

Liquids from Germany fulfilled requirements presented in the European Tobacco Directive. The product packaging had appropriate health warnings and a list of ingredients. Manufacturers indicated a nicotine concentration per ml on each label; however, information about total nicotine content was only on four of them, and did not consider the delivery dose. The nicotine level of all tested liquids from Germany was less than or equal to 20 mg/mL, and the volume of their refill bottles did not exceed 10 mL. Liquids in this study did not contain other addictive substances, except for nicotine. Health warnings like "this product contains nicotine which is a highly addictive substance" or "the product must be kept out of reach of children" or symbols indicating toxicity or danger appeared on the package or on the bottle label.

3.1.2. United Kingdom

From 24 tested liquids from the UK, only eight (33.3%) of them placed information about the total nicotine concentration on the package or bottle. We observed the nicotine concentration per dosage only on seven (29.2%) liquids from the UK, which participated in this survey. The nicotine level of all tested liquids from the UK, like in liquids from Germany, were less than or equal to 20 mg/mL, and the volume of their refill bottles did not exceed 10 mL. Liquids in this study did not contain other addictive substances, except for nicotine. Health warnings were present on all tested liquids, even on products without nicotine. Information placed on liquids by producers mostly concerned things like keeping it out of the reach of children, not allowing it for pregnant women, and information about the concentration of nicotine and the addictive properties of this substance. On liquids which did not contain nicotine, producers placed information about propylene glycol. All tested products from the UK have symbols about possible risks, toxicity, and danger after usage.

3.1.3. Poland

From 28 liquids with nicotine from Poland, on 10 (35.7%) of them, information about total nicotine amount was present; however, on 16 (57.1%) of them, information about nicotine level per dosage was found. The nicotine level of all tested liquids from Poland was less than or equal to 20 mg/mL, and the volume of their refill bottles did not exceed 10 mL. Except nicotine, there were no other addictive substances in the liquid components listed. Eight (28.6%) of all participating liquids in this study had textual information about keeping it out of the reach of children; however, these products had marks which symbolized it being banned for adolescents. On 8 (22.8%) of 35 tested liquids from Poland, manufacturers did not place symbols about toxicity and banned usage for children.

3.1.4. Croatia

On every liquid from Croatia, the manufacturer placed information about the nicotine concentration per ml and per dosage; however, they did not include the total nicotine level per bottle. The nicotine concentration in refill bottles of all tested liquids from Croatia was less than or equal to 20 mg/mL, and their volume did not exceed 10 mL. Nicotine was the only addictive substance which was included in the compounds section on the label. All tested liquids with nicotine from Croatia had information or symbols about toxicity, danger, harmful effects after ingestion, or being banned for adolescents. The team observed a notification about the product's harmful effects on pregnant women only on three of them.

3.1.5. Czech Republic

On all liquids from the Czech Republic which participated in this study, producers placed information about the nicotine concentration per mL. On three of them, manufacturers placed information about the total nicotine amount per bottle, and the team observed information about the nicotine level per dosage on none of them. All liquids from the Czech Republic had a nicotine concentration lower than or equal to 20 mg/mL, and the volume of refill containers did not exceed 10 mL. Nicotine was the only addictive substance placed by manufacturers on the label. All tested products from the Czech Republic had symbols about the possible risks, toxicity, and danger after usage; however, three of them had information and symbols only on the external carton package. On every package, information about it being banned for children and pregnant women was present.

3.1.6. Italy and France

Liquids from Italy had information about the nicotine concentration per ml and total nicotine amount per bottle, except for the nicotine level per dosage. Their refill containers did not exceed 10 mL, and their nicotine concentration was lower than 20 mg/mL. Producers placed information and symbols about toxicity, danger, and the product being banned for children and adolescents. The same information was observed on labels on liquids from France; however, the manufacturers did not place notifications about the total nicotine amount per bottle, and as in Italy, there were no symbols or information about the product being banned for pregnant women.

All tested liquids presented in this survey fulfilled the requirements presented in the European Tobacco Directive; however, the team observed differences between the tested samples. The differences in most cases depended on the liquid manufacturer, not the origin of the liquid. Some producers placed additional information, like the total nicotine amount or nicotine level per dosage, but there were no requirements about these parameters in the directive or local regulations. The divergences observed mainly concerned the type of symbols and their meanings. On some labels, the producers only placed symbols about danger, and on others, they included pictograms related to toxicity. Some manufacturers put information or symbols about its harmful effects on pregnant women, and others did not. In some cases, the team noticed very specific and accurate information about health risks connected with the liquid's usage; however, in most of the samples, there were only general notifications about its effects on user health. Some liquids without nicotine had information about risks and health effects if swallowed, or information about it not being allowed for pregnant women and children, while others only had information about keeping away from adolescents. The main purpose of the European Tobacco Directive was to unify regulations concerning liquids in European countries; however, these guidelines are still not precise and provide the possibility to obtain liquids with the same nicotine concentration, but with different health warning symbols and textual warnings.

Because liquids do not have standardized guidelines, we used the USP and ICH guidelines for the liquid analysis with the acceptance criteria of $\pm 2\%$ for and $\pm 10\%$, as followed by pharmaceutical manufacturers for labeling claims. From all tested products, only two of them which were manufactured in China and available in Poland met the $\pm 2\%$ criteria. The $\pm 10\%$ criteria was fulfilled by liquids from Italy and Czech Republic. In two nicotine-free liquids, nicotine was present—one from Poland with 0.02 mg/mL nicotine content, and the second one from Croatia, with 0.05 mg/mL nicotine concentration. Sixty-two of the tested products had a higher deviation than $\pm 2\%$. Thirty-nine of them were with a nicotine concentration between >0 to 6 mg/mL (Group I). A total of 11 liquids which exceeded a $\pm 2\%$ deviation range were from a group with a nicotine level from 9 to 12 mg/mL (Group II). In the group with the highest nicotine range between 16 and 18 mg/mL (Group III), 12 marked liquids had not met the $\pm 2\%$ criteria. In the $\pm 10\%$ deviation, the lowest nicotine concentration group (Group I) had the highest number of exceeded samples. In the second group (Group II), from 15 tested liquids, three of them failed to meet the $\pm 10\%$ criteria. In the last group (Group III), none of those which participated in this study exceeded the 10% range. From all tested liquids in this survey, six liquids had a nicotine concentration higher than the labeled claim. Three of them were in the group with the lowest nicotine level. One of the exceeded samples was part of a group with a nicotine concentration between 9 and 12 mg/mL (Group II). In the last group (Group III), only two liquids had higher nicotine levels than declared by the manufacturers on the label. The lowest nicotine concentration was investigated in 56 of all liquids which participated in this study. Thirty-six of them were a part of the lowest nicotine content group (Group I). In the second and third groups (Group II and III), there were 10 samples with a lower nicotine level compared to the label.

In samples obtained from Italy, both tested liquids had a different nicotine concentration than the content presented on the label. One with 9 mg/mL nicotine had lower nicotine content by 13.2%. In the second one, the nicotine level was higher by 3%. Italian liquids failed to meet the ±2% criteria, and the liquid labeled as 18 mg/mL passed the ±10% criteria. All samples from France had a lower concentration of nicotine (by 15.4 ± 3.9%, $n = 3$) compared to the content declared by the producers on the packaging (m). Samples from this country did not meet the criteria of ±2% and the criteria of ± 10%. Three marked liquids from Germany had a higher nicotine level by (1.6 ± 2.21%, $n = 3$). For five German samples, the team found there was a lower nicotine level than that declared (8.3 ± 6.5%, $n = 5$). Five liquids from Germany failed the ±2% criteria, and for one, the ±10%. All samples from the Czech Republic had a lower nicotine concentration than that declared on average by 4.1 ± 1.9%; $n = 6$. All liquids from this country failed to meet the 2% criteria; however, all of them passed the 10% criteria. In the case of liquids from Croatia, six of them exceeded the ±2% limit, and one of them also did not meet the ±10% limit. All marked samples had a lower nicotine concentration than the declared value (mean 8.6 ± 5.8%, $n = 6$). For Polish liquids, 23 (65.7%) of 35 samples had a lower nicotine concentration than the content on the labels by (14.6 ± 19.9%, $n = 23$). Five liquids had a higher nicotine level in comparison to the value on the package (4.5 ± 3.8%, $n = 5$). The 2% criteria was unacceptable in 24 (68.6%) liquids, and 9 (25.7%) did not pass the 10% criteria. Samples from the United Kingdom revealed a lower nicotine concentration than the level presented by producers on labels (11.6 ± 11.7%, $n = 17$). Two of all liquids from this country had higher nicotine content compared to the concentration placed on the package (higher by 142.09% and 0.083%). The criteria of ±2% and ±10% did not pass 16 and 7 samples, respectively.

3.2. Nicotine Content

The comparison of labeled and calculated nicotine concentration was performed for all 86 e-liquids. Fourteen chosen liquids from four countries had a nicotine concentration labeled as 0 mg/mL. Twelve had no detectable nicotine level, and the remaining two liquids had a determined nicotine level of 0.02 and 0.05 mg/mL from Poland and Croatia, respectively. From all tested products, eight of them from Germany, Poland, and the UK (from 3 to 18 mg/mL) met the ±2% criteria. The ±10% criteria fulfilled 50 (58.1%) liquids from all countries excluding France, where only two liquids were tested, with a quantified concentration lower by 14.3% and 19.9% (both labeled as 4 mg/mL). Only one liquid had a concentration higher than that claimed by more than 10%, where the quantified concentration for this liquid was 3.63 and labeled 1.5 mg/mL. Twenty-one liquids had a concentration lower by more than 10%, with one liquid with a labeled nicotine concentration of 6 mg/mL with no traces of nicotine in it (liquid from Poland). The mean difference of quantified nicotine versus the label for 72 liquids, which had a labeled nicotine level of 1.5 or higher, was −7.5 ± 22.7%. There was no statistical difference in the relative difference between countries or labeled nicotine ($p > 0.05$), probably due to the small sample amounts of 1.5 mg/mL and 16 mg/mL. In Tables 1 and 2, the mean values for relative differences are presented in relation to labeled nicotine and country of origin. In Supplementary Table S2, we present the results for non-nicotine e-liquids, as those were not statistically analyzed.

3.3. Freebase Nicotine Content

Among 71 liquids which contain nicotine (one e-liquid labeled as 6 mg/mL had no nicotine level quantified), the amount of freebase nicotine differed from 0 to 97.8%, with a mean value of 56.5 ± 35.7. None of the tested liquids contained nicotine salt, so a low level of freebase nicotine in some liquids was achieved probably by added flavorings. Fifty percent of tested liquids had a freebase nicotine level higher than 74.4%, 25% lower than 17.2%, or higher than 86.7%.

Table 1. Mean difference in nicotine content divided into countries in e-liquids with labeled nicotine level above 0 mg/mL.

Country	N	Relative Difference (%) Mean ± SD	Freebase Nicotine (%) Mean ± SD	pH Mean ± SD
Croatia	6	−8.65 ± 5.84	40.4 ± 40.1	7.65 ± 1.67
Czech Republic	6	−4.38 ± 1.42	81.8 ± 9.4	8.63 ± 0.26
France	3	−15.42 ± 3.88	4.2 ± 3.4	6.51 ± 0.83
Germany	8	−4.53 ± 7.23	88.8 ± 5.5	9.12 ± 0.25
Italy	2	−5.11 ± 11.47	72.5 ± 20.1	8.65 ± 0.47
Poland	28	−11.23 ± 19.40	61.9 ± 30.0 *	8.26 ± 1.16
United Kingdom	19	−2.88 ± 36.89	38.9 ± 39.2	7.46 ± 1.40

Note: * n = 27 due to one e-liquid with nicotine undetected.

Table 2. Mean difference in nicotine content of different nicotine labeled refill solutions and freebase nicotine content in e-liquids with labeled nicotine level above 0 mg/mL.

Labeled Nicotine Concentration (mg/mL)	N	Relative Difference (%) Mean ± SD	Freebase Nicotine (%) Mean ± SD	pH Mean ± SD
1.5	3	30.27 ± 96.91	0.5 ± 0.4	5.38 ± 1.10
3	23	−10.40 ± 11.57	35.0 ± 34.9	7.38 ± 1.35
4	3	−15.42 ± 3.88	4.2 ± 3.4	6.51 ± 0.83
6	15	−12.96 ± 24.66	67.6 ± 28.1 *	8.50 ± 0.70
9	1	−13.22	58.3	8.32
12	14	−5.96 ± 7.41	77.9 ± 16.0	8.83 ± 0.44
16	2	−5.59 ± 0.66	81.8 ± 5.7	8.83 ± 0.17
18	11	−3.92 ± 4.38	84.9 ± 15.3	9.04 ± 0.43

Note: * n = 14 for mean and SD analysis due to one e-liquid with undetected nicotine.

Liquids from France and Italy (as only liquids with 4 and 9 mg/mL), as well as 16 mg/mL e-liquids were excluded from statistical analysis for association of nicotine content on the freebase nicotine level due to a small sample size. Detailed freebase nicotine ratios broken into countries or labeled nicotine are presented in Tables 1 and 2. There were no statistical differences between countries in freebase nicotine content ($p > 0.05$), in contrast to types of flavor and labeled nicotine ($p < 0.001$ and $p = 0.0012$, respectively). Details can be found in Figures 2 and 3 and Tables 1 and 2. Sweet types of liquids differed statistically from fruity, menthol, and tobacco flavors; fruity liquids differed from tobacco-type liquids in freebase nicotine content (both $p < 0.05$). There was no statistical difference in relation to freebase nicotine between countries and concentrations > 0.05. In Table 3, detailed results for freebase nicotine content in different flavoring groups can be found.

Table 3. Mean freebase nicotine content of different nicotine labeled refill solutions.

Type of Flavor	Number of E-Liquids in a Group	Number of E-Liquids with Nicotine	Freebase Nicotine (%) Mean ± SD *	pH Mean ± SD *
Fruit	34	26	60.7 ± 27.9%	8.22 ± 1.18
Sweet	22	20	17.9 ± 30.8%	6.83 ± 1.23
Tobacco	24	19	86.8 ± 7.5%	9.05 ± 0.31
Menthol	5	5	72.1 ± 20.9%	8.67 ± 0.47
Unassigned	1	1	66.7%	8.47

Note: * Calculated only for e-liquids containing nicotine.

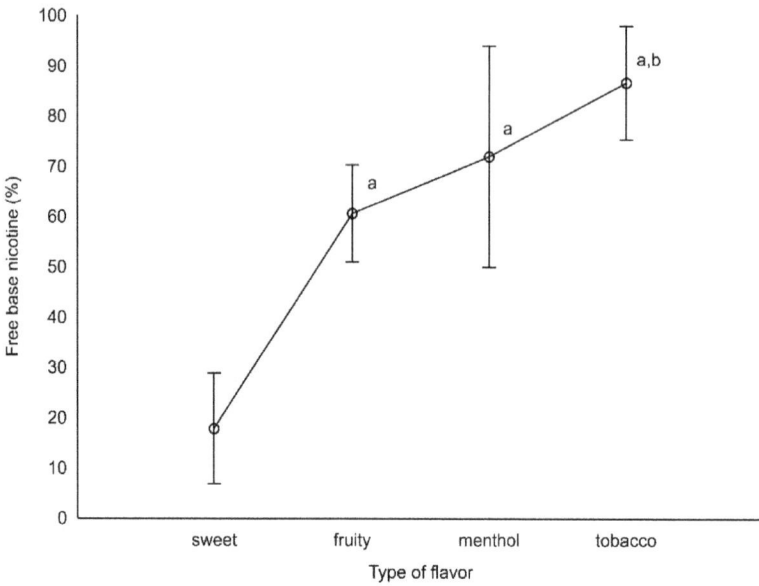

Figure 2. Differences in freebase nicotine content between different types of flavors. Liquids which differ statistically from sweet or fruity liquids were marked as a and b, respectively ($p < 0.05$, Scheffe test).

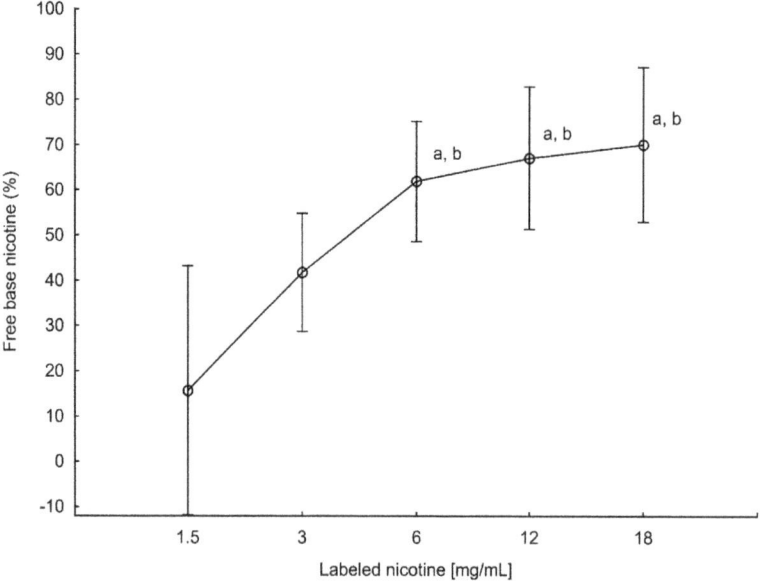

Figure 3. Differences in freebase nicotine content between different labeled nicotine concentrations. Liquids which differed statistically from 1.5 mg/mL nicotine liquids or 3 mg/mL liquids were marked as a and b, respectively ($p < 0.05$, Scheffe test).

4. Discussion

All tested liquids presented in this study were generally compliant with the European Tobacco Directive. However, the team observed differences between the samples tested in some areas. In most cases, these differences depended on the producer of the liquid, not the origin of the liquid. Some manufacturers provided additional information, such as the total nicotine level per dose, although there are no requirements for these parameters in the directive or local legislation. The observed discrepancies mainly regarded the type of symbols and their marks. Some labels had only symbols of danger, while others had pictograms related to toxicity. Some producers included information or symbols of the product's harmful effects on pregnant women, while others did not. In some cases, very detailed and accurate information about the health risks of using the liquids were present; however, only general notifications about the health effects of users appeared in most samples. Some of the nicotine-free liquids contained information about risks and health effects if swallowed, or prohibition of use for pregnant women and children, while others merely contained information about keeping away from adolescents. The main goal of the European Tobacco Directive was to harmonize the regulations on liquids in European countries, but for the time being, these guidelines are still not precise and allow consumers to purchase liquids with the same nicotine concentration, but with different warning symbols and text warnings.

In our study, all tested packages of liquids contained information about the nicotine content in mg/mL (100%) if nicotine was present. Approximately 31% of them also contained information about the amount of nicotine delivered per dose; however, the information about the content in mg/mL and per dose was present in only 16.3% of tested liquids. In the outer packaging, warning information about the nicotine content was observed on each of the tested samples, while the percentage of warning symbols on the outer packaging constituted 79.6%. On bottle labels of 80.5% of the tested liquids, information was present about the concentration of nicotine, and on 77.9%, there were warning symbols. There was no warning text (4.6%) on the labels of the four bottles. The percentage of leaflets in the case of the tested samples was 46.5%.

Our observations regarding the discrepancy in the characteristics of liquids were consistent with the results obtained by other authors. Girvalaki et al. [42] observed that after the introduction of the European Tobacco Directive, the compliance of the volume of liquid refilling bottles ($\leq$10 mL in vials) increased from 86.9% to 94.4%, $p = 0.008$. They also observed compliance with the maximum levels of nicotine concentration (100.0%) in the tested samples, while the percentage of products reporting nicotine delivery per dose increased from 0.9% to 43.9%, $p < 0.001$. The percentage of products containing a package leaflet also increased from 26.2% to 53.3%, $p < 0.001$. Additionally, the number of warnings on a bottle, box, or leaflet increased significantly after the introduction of the Directive. The presence of textual warnings on the box increased from 2.8% to 72.0%, $p < 0.001$, on bottles from 19.6% to 32.7%, $p = 0.022$, and on the leaflet from 13.1% to 42.1%, $p < 0.001$. Eighty-six percent of the tested products had some form of warnings in the period after the introduction of the directive, compared with 32.7% of products before the implementation of the directive ($p < 0.001$).

Very important information for the user is the amount of nicotine concentration placed on the package. This is due to the fact that the actual lower concentration of nicotine by the concentration declared by the manufacturer may, for some e-cigarette users, be associated with a compensatory effect of deeper and more frequent puffs. It is related to inhalation of a larger number of toxic compounds that may be degradation products of the liquid. As a result, a higher nicotine concentration in the liquid than the declared value may increase the potential of nicotine addiction.

Our research shows that among all tested liquids, in 7% of them, the marked nicotine concentrations were higher than the declared content by the manufacturer. Lower content was determined in the case of 77.8% of liquids. The difference between the quantified nicotine content and the manufacturer's was declared for 72 liquids, where a nicotine level described on the packaging of 1.5 mg/mL or higher was $-7.5 \pm 22.7\%$.

Our observations about the differentiation of nicotine concentration provided by the manufacturer and its actual concentration confirmed the previous results obtained by other research teams. A retrospective analysis of 23 studies from 2013–2020 showed that out of 545 liquids, 107 contained nicotine at a level above 20 mg/mL. Importantly, many of these liquids came from the USA, where there is no legal upper limit of nicotine concentration in liquids. Only 15 liquids in this group came from countries with a nicotine limit of 20 mg/mL (Great Britain, Greece, France, and Poland). The most common case of mislabeling was 0% to 5% of the nicotine concentration stated by the manufacturer. The second largest frequency of mislabeling was in the range of 10–20% [43].

Over the past few years, e-liquids have started to be advertised as liquids containing nicotine salts. This approach not only masks the irritating taste of nicotine, but can also affect the intensity of nicotine absorption into the bloodstream. This is due to the form in which it is absorbed into the body.

According to Pankow's theory, nicotine in aerosols occurs in the form of a freebase or in protonated form (salt), depending on the chemical composition of the aerosol, which, in the case of e-cigarettes, is closely related to the composition of the liquid. Freebase, due to its volatility, occurs mainly in the gaseous state, while protonated nicotine occurs mainly in the form of solid particles (droplets) [44]. Recently, David et al. experimentally proved that protonated nicotine remains in the aerosol droplets by use of ion-trapping and the Raman scattering technique [45]. Therefore, nicotine has a better chance of reaching the lungs where it dissociates, and the freebase form is absorbed by alveolar cells [46,47]. The volatility of free nicotine and its gaseous presence means that it is more likely to remain in the upper respiratory tract; hence, the absorption of nicotine is slower than that from the lungs [48]. Additionally, there is a greater chance of exhaling the gas fraction containing nicotine as a freebase [39,49]. In summary, the amount of nicotine reaching the lungs influences the plasma concentration of nicotine, and the amount of nicotine reaching the lungs is influenced by the form of inhaled nicotine. Consequently, two liquids with the same total nicotine concentration but with a different form of nicotine (free versus salt) can potentially cause significant variations in plasma nicotine levels. We would observe a higher concentration of nicotine in the plasma with a large amount of protonated form.

The observed differences in the pH of liquids for different nicotine concentrations declared by the manufacturer (range $5.38 \pm 1.10 \div 9.04 \pm 0.43$) were the basis for a hypothesis about the effect on the pH of flavorings added to liquids. Consequently, in the tested liquids, nicotine occurred in both discussed forms, but in a different quantitative ratio. The smallest amount of free nicotine was found in sweet liquids and increased in the following order: fruit, menthol, tobacco.

This work has some limitations. First is the method for quantifying the free nicotine base in e-cigarettes. It was limited by factors such as the arbitrary dilution factor and the unknown H 'activity factor due to unknown ion concentrations. However, we believe that the impact of these restrictions is negligible [39,40]. Secondly, the division into flavor groups was based on the description on the packaging. In approximately 12, the description did not allow assignment of the liquid to the appropriate group. Finally, experienced vapers were included whom, after using it, assigned the liquid to one of four groups; however, this could be considered subjective.

To fully confirm our hypothesis, clinical trials are needed to determine the level of nicotine in the plasma of vapers using liquids with the same starting concentration but a different ratio of nicotine freebase and protonated nicotine (different flavors). Additionally, it is important to understand the absorption profile of both forms of nicotine under different vaping conditions [50]. Recently, Gholap et al. described various factors that can affect the freebase/protonated nicotine yields from the e-cigarettes in detail. Such research acts an important stepping-stone towards understanding the absorption profiles of nicotine under various user conditions. Therefore, future research should be conducted considering a multidimensional approach to aid in better regulation of e-cigarettes.

5. Conclusions

All tested liquids presented in this study met the basic requirements of TPD. There were differences in the scope of information about harmfulness, the type of warning on the packaging, attaching leaflets, the placement of graphic symbols, and discrepancies between the declared nicotine concentrations and its actual concentration. An important aspect of this work is the demonstration that flavoring substances were associated with different ratios of the form of nicotine, which may have an impact on inhaled nicotine form and plasma nicotine levels and hence, on addiction, which requires further research. We believe this aspect of the work is important in the context policy and practice in the field of tobacco control, especially as the use of nicotine salts and modified wicks has been found to be associated with higher rates of addiction [51].

Supplementary Materials: The following are available online at https://www.mdpi.com/article/10.3390/toxics10020051/s1, Table S1: Detailed e-liquid data, Table S2: Results for e-liquids with nicotine level labeled as 0 or with no quantified nicotine level.

Author Contributions: Conceptualization, L.K., A.S., P.K.B. and M.H.; methodology, L.K., V.G., M.H. and A.S.; Validation, V.G. and M.H.; sample collection P.K.B.; analytical analysis, V.G., M.H. and L.K.; statistical analysis, L.K., A.S. and P.K.B.; writing—original draft preparation, L.K., P.K.B. and A.S.; writing—review and editing, all authors; funding acquisition, A.S. All authors have read and agreed to the published version of the manuscript.

Funding: The study has been supported by internal Medical University of Silesia funding grant number: PCN-1-002/N/1/F. In addition, Dr. Matthew Halquist is supported by the National Institute of Health (NIH) Center for Drug Abuse grant P30DA033934.

Institutional Review Board Statement: Not applicable.

Informed Consent Statement: Not applicable.

Data Availability Statement: The datasets generated during and/or analyzed during the current study are available from the corresponding author on reasonable request.

Conflicts of Interest: Authors have no conflicts to declare.

References

1. Frank, C.; Budlovsky, T.; Windle, S.B.; Filion, K.B.; Eisenberg, M.J. Electronic cigarettes in North America: History, use, and implications for smoking cessation. *Circulation* **2014**, *129*, 1945–1952. [CrossRef] [PubMed]
2. Vapex. The Evolution of Vaping. Available online: https://vapex.co/guide/beginners-guide-to-vaping/ch-1-history-of-vaping/ (accessed on 28 October 2016).
3. VapourArt. Which are the Benefits of Electronic Cigarettes over Tobacco Cigarettes. Available online: http://www.vapourart.com/en/faqitem/which-are-benefits-electronic-cigarettes-over-tobacco-cigarettes (accessed on 16 April 2015).
4. Drug & Therapeutics Bulletin. Republished: Nicotine and health. *BMJ* **2014**, *349*, 8.
5. National Institute for Health and Care Excellence. *PH45 Tobacco: Harm-Reduction Approaches to Smoking*; NICE: London, UK, 2013.
6. Kośmider, L.; Knysak, J.; Goniewicz, M.Ł.; Sobczak, A. Electronic cigarette—A safe substitute for tobacco cigarette or a new threat? *Przeglad Lekarski.* **2012**, *69*, 1084–1089. [PubMed]
7. Schober, W.; Szendrei, K.; Matzen, W.; Osiander-Fuchs, H.; Heitmann, D.; Schettgen, T.; Jörres, R.A.; Fromme, H. Use of electronic cigarettes (e-cigarettes) impairs indoor air quality and increases FeNO levels of e-cigarette consumers. *Int. J. Hyg. Environ. Health* **2014**, *217*, 628–637. [CrossRef] [PubMed]
8. Soule, E.K.; Maloney, S.F.; Spindle, T.R.; Rudy, A.K.; Hiler, M.M.; Cobb, C.O. Electronic cigarette use and indoor air quality in a natural setting. *Tob. Control* **2017**, *26*, 109–112. [CrossRef] [PubMed]
9. McNeill, A.; Etter, J.-F.; Farsalinos, K.; Hajek, P.; le Houezec, J.; McRobbie, H. A critique of a WHO-commissioned report and associated article on electronic cigarettes. *Addiction* **2014**, *109*, 2128–2134. [CrossRef]
10. Ruprecht, A.A.; De Marco, C.; Pozzi, P.; Munarini, E.; Mazza, R.; Angellotti, G.; Turla, F.; Boffi, R. Comparison between particulate matter and ultrafine particle emission by electronic and normal cigarettes in real-life conditions. *Tumori J.* **2014**, *100*, 24–27. [CrossRef] [PubMed]

11. Fernandez, E.; Ballbe, M.; Sureda, X.; Fu, M.; Saltó, E.; Martínez-Sánchez, J.M. Particulate matter from electronic cigarettes and conventional cigarettes: A systematic review and observational study. *Curr. Environ. Health Rep.* **2015**, *2*, 423–429. [CrossRef] [PubMed]
12. Grana, R.; Benowitz, N.; Glantz, S.A. *Background Paper on E-Cigarettes (Electronic Nicotine Delivery Systems)*; World Health Organization report; World Health Organization: Geneva, Switzerland, 2013; Available online: http://escholarship.org/uc/item/13p2b72n (accessed on 6 August 2014).
13. Grana, R.; Benowitz, N.; Glantz, S.A. E-cigarettes: A scientific review. *Circulation* **2014**, *129*, 1972–1986. [CrossRef]
14. The ASPECT Consortium. Tobacco or Health in the European Union. Past, Present and Future. Brussels. 2004. Available online: http://ec.europa.eu/health/ph_determinants/life_style/Tobacco/Documents/tobacco_fr_en.pdf (accessed on 9 April 2014).
15. Cairney, P.; Studlar, D.T.; Mamudu, H.M. European Countries and the EU. In *Global Tobacco Control. Power, Policy, Governance and Transfer*; Palgrave McMillan: Basingstoke, UK, 2012; pp. 72–98.
16. European Commission. Proposal for a Directive of the European Parliament and of the Council on the Approximation of the Laws, Regulations and Administrative Provisions of the Member States Concerning the Manufacture, Presentation and Sale of Tobacco and Related Products. Brussels. 2012. Available online: http://ec.europa.eu/health/tobacco/products/revision/index_en.htm (accessed on 7 January 2013).
17. Gilmore, A.; McKee, M. Tobacco-Control Policy in the European Union. In *Unfiltered. Conflicts over Tobacco Policy and Public Health*; Feldman, E.A., Bayer, R., Eds.; Harvard University Press: Cambridge, MA, USA, 2004; pp. 219–254.
18. Huang, L.L.; Baker, H.M.; Meernik, C.; Ranney, L.M.; Richardson, A.; O Goldstein, A. Impact of non-menthol flavours in tobacco products on perceptions and use among youth, young adults and adults: A systematic review. *Tob. Control* **2017**, *26*, 709–719. [CrossRef]
19. Bold, K.W.; Kong, G.; Camenga, D.R.; Simon, P.; Cavallo, D.A.; Morean, M.E.; Krishnan-Sarin, S. Trajectories of e-cigarette and conventional cigarette use among youth. *Pediatrics* **2018**, *141*, 20171832. [CrossRef] [PubMed]
20. Chaffee, B.W.; Watkins, S.L.; Glantz, S.A. Electronic cigarette use and progression from experimentation to established smoking. *Pediatrics* **2018**, *141*, 20173594. [CrossRef] [PubMed]
21. Tierney, P.A.; Karpinski, C.D.; Brown, J.E.; Luo, W.; Pankow, J.F. Flavour chemicals in electronic cigarette fluids. *Tob. Control* **2016**, *25*, 10–15. [CrossRef] [PubMed]
22. Kosmider, L.; Sobczak, A.; Prokopowicz, A.; Kurek, J.; Zaciera, M.; Knysak, J.; Smith, D.; Goniewicz, M.L. Cherry-flavoured electronic cigarettes expose users to the inhalation irritant, benzaldehyde. *Thorax* **2016**, *71*, 376–377. [CrossRef] [PubMed]
23. Kaur, G.; Muthumalage, T.; Rahman, I. Mechanisms of toxicity and biomarkers of flavoring and flavor enhancing chemicals in emerging tobacco and non-tobacco products. *Toxicol. Lett.* **2018**, *288*, 143–155. [CrossRef]
24. Leigh, N.J.; Lawton, R.I.; Hershberger, P.A.; Goniewicz, M.L. Flavourings significantly affect inhalation toxicity of aerosol generated from electronic nicotine delivery systems (ENDS). *Tob. Control* **2016**, *25*, 81–87. [CrossRef]
25. St Helen, G.; Dempsey, D.A.; Havel, C.M.; Jacob, P., III; Benowitz, N.L. Impact of e-liquid flavors on nicotine intake and pharmacology of e-cigarettes. *Drug Alcohol Depend.* **2017**, *178*, 391–398. [CrossRef] [PubMed]
26. St Helen, G.; Shahid, M.; Chu, S.; Benowitz, N.L. Impact of e-liquid flavors on e-cigarette vaping behavior. *Drug Alcohol Depend.* **2018**, *189*, 42–48. [CrossRef]
27. McNeill, A.; Brose, L.S.; Calder, R.; Hitchman, S.C.; Hajek, P.; McRobbie, H. *E-Cigarettes: An Evidence Update*; Public Health: London, UK, 2015. Available online: https://www.gov.uk/government/uploads/system/uploads/attachment_data/file/457102/Ecigarettes_an_evidence_update_A_report_commissioned_by_Public_Health_England_FINAL.pdf (accessed on 24 March 2017).
28. Medicines and Healthcare Products Regulatory Agency. E-Cigarettes: Regulations for Consumer Products. Available online: https://www.gov.uk/guidance/e-cigarettes-regulations-for-consumer-products#history (accessed on 6 February 2017).
29. New Rules for Nicotine-Containing E-Cigarettes and Refill Containers. Available online: https://laegemiddelstyrelsen.dk/en/licensing/definition-of-a-medicine/special-classifications/new-rules-for-nicotine-containing-e-cigarettes-and-refill-containers/ (accessed on 9 June 2016).
30. Cross-Border or Distance Sales of Tobacco and E-Cigarettes in Norway. Available online: https://helsedirektoratet.no/english/tobacco-control#cross-border-or-distance-sales-of-tobacco-and-e-cigarettes-in-norway (accessed on 9 February 2018).
31. Court Overturns Swiss Ban on E-Cigarettes. Available online: https://www.swissinfo.ch/eng/business/immediate-effect_court-overturns-swiss-ban-on-e-cigarettes/44082174 (accessed on 28 April 2018).
32. Swedish Court Stubs out Right to Ban E-Cigarettes. Available online: https://www.thelocal.se/20160217/swedish-court-stubs-out-right-to-ban-e-cigs-smoking (accessed on 17 February 2016).
33. Prohibition on Certain Products. Available online: http://www.hsa.gov.sg/content/hsa/en/Health_Prod-ucts_Regulation/Tobacco_Control/Overview/Tobacco_Legislation/Prohibition_on_Certain_Products.html (accessed on 1 February 2018).
34. Kennedy, R.D.; Awopegba, A.; Leon, E.D.; Cohen, J.E. Global approaches to regulating electronic cigarettes. *Tob. Control* **2017**, *26*, 440–445. [CrossRef]
35. Report from the Commission to the European Parliament. Available online: https://eur-lex.europa.eu/legal-content/EN/TXT/?uri=COM:2021:249:FIN (accessed on 20 May 2021).
36. Bowen, A.; Xing, C. Nicotine Salt Formulations for Aerosol Devices and Methods Thereof. U.S. Patent 9,215,895 B2, 22 December 2015.

37. Gholap, V.; Halquist, M.S. Historical Perspective of Proactive and Reactive Regulations of E-cigarettes to Combat Nicotine Addiction. *J. Addict. Med.* **2020**, *14*, 443–445. [CrossRef]
38. Yingst, J.M.; Hrabovsky, S.; Hobkirk, A.; Trushin, N.; Richie, J.P., Jr.; Foulds, J. Nicotine Absorption Profile Among Regular Users of a Pod-Based Electronic Nicotine Delivery System. *JAMA Netw. Open* **2019**, *2*, e1915494. [CrossRef] [PubMed]
39. Gholap, V.V.; Kosmider, L.; Golshahi, L.; Halquist, M.S. Nicotine forms: Why and how do they matter in nicotine delivery from electronic cigarettes? *Expert Opin. Drug Deliv.* **2020**, *17*, 1727–1736. [CrossRef] [PubMed]
40. Gholap, V.V.; Heyder, R.S.; Kosmider, L.; Halquist, M.S. An Analytical Perspective on Determination of Free Base Nicotine in E-Liquids. *J. Anal. Methods Chem.* **2020**, *10*, 6178570. [CrossRef] [PubMed]
41. Gholap, V.V.; Kosmider, L.; Halquist, M.S. A Standardized Approach to Quantitative Analysis of Nicotine in e-Liquids Based on Peak Purity Criteria Using High-Performance Liquid Chromatography. *J. Anal. Methods Chem.* **2018**, *2018*, 1720375. [CrossRef] [PubMed]
42. Girvalaki, C.; Vardavas, A.; Tzatzarakis, M.; Kyriakos, C.N.; Nikitara, K.; Tsatsakis, A.M.; Vardavas, C.I. Compliance of e-cigarette refill liquids with regulations on labelling, packaging and technical design characteristics in nine European member states. *Tob. Control* **2020**, *29*, 531–536. [CrossRef] [PubMed]
43. Taylor, A.; Dunn, K.; Turfus, S. A review of nicotine-containing electronic cigarettes—Trends in use, effects, contents, labelling accuracy and detection methods. *Drug Test Anal.* **2021**, *13*, 242–260. [CrossRef]
44. Pankow, J.F. A consideration of the role of gas/particle partitioning in the deposition of nicotine and other tobacco smoke compounds in the respiratory tract. *Chem. Res. Toxicol.* **2001**, *14*, 1465–1481. [CrossRef]
45. David, G.; Parmentier, E.A.; Taurino, I.; Signorell, R. Tracing the composition of single e-cigarette aerosol droplets in situ by laser-trapping and Raman scattering. *Sci. Rep.* **2020**, *10*, 1–8. [CrossRef]
46. Seeman, J.I.; Carchman, R.A. The possible role of ammonia toxicity on the exposure, deposition, retention, and the bioavailability of nicotine during smoking. *Food Chem. Toxicol.* **2008**, *46*, 1863–1881. [CrossRef]
47. Caldwell, B.; Sumner, W.; Crane, J. A systematic review of nicotine by inhalation: Is there a role for the inhaled route? *Nicotine Tob. Res.* **2012**, *14*, 1127–1139. [CrossRef]
48. Cipolla, D.; Gonda, I. Inhaled nicotine replacement therapy. *Asian J. Pharm. Sci.* **2015**, *10*, 472–480. [CrossRef]
49. Jabbal, S.; Poli, G.; Lipworth, B. Does size really matter?: Relationship of particle size to lung deposition and exhaled fraction. *J. Allergy Clin. Immunol.* **2017**, *139*, 2013–2014.e1. [CrossRef] [PubMed]
50. Gholap, V.V.; Pearcy, A.C.; Halquist, M.S. Potential factors affecting free base nicotine yield in electronic cigarette aerosols. *Expert Opin. Drug Deliv.* **2021**, *18*, 979–989. [CrossRef] [PubMed]
51. Mallock, N.; Trieu, H.L.; Macziol, M.; Malke, S.; Katz, A.; Laux, P.; Henkler-Stephani, F.; Hahn, J.; Hutzler, C.; Luch, A. Trendy e-cigarettes enter Europe: Chemical characterization of JUUL pods and its aerosols. *Arch. Toxicol.* **2020**, *94*, 1985–1994. [CrossRef] [PubMed]

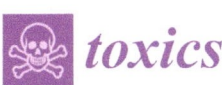

Article

The Use of E-Cigarettes among High School Students in Poland Is Associated with Health Locus of Control but Not with Health Literacy: A Cross-Sectional Study

Mariusz Duplaga * and Marcin Grysztar

Department of Health Promotion and e-Health, Institute of Public Health, Faculty of Health Sciences, Jagiellonian University Medical College, Skawinska Str. 8, 31-066 Krakow, Poland; marcin.grysztar@uj.edu.pl
* Correspondence: mariusz.duplaga@uj.edu.pl

Abstract: Since their introduction, the use of electronic cigarettes has increased considerably in the population and among adolescents. Determinants of smoking conventional cigarettes were thoroughly studied in various social groups. However, we know less about the predictors of the use of e-cigarettes in younger generations. The main aim of this study was the assessment of the factors associated with the use of electronic cigarettes among high school students. Specifically, the roles of health literacy (HL) and health locus of control (HLC) were addressed. The analysis was based on the data from a 'pen-and-pencil' survey performed in a large sample of 2223 high school students from southern Poland. The tools used in the survey encompassed 133 items, including a 47-item European Health Literacy Survey questionnaire, an 18-item Multidimensional Health Locus of Control Scale, and a set of questions asking about the health behaviors, and sociodemographic and economic characteristics of respondents. In the study sample, 47.5% of the respondents had used e-cigarettes in the past, and 18.6% had used them in the last month. HL was not significantly associated with dependent variables reflecting the use of e-cigarettes. Two types of external HLC were associated with using e-cigarettes in the past, and 'Chance' HLC (CHLC) was also associated with their use in the last month. Males, students of schools providing vocational training, and students declaring more Internet use during the week showed a higher likelihood of ever using e-cigarettes or using them in the last month. Students smoking conventional cigarettes were also more prone to use e-cigarettes. To sum up, it was an unexpected result that HL is not associated with the use of e-cigarettes. A greater likelihood of using e-cigarettes was positively associated with higher CHLC scores, as in the case of smoking traditional cigarettes.

Keywords: electronic cigarettes; e-cigarettes; high school students; adolescents; health literacy; health locus of control; European Health Literacy Survey questionnaire; pen and pencil interviewing; logistic regression

Citation: Duplaga, M.; Grysztar, M. The Use of E-Cigarettes among High School Students in Poland Is Associated with Health Locus of Control but Not with Health Literacy: A Cross-Sectional Study. *Toxics* **2022**, *10*, 41. https://doi.org/10.3390/toxics10010041

Academic Editors: Andrzej Sobczak and Leon Kośmider

Received: 29 December 2021
Accepted: 13 January 2022
Published: 17 January 2022

Publisher's Note: MDPI stays neutral with regard to jurisdictional claims in published maps and institutional affiliations.

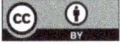

Copyright: © 2022 by the authors. Licensee MDPI, Basel, Switzerland. This article is an open access article distributed under the terms and conditions of the Creative Commons Attribution (CC BY) license (https://creativecommons.org/licenses/by/4.0/).

1. Introduction

The use of e-cigarettes by youth has increased considerably in the last decade [1]. According to Fadus et al. [2], the use of e-cigarettes among youth has increased from 1.5% in 2011 to 20.8% in 2018. The growing use of e-cigarettes among this population has been explained by various factors, including advertising exposure, the availability of flavors attractive to youth, the introduction of easily concealable devices with high nicotine content, their user-friendly function, and their ability to be used discreetly in places where smoking is prohibited [2,3].

A USA study has shown that a significant increase in e-cigarettes sales was accompanied by only a small decrease in conventional cigarette sales during the period of 2011–2015 [4]. Although e-cigarettes were marketed as a smoking cessation means, the results of a large study showed that there has been only a marginal decline of regular smoking among youth since 2010 when e-cigarettes emerged on the market [5]. Fadus et al. suggested that, on the contrary, the use of e-cigarettes may have a "gateway" effect for combustible cigarettes and cannabis use [2]. The observations from Poland tend to confirm these claims. Smith et al. have found that exclusive use of e-cigarettes among adolescents 15–19 years old in Poland increased from 2.0% in 2010–2011 to 11% in 2015–2016 [6]. However, dual-use also increased, from 4% in 2010–2011 to 23% in 2015–2016 [6]. Interestingly, as many as 76% of dual users confirmed (in the study from 2015–2016) that they had used cigarettes before trying e-cigarettes. According to the cross-sectional study performed in two waves between 2014 and 2018 by Kaleta and Polanska [7], the percentage of secondary school girls using e-cigarettes increased from 20.7% to 31.7%. Furthermore, the smoking of traditional cigarettes has been stable in the period covered by the study and has remained on the level from 25.1% to 27.9%. There was a significant increase of dual use among older boys from 45.7% in 2014–2015 to 56.8% in 2017–2018 [7]. Another study, performed in Poland within the Global Youth Tobacco Survey among 11–17 year old youth in 2016, revealed that 31.5% of boys and 21.8% of girls were current e-cigarette users and 21.8% of boys and 19.9% of girls smoked traditional cigarettes [8]. Dual uses made up 14% of the respondents in this study group. All these reports indicate that the use of e-cigarettes among adolescents has become an urgent public health issue requiring adequate attention.

According to Wallston [9], health locus of control (HLC) reflects the degree to which individuals believe that their health status remains under their own control or is influenced by factors external to themselves, e.g., other people, fate, chance, or some undefined 'higher power'. In 1978, Wallston et al. developed the Multidimensional Health Locus of Control (MHLC) scale measuring three dimensions of HLC, internal (IHLC) and two external called 'Powerful Other' (OHLC) and "Chance" HLC (CHLC) [10]. People with higher IHLC are convinced that they can control their health through appropriate behaviors. Higher external HLC shows that a person is more inclined to attribute their health status either to other people or to chance factors. It has been demonstrated in various populations that the MHLC score may be associated with health behaviors [11–14], quality of life [15], and self-assessed health [16]. Many authors have also reported a significant relationship between HLC and smoking, indicating that high CHLC predicted active smoking or resuming smoking after control programs [17–23]. It remains in line with the theory of HLC that explains that people with high CHLC believe that health is independent of their personal health behaviors.

In 1982, Clarke et al. reported that adolescents with an external locus of control were the group at the greatest risk that they would start smoking early, smoke at a high frequency, and continue smoking behavior [24]. Eiser et al. observed, among a large group of school students 11–16 years old, that smokers, compared to non-smokers, showed lower OHLC and IHLC and higher belief in the importance of a "chance" influence on their health outcomes [25]. Many more recent studies confirmed a significant association between external HLC and smoking habits among youths and young adults [26–29]. Unfortunately, the relationship between HLC and the proclivity towards the use of e-cigarettes has not been reported on yet.

There are many definitions of health literacy (HL). According to the World Health Organization, HL may be perceived as the cognitive and social skills resulting in individuals' motivation and ability to access, understand, and use information to promote health [30]. The level of HL may be assessed with general-purpose or domain-specific instruments. Currently, the questionnaire developed within the European Health Literacy Survey (EHLS) is one of the most popular tools used to assess general HL in population studies [31]. Its basic form consists of 47 items (HLS-EU-Q47) evaluating the abilities to access, understand, appraise, and apply health information in the domains of health promotion, disease prevention, and health care [31]. It was evidenced that HL is one of the key factors associated with health behaviors, utilization of health services, and the ability to communicate with health care providers [32–34]. Although the association between HL and smoking traditional cigarettes has frequently been studied, reports on e-cigarettes are relatively rare.

The survey performed in several European countries by the EHLS project team revealed that HL is significantly associated with smoking and other health behaviors. However, the study conducted among the Polish population in 2016 did not show a significant association between HL and smoking [35]. A recent survey carried out by Clifford et al. revealed that respondents with higher levels of oral HL were less likely to be current dual users of e-cigarettes and conventional cigarettes [36]. Interestingly, these authors did not find a significant association between written HL and either the smoking of traditional cigarettes or the use of e-cigarettes. As for the adolescents, the study performed in the Netherlands, Germany, and Finland among adolescents 14–16 years old revealed that HL was not associated with smoking. Still, it was positively related to beliefs about the consequences of smoking [37]. The fact that the use of e-cigarettes became an issue in public health seems to be supported by the recent development of the e-Cigarette Use Health Literacy scale [38].

The main aim of this study was to assess the association of socio-demographic and economic factors, HL and HLC, with the use of e-cigarettes among high school students from southern Poland. Furthermore, the relationship between the use of e-cigarettes and conventional cigarettes among this population was analyzed.

2. Materials and Methods
2.1. Survey

The study reports the analysis of data obtained from a sample of high school students from a district (Malopolska Voivodship) in southern Poland. The survey was performed with the 'pen-and-paper' technique. The respondents were selected as the result of cluster two-stage random sampling. In the first stage, twenty high schools located in the Malopolska Voivodship were randomly selected from the repository of schools maintained by the Board of Education. The directors of these schools were invited to the study; nine responded positively. In each of these schools, 5–10 classes were randomly selected for the survey, considering grades and profiles. The parents of students attending selected classes were informed about the study aims and procedures. Parents of students younger than 18 years old were asked for consent to include their child in the survey. All students attending the selected classes were informed about the study and asked for their informed consent. Data were collected in the period from September to October 2017.

The study was conducted after receiving consent from the Bioethical Committee of Jagiellonian University issued on 25 September 2014 (KBET/193/B/2014).

The questionnaire used in the survey encompassed 130 individual items, including questions exploring the health behaviors and socioeconomic status of respondents, the questionnaire developed within the EHLS project consisting of 47 items (HLS-EU-Q47) [39], and the MHLC scale composed of 18 items [40]. Only the Polish version of the questionnaire was applied. The items used in the analysis in this paper (apart from earlier validated tools such as HLS-EU-Q47 and MHLC scale) have been translated to English and are available in the Supplementary Materials file.

2.2. Dependent and Independent Variables

Two dichotomous variables reflecting the use of electronic cigarettes were applied as dependent variables in univariate and multivariate logistic regression models. They were derived from items asking if respondents had ever used e-cigarettes (yes coded as '1' vs. no coded as '0') and about their use in the last month (yes coded as '1' vs. no coded as '0').

In the univariate and multivariate logistic regression models, the following independent variables were applied:
- Sociodemographic variables: gender, attended class in school (treated as a proxy of respondent's age), place of residence, marital status of parents, the levels of education

of the mother and farther, the number of siblings, the category of school (including vocational training or not);
- Variables reflecting the financial situation of the respondent's family: receiving external help, self-assessment of family economic status, and monthly expenses for a mobile phone;
- The use of information technology—variables indicating the time spent on the Internet per week;
- Health literacy score based on the HLS-EU-Q47.

The HL score was established according to the guidelines from the EHLS project team; responses to each item included in the HLS-EU-Q47 were transformed to individual scores from 1 to 4 [39]. If the respondent was not decided or missed the response for a particular item, it was treated as a missing value. A percentage of missing values surpassing 20% in the HLS-EU-Q47 questionnaire precluded calculating the general score for the respondent.

- Three subscores of the MHLC scale measuring IHLC, OHLC, and CHLC.

As recommended by the authors of the scale [10,40], the responses obtained according to the Likert scale from strongly disagree to strongly agree were assigned numerical values from 1 to 6. Subscales reflecting IHLC, OHLC, and CHLC were calculated as sums of six relevant items. As a result, subscales' scores could range from 6 to 36. Wallston et al. [10] explained that each type of HLC is not mutually exclusive; therefore, all three scores were applied in multivariate regression modeling.

The variables showing 'ever used' and 'used in the last month' of conventional cigarettes were utilized to analyze their association with the use of electronic cigarettes.

2.3. Statistical Analysis

The software package IBM SPSS Statistics v.26 (IBM Corp., Armonk, NY, USA) was utilized for statistical assessment. Relative and absolute frequencies were used to describe categorical variables and the mean and standard deviation (SD) for continuous numerical variables.

The roles of potential predictors of the use of e-cigarettes were assessed with univariate and multivariate logistic regression models. Each model was characterized with the Hosmer–Lemeshow test. Furthermore, for all regression models, Nagelkerke R^2 was also established. In the Result section, the effect of independent variables was presented as the odds ratio (OR), 95% confidence interval (95% CI), and p-values in the case of univariate models and adjusted OR (aOR), 95% CI and p-value for multivariate models. Statistical significance was established as $p < 0.05$.

3. Results

3.1. Characteristics of the Study Group

The number of questionnaires included in the final analysis after quality control was 2223 (response rate 95.4%). Girls made 66.3% ($n = 1457$) of the study group, students of high schools providing general education—82.3% ($n = 1829$). The average age of the study participant was 17.01 years (SD = 0.97). Students attending I class were 37.0% ($n = 1457$), II class—28.8% ($n = 630$) and III or IV class—34.2% (748). The average HL score was 34.76% (SD = 6.13), IHLC 25.04 (SD = 4.59), OHLC—20.60 (SD = 4.99) and CHLC—19.89 (SD = 5.29). Detailed characteristics of the study group have already been published [41].

3.2. The Use of E-Cigarettes and Smoking of Conventional Cigarettes

It was shown that the use of e-cigarettes in the past and the use in the last 30 days are significantly associated with smoking traditional cigarettes in the past and smoking in the previous 30 days (Table 1). Among respondents who have ever used e-cigarettes, 87.6% ($n = 923$) had smoked traditional cigarettes in the past. The percentage of respondents who had ever smoked traditional cigarettes among those who had never used e-cigarettes was only 22.0% ($n = 249$) (Fisher exact test, $p < 0.001$). The percentages of the respondents who had smoked traditional cigarettes in the last 30 days among those who had ever used and never used e-cigarettes were 55.4% (586) and 8.8% (n = 102), respectively (Fisher exact test, <0.001). Furthermore, the percentage of respondents who had ever smoked traditional cigarettes, among those who had used and had not used e-cigarettes in the last 30 days, was 92.7% (n = 381) and 44.6% (n = 795), respectively (Fisher exact test, $p < 0.001$). Finally, respondents who had smoked traditional cigarettes in the last 30 days, among those who had or had not used e-cigarettes in the previous 30 days, were 72.4% (n = 299) and 21.7% (n = 392), respectively (Fisher exact test, $p < 0.001$).

Table 1. Association between using e-cigarettes and smoking conventional cigarettes.

Variables			Using E-Cigarettes				
		Ever Used E-Cigarettes			Used E-Cigarettes in the Last 30 Days		
Smoking Conventional Cigarettes		no % (n)	yes % (n)	p	no % (n)	yes % (n)	p
ever smoked	no	78.0 (885)	12.4 (131)	<0.001	55.4 (989)	73 (30)	<0.001
	yes	22.0 (249)	87.6 (923)		44.6 (795)	92.7 (381)	
smoked in last 30 days	no	91.2 (1051)	44.6 (471)	<0.001	78.3 (1418)	27.6 (114)	<0.001
	yes	8.8 (102)	55.4 (586)		21.7 (392)	72.4 (299)	

Abbreviations: p—Fisher exact test.

3.3. Predictors of Having Ever Used E-Cigarettes in the Past

High school students who had ever used e-cigarettes in the past were 47.5% (n = 1057). Univariate logistic regression revealed that significant predictors of having ever used e-cigarettes in the past included gender, the type of school, attended class (year of high school) at the moment of the survey, size of the accommodation, the number of siblings, marital status of parents, the expenses on mobile phone, the weekly duration of Internet use, the number of books at home, PHLC, and CHLC (Table 2). Boys were more likely to use e-cigarettes than girls (OR, 95%CI: 1.28, 1.07–1.52). Students of vocational education schools were as much as 2.28 times more likely to use e-cigarettes than those from general education schools (OR, 95%CI: 2.28, 1.82–2.86). Furthermore, the oldest students were more likely than the youngest (attending III or IV class in comparison to attending I class, OR, 95% CI: 1.47, 1.20–1.80), those whose parents were divorced or separated than those whose parents were married (OR, 95% CI: 1.45, 1.10–1.92), and those spending the most on the mobile phone were more likely than those spending the least (OR, 95% CI: 2.11, 1.39–3.22), to use e-cigarettes. More frequent use of the Internet has also been associated with a higher likelihood of using e-cigarettes (OR, 95% CI: 2.20, 1.56–3.09). Higher CHLC was also a predictor of more frequent use of e-cigarettes (OR, 95%CI: 1.21, 1.10–1.33). Having more than two siblings rather than no siblings (OR, 95% CI: 0.65, 0.46–0.91), living in the largest home rather than in the smallest (OR, 95% CI: 0.74, 0.55–0.99), and having at home more than 50 books rather than having less than 25 books (OR, 95% CI for comparison between those having the smallest and greatest number of books: 0.50, 0.34–0.72) was associated with less frequent use of e-cigarettes. A higher rather than a lower OHLC score was also related to less frequent use (OR, 95% CI: 0.86, 0.78–0.95).

In the multivariate regression model, a significant association was maintained only for gender, type of school, attended class, mobile phone expenses, Internet use duration, OHLC, and CHLC (Table 2). The association between the use of e-cigarettes and duration of Internet use became significant for all but one category of longer Internet use in the multivariate model.

Table 2. Uni- and multivariate logistic regression models for the use of e-cigarettes in the past.

Variables	Categories	The Use of E–Cigarettes Ever in Past			
		OR (95% CI)	p	aOR (95% CI)	p
Gender	Female *				
	male	1.28 (1.07–1.52)	0.007	1.44 (1.17–1.79)	0.001
Type of school	general education				
	vocational training	2.28 (1.82–2.86)	<0.001	2.16 (1.63–2.86)	<0.001
Attended class in school	class I *				
	class II	1.16 (0.94–1.44)	0.155	1.17 (0.91–1.50)	0.216
	class III or IV	1.47 (1.2–1.8)	<0.001	1.45 (1.15–1.83)	0.002
Mother's level of education	lower than secondary *				
	secondary	1.21 (0.97–1.5)	0.090	1.18 (0.90–1.55)	0.233
	university	1.06 (0.86–1.32)	0.574	1.20 (0.88–1.62)	0.246
Father's level of education	lower than secondary *				
	secondary	1.08 (0.88–1.31)	0.455	0.95 (0.74–1.22)	0.702
	university	0.84 (0.68–1.03)	0.101	0.83 (0.61–1.12)	0.219
Place of residence	Rural *				
	urban ≤10,000	1.15 (0.8–1.65)	0.447	1.00 (0.65–1.53)	0.992
	urban > 10,000 to 200,000	1.13 (0.91–1.41)	0.278	0.99 (0.75–1.30)	0.919
	urban >200,000	0.98 (0.79–1.20)	0.825	0.82 (0.61–1.11)	0.199
Size of home	≤50 m² *				
	>50 m²–70 m²	0.85 (0.6–1.20)	0.362	0.97 (0.65–1.46)	0.883
	>70 m²–90 m²	0.72 (0.5–1.03)	0.074	0.73 (0.47–1.13)	0.162
	>90 m²	0.74 (0.55–0.99)	0.041	0.79 (0.54–1.15)	0.215
Number of siblings	0 *				
	1	0.95 (0.77–1.16)	0.620	1.09 (0.85–1.40)	0.495
	2	0.9 (0.70–1.16)	0.421	1.20 (0.87–1.64)	0.271
	>2	0.65 (0.46–0.91)	0.011	0.76 (0.50–1.17)	0.210
Marital status	Married *				
	divorced or separated	1.45 (1.10–1.92)	0.009	1.37 (0.97–1.92)	0.072
	one or both parents dead	1.04 (0.65–1.67)	0.875	1.06 (0.60–1.89)	0.842
External help	No *				
	yes	1.16 (0.98–1.38)	0.084	1.03 (0.83–1.28)	0.792
The self–assessed financial situation of the family	worse than good *				
	good	1.01 (0.79–1.30)	0.919	1.06 (0.79–1.44)	0.683
	very good	1.04 (0.79–1.36)	0.786	1.19 (0.85–1.66)	0.308
Monthly expenses on mobile phone	≤5 PLN *				
	>5–10 PLN	0.73 (0.43–1.22)	0.223	0.96 (0.53–1.75)	0.894
	>10–30 PLN	1.13 (0.76–1.70)	0.543	1.37 (0.85–2.20)	0.202
	>30–50 PLN	1.39 (0.93–2.08)	0.111	1.59 (0.99–2.56)	0.056
	>50 PLN	2.11 (1.39–3.22)	<0.001	2.34 (1.42–3.86)	0.001
Books at home	≤25 *				
	26–50	0.75 (0.55–1.02)	0.067	0.88 (0.61–1.27)	0.502
	51–100	0.74 (0.55–0.99)	0.041	0.81 (0.58–1.14)	0.230
	101–500	0.66 (0.50–0.87)	0.003	0.73 (0.52–1.02)	0.067
	>500	0.50 (0.34–0.72)	<0.001	0.68 (0.44–1.06)	0.087
Duration of Internet use per week	not more than 2 h *				
	>2–7 h	1.48 (1.05–2.07)	0.025	1.67 (1.12–2.48)	0.012
	>7–14 h	1.36 (0.96–1.92)	0.083	1.63 (1.09–2.45)	0.018
	>14–21 h	1.21 (0.85–1.72)	0.299	1.35 (0.89–2.04)	0.158
	>21–35 h	1.37 (0.96–1.95)	0.085	1.52 (1.00–2.29)	0.048
	>35 h	2.2 (1.56–3.09)	<0.001	2.38 (1.59–3.57)	<0.001
HL		1.00 (0.99–1.02)	0.648	1.01 (0.99–1.02)	0.509
IHLC		1.00 (0.99–1.02)	0.700	1.01 (0.99–1.03)	0.329
OHLC		0.98 (0.96–0.99)	0.003	0.96 (0.94–0.98)	<0.001
CHLC		1.03 (1.02–1.05)	<0.001	1.05 (1.03–1.07)	<0.001

Abbreviations: *—referential category, OR—odds ratio, 95%CI—95% confidential interval, p—p-value for uni- and multivariate logistic regression model, HL—health literacy, IHLC—internal health locus of control, OHLC—'powerful other' health locus of control, CHLC—'chance' health locus of control.

3.4. Predictors of Regular Use of E-Cigarettes

18.6% (n = 413) of the study participants had used e-cigarettes in the last month. The regression model developed for the use of e-cigarettes in the previous month revealed similar relationships as for their ever having been used in the past for gender, type of school, marital status of parents, the number of books at home, the duration of weekly Internet use, and CHLC (Table 3). However, no significant association has been confirmed between use of e-cigarettes in the last 30 days and the year in high school, the number of siblings, the size of home, and OHLC. Interestingly, new relationships have been revealed. Having a mother with higher levels of attained education rather than the lowest was associated with more frequent use of e-cigarettes (OR, 95% CI: 1.47, 1.10–1.98 and 1.60, 1.19–2.15, respectively). Furthermore, inhabitants of more populated urban areas were more prone to use e-cigarettes than those living in rural areas (OR, 95% CI: 1.40, 1.07–1.84). In the multivariate regression model, the significant association of using e-cigarettes in the previous 30 days was maintained for the same independent variables as in univariate regression models (Table 3).

Table 3. Uni- and multivariate logistic regression models for the use of cigarettes in the last month.

Variables	Categories	The Use of Cigarettes in the Last Month			
		OR (95% CI)	p	aOR (95% CI)	p
Gender	Female *				
	male	1.93 (1.55–2.40)	<0.001	1.96 (1.51–2.54)	<0.001
Type of school	general education *				
	vocational training	2.42 (1.89–3.10)	<0.001	2.34 (1.71–3.19)	<0.001
Attended class in school	class I *				
	class II	0.98 (0.75–1.28)	0.87	1.16 (0.85–1.58)	0.354
	class III or IV	0.95 (0.74–1.23)	0.711	1.00 (0.74–1.34)	0.981
Mother's level of education	lower than secondary *				
	secondary	1.60 (1.19–2.14)	0.002	1.49 (1.04–2.13)	0.030
	university	1.47 (1.09–1.98)	0.011	1.72 (1.16–2.55)	0.007
Father's level of education	lower than secondary *				
	secondary	1.12 (0.87–1.44)	0.385	0.88 (0.64–1.2)	0.413
	university	1.04 (0.79–1.36)	0.782	0.82 (0.56–1.19)	0.292
Place of residence	Rural *				
	urban ≤10,000	1.11 (0.69–1.78)	0.679	1.17 (0.67–2.04)	0.582
	urban >10,000 to 200,000	1.56 (1.19–2.06)	0.002	1.53 (1.09–2.14)	0.015
	urban >200,000	1.41 (1.08–1.83)	0.011	1.41 (0.98–2.03)	0.065
Size of home	≤50 m^2 *				
	>50 m^2–70 m^2	1.08 (0.71–1.66)	0.706	1.33 (0.80–2.19)	0.271
	>70 m^2–90 m^2	0.99 (0.63–1.56)	0.96	1.36 (0.79–2.35)	0.261
	>90 m^2	0.84 (0.58–1.21)	0.344	1.31 (0.82–2.11)	0.257
Number of siblings	0 *				
	1	1.12 (0.86–1.45)	0.391	1.26 (0.92–1.72)	0.143
	2	0.82 (0.58–1.14)	0.240	1.09 (0.72–1.64)	0.695
	>2	0.83 (0.53–1.29)	0.409	1.18 (0.68–2.04)	0.559
Marital status	Married *				
	divorced or separated	1.53 (1.11–2.11)	0.010	1.53 (1.04–2.26)	0.033
	one or both parents dead	0.84 (0.43–1.61)	0.591	0.64 (0.27–1.48)	0.297
External help	No *				
	yes	1.10 (0.88–1.37)	0.390	1.14 (0.87–1.51)	0.334
Self–assessed financial situation of the family	worse than good *				
	good	0.96 (0.70–1.33)	0.816	1.12 (0.76–1.65)	0.556
	very good	0.97 (0.69–1.37)	0.864	1.01 (0.66–1.55)	0.967

Table 3. Cont.

Variables	Categories	The Use of Cigarettes in the Last Month			
Monthly expenses on mobile phone	≤5 PLN *				
	>5–10 PLN	0.59 (0.31–1.14)	0.115	0.66 (0.31–1.41)	0.281
	>10–30 PLN	0.70 (0.43–1.15)	0.159	0.86 (0.49–1.53)	0.612
	>30–50 PLN	0.83 (0.51–1.35)	0.457	0.98 (0.56–1.73)	0.952
	>50 PLN	1.09 (0.66–1.80)	0.73	1.44 (0.80–2.58)	0.223
Books at home	≤25 *				
	26–50	0.81 (0.56–1.18)	0.277	1.00 (0.65–1.52)	0.987
	51–100	0.74 (0.52–1.04)	0.087	0.64 (0.43–0.96)	0.031
	101–500	0.63 (0.45–0.89)	0.008	0.58 (0.39–0.88)	0.009
	>500	0.55 (0.35–0.89)	0.014	0.6 (0.35–1.04)	0.070
Duration of Internet use in a week	not more than 2 h *				
	>2–7 h	1.14 (0.73–1.80)	0.560	1.05 (0.62–1.76)	0.865
	>7–14 h	1.36 (0.86–2.14)	0.187	1.55 (0.93–2.59)	0.094
	>14–21 h	0.99 (0.61–1.60)	0.972	0.90 (0.52–1.56)	0.714
	>21–35 h	1.01 (0.63–1.64)	0.952	1.02 (0.60–1.74)	0.945
	>35 h	1.88 (1.21–2.92)	0.005	1.8 (1.09–2.96)	0.021
HL		1.01 (0.99–1.02)	0.487	1.01 (0.99–1.03)	0.371
IHLC		1.00 (0.98–1.03)	0.841	1.00 (0.97–1.03)	0.981
OHLC		0.99 (0.97–1.01)	0.399	0.98 (0.95–1.00)	0.073
CHLC		1.03 (1.01–1.05)	0.003	1.04 (1.02–1.07)	0.001

Abbreviations: *—referential category, OR—odds ratio, 95%CI—95% confidential interval, p—p-value for uni- and multivariate logistic regression model, HL—health literacy, IHLC—internal health locus of control, OHLC—'powerful other' health locus of control, CHLC—'chance' health locus of control.

4. Discussion

In our study, we have analyzed the data from a survey on a large sample of 2223 students of high schools located in urban and rural areas of a voivodship in southern Poland. We have addressed the problem of the use of e-cigarettes within a broader survey focused on the health behaviors of Polish adolescents and their relationships with selected potential predictors. We have assumed that HLC may serve as a construct to explain, to some extent, the mechanisms leading to the use of e-cigarettes in this group. The decision to include HL assessment in our survey was dictated by our attempt to measure the level of HL in the adolescent population (as this has not been done before) and understand if adequate HL protects against potentially risky health behaviors in this group.

We have shown that the likelihood that respondents have ever used e-cigarettes was higher among boys than girls, among students of schools providing vocational training than only general education, among older students than younger students, among respondents who spend the most on mobile phones than those paying the least as well as among the respondents using the Internet for the longest time per week than among those using it for the shortest time. The level of HL was not significantly associated with the likelihood of using e-cigarettes. Finally, it was significantly lower among persons with higher OHLC scores and higher among persons with greater CHLC. The multivariate logistic regression model has shown a similar pattern of interrelationships between the use of e-cigarettes in the last 30 days and gender, type of school, weekly duration of Internet use, and CHLC, but not with attended class, expenses on mobile phone and OHLC. We have also observed that recent use of e-cigarettes was significantly associated with the level of education attained by respondents' mothers, place of residence, marital status, and the number of books at home.

The higher prevalence of the use of electronic cigarettes among males than females has been reported in many previous studies [42–46]. Additionally, older adolescents in the studied groups showed higher use of e-cigarettes [42,47,48]. Vuolo et al. reported a higher likelihood of using e-cigarettes among 17 years old adolescents from families with only one parent or whose parents were divorced [44]. Contrary to our findings, the study published recently by Janik-Koncewicz et al. showed that the use of e-cigarettes among

Polish students was higher among those living in rural rather than urban areas [8]. In turn, Vuolo et al. found that youths from larger cities were more prone to use e-cigarettes [44]. A higher incidence of vocational students using e-cigarettes has been seen by Surís et al. [46].

We have used the expenses on mobile phones as an indicator of the economic status of the family of the respondent. The respondents who spent the most on their mobile phones have exhibited a higher likelihood of using e-cigarettes than those paying the least. The relationships with other variables that could be treated as indicators of economic status of a given respondent and the use of e-cigarettes have also been observed by other authors [48].

In our study, we have found that using e-cigarettes is significantly associated with the smoking of conventional cigarettes. The percentage of respondents who smoked cigarettes among the recent users of e-cigarettes was about 72%. In the study performed by Janik-Koncewicz et al., this percentage was 55% [8]. In turn, we have found that among current smokers of conventional cigarettes, 43% also used e-cigarettes, and in the study of Janik-Koncewicz et al., 69% did [8]. Many other authors have studied and confirmed the relationship between smoking conventional cigarettes and using e-cigarettes [42,44,45].

More Internet use during the week was associated with higher odds of using e-cigarettes among Polish adolescents. Interestingly, Lee et al. observed in South Korean youth that the respondents not using the Internet were more prone to use all types of tobacco products and e-cigarettes [49]. Other authors have suggested a significant association between the use of electronic cigarettes and the use of the Internet or information-seeking behaviors online [50,51]. One possible explanation for the relationship between more intensive Internet use and online information search behaviors and the use of e-cigarettes is the positive sentiment toward e-cigarettes on the Internet and especially social media [52].

The importance of HLC as a predictor of the smoking of conventional cigarettes among the general population and adolescents has been reported earlier by many authors [21–27,29]. Usually, they confirmed that higher CHLC was related to the higher likelihood of smoking. Our study is probably one of the first to confirm that CHLC is also consistently associated with the likelihood of using e-cigarettes either ever in the past or during the last 30 days before the survey. This finding may suggest that, to some extent, similar mechanisms, as in the case of conventional cigarettes, are responsible for initiating and maintaining the use of e-cigarettes in youths.

There was no significant relationship between HL and the use of e-cigarettes in Polish high school students. Previous studies analyzing the association between the level of HL and health behaviors have yielded unambiguous results. Sørensen et al. reported that among the population 15–75 years old, HL, as measured with HLS–EU–Q47, has been significantly associated with smoking conventional cigarettes, but the correlation was rather low [31]. The study performed in 2016 among the adult Polish population with a short, 16-item version of the HLS–EU questionnaire did not show a significant association between HL and smoking [35]. Only a few studies indicate a relationship between HL and the use of e-cigarettes. Recently, Clifford et al. found no significant relationship between HL and conventional cigarettes, e-cigarettes, or dual-use among the large sample of respondents recruited for the 2016 Behavioral Risk Factor Surveillance System [36]. It seems that our study is the first to report the results of the analysis of the association between the levels of HL and the use of electronic cigarettes by adolescents. The lack of a significant relationship between HL and the use of e-cigarettes among Polish adolescents may be an important indication that interventions increasing health-related knowledge and skills, especially those provided at schools, should put more emphasis on the aspects related to smoking and the use of e-cigarettes. Currently, these aspects are not adequately covered by health education focused on younger generation.

Due to its limitations, in our study, we have not been able to address many other determinants reported by other authors, including opinions about the social acceptability of e-cigarettes and the sensory experience [53], daily cannabis use and frequent alcohol use [44], exposure to secondhand smoking in various places [45] or early sexual experience [44].

Limitations

Our study was aimed at the assessment of many types of health behaviors. Therefore, we have included only a limited set of items asking about using e-cigarettes. Due to the broad scope of potential determinants addressed in the survey, our analysis covers variables reflecting the socio-demographic and financial status of respondents and HLC and HL.

However, it should be noted that the study reported here has not addressed many potential factors that can influence the acceptability and use of e-cigarettes. In their review, Trucco et al. mention several attributes increasing the appeal of e-cigarettes to youth, such as flavor variety, device modifiability, the ability to perform tricks, and concealment from authority figures [54]. It is also well known that adolescents have high positive expectations about e-cigarettes associated with personal enjoyment, social benefits, and perceived safety [54].

The number of students who refused to participate in the survey was 107 (4.56% of all the approached students). It seems that this fraction should not considerably influence the results reported in the paper. The questionnaire applied in the survey consisted of about 130 individual items and this could result in a lower quality of response. However, we have not observed a high number of missing responses. In the case of the HL score, we were not able to calculate it for only 6.3% of the returned questionnaires, partially due to the fact that some of the respondents selected the response option 'not applicable'. The number of missing responses in the HLC scale was very low, not surpassing 1.0% of the questionnaires.

This study was carried out in only one district of southern Poland, and it would be risky to extend the obtained results to the whole Polish population of adolescents. On the other hand, good representation of urban and rural communities and various types of included schools allows the assessment of multiple factors that could influence the use of e-cigarettes.

The analysis reported here has been performed on data collected in 2017, and the obtained results should be treated cautiously as the trends in the use of e-cigarettes and other emerging nicotine delivery products are changing quickly.

5. Conclusions

Adolescents have become one of the main groups of users of new nicotine delivery products, including e-cigarettes. Contrary to marketing slogans, e-cigarettes can hardly be treated as a tool used to limit the use of conventional cigarettes among this population. Similar to other reports, our study clearly shows that the users of e-cigarettes are also frequently smokers of traditional cigarettes. We have found that among the sociodemographic factors, gender is the main predictor of the use of electronic cigarettes. Some effects, especially on the recent use of e-cigarettes, have also been found for the place of residence, marital status of parents, and the level of education of the mothers but not the fathers of respondents. Unexpectedly, respondents whose mothers have attained higher levels of education showed a more increased risk of using e-cigarettes. It also seems that respondents living in urban areas are more prone to use e-cigarettes than inhabitants of rural areas. This study showed that intensive Internet users show a higher proclivity toward electronic cigarettes than those using the Internet for a shorter time weekly. Finally, HL did not affect the use of e-cigarettes, but CHLC was a consistent predictor.

The results of this study also suggest directions for future research. It should be explained why general HL is not associated with a cautious approach to smoking e-cigarettes. Furthermore, health educators should be aware that there are strong interrelations between smoking traditional cigarettes and the use of e-cigarettes. This implies that e-cigarettes cannot be treated as a means of preventing the initiation of smoking cigarettes or a contingency measure, at least among adolescents.

In practical terms, health promotion interventions focused on improving the HL of children and adolescents should strive for better understanding of the potential adverse effects of e-cigarettes as well as the relationships between their use and smoking conventional cigarettes. It also seems that the use of e-cigarettes by adolescents has become an important public health issue. Still, neither the mechanisms nor consequences of this phenomenon are sufficiently understood or adequately addressed in public health policies.

Supplementary Materials: The following are available online at https://www.mdpi.com/article/10.3390/toxics10010041/s1, items of the questionnaire used in the analysis in this paper.

Author Contributions: Conceptualization, M.D. and M.G.; methodology, M.G and. M.D.; questionnaire development, M.G., and M.D.; data collection, M.G.; survey supervision, M.D.; data curation, M.D.; statistical analysis, M.D.; writing—original draft preparation, M.D.; writing—review and editing, M.D. All authors have read and agreed to the published version of the manuscript.

Funding: This research was conducted within statutory projects funded by the Jagiellonian University Medical College, titled "The determinants of health behaviours of high school students in Poland" (grant number N43/DBS/000154) and "Modern health promotion strategies focused on the change of health behaviors and the development of health literacy" (grant number N43/DBS/000167).

Institutional Review Board Statement: The study was conducted according to the guidelines of the Declaration of Helsinki and approved by the Bioethical Committee of Jagiellonian University (No. KBET/193/B/2014 issued 25 September 2014).

Informed Consent Statement: Informed consent was obtained from all subjects involved in the study and, in the case of subjects below 18 years of age, additionally from their parents or legal guardians.

Data Availability Statement: The data that support the findings of this study are available on request from the corresponding author. The data are not publicly available due to privacy and ethical restrictions. The authors did not inform participants that public access to the survey data may be considered. Access to the data will be granted on a case-by—case basis, following a justified request after receiving consent from the Bioethical Committee at Jagiellonian University.

Acknowledgments: The authors thank Glen Cullen for proofreading of the manuscript.

Conflicts of Interest: The authors declare no conflict of interest.

References

1. Durmowicz, E.L. The Impact of Electronic Cigarettes on the Paediatric Population. *Tob. Control* **2014**, *23*, ii41–ii46. [CrossRef] [PubMed]
2. Fadus, M.C.; Smith, T.T.; Squeglia, L.M. The Rise of E-Cigarettes, Pod Mod Devices, and JUUL among Youth: Factors Influencing Use, Health Implications, and Downstream Effects. *Drug Alcohol Depend.* **2019**, *201*, 85–93. [CrossRef] [PubMed]
3. Office of the US Surgeon General. *E-Cigarette Use among Youth and Young Adults: A Report of the Surgeon General*; Office of the US Surgeon General: Rockville, MD, USA, 2016.
4. Marynak, K.L.; Gammon, D.G.; King, B.A.; Loomis, B.R.; Fulmer, E.B.; Wang, T.W.; Rogers, T. National and State Trends in Sales of Cigarettes and E-Cigarettes, U.S., 2011–2015. *Am. J. Prev. Med.* **2017**, *53*, 96–101. [CrossRef] [PubMed]
5. Hallingberg, B.; Maynard, O.M.; Bauld, L.; Brown, R.; Gray, L.; Lowthian, E.; MacKintosh, A.M.; Moore, L.; Munafo, M.R.; Moore, G. Have E-Cigarettes Renormalised or Displaced Youth Smoking? Results of a Segmented Regression Analysis of Repeated Cross Sectional Survey Data in England, Scotland and Wales. *Tob. Control* **2020**, *29*, 207–216. [CrossRef] [PubMed]
6. Smith, D.M.; Gawron, M.; Balwicki, L.; Sobczak, A.; Matynia, M.; Goniewicz, M.L. Exclusive versus Dual Use of Tobacco and Electronic Cigarettes among Adolescents in Poland, 2010–2016. *Addict. Behav.* **2019**, *90*, 341–348. [CrossRef]
7. Kaleta, D.; Polanska, K. Trends of E-Cigarettes and Tobacco Use among Secondary and High School Students from Poland over Three Years Observation. *Tob. Induc. Dis.* **2021**, *19*, A72. [CrossRef]
8. Janik-Koncewicz, K.; Parascandola, M.; Bachand, J.; Zatoński, M.; Przewoźniak, K.; Zatoński, W. E-Cigarette Use among Polish Students: Findings from the 2016 Poland Global Youth Tobacco Survey. *J. Health Inequal.* **2020**, *6*, 95–103. [CrossRef]
9. Wallston, K. Multidimensional Health Locus of Control Scales. In *Encyclopedia of Behavioral Medicine*; Gellman, G.D., Turner, J.R., Eds.; Springer: New York, NY, USA, 2013; pp. 1266–1269.
10. Wallston, K.A.; Wallston, B.S.; DeVellis, R. Development of the Multidimensional Health Locus of Control (MHLC) Scales. *Health Educ. Behav.* **1978**, *6*, 160–170. [CrossRef] [PubMed]
11. Gacek, M.; Wojtowicz, A. Personal Resources and Nutritional Behavior of Polish Basketball Players. *J. Phys. Educ. Sport* **2021**, *21*, 130–139. [CrossRef]
12. Lee, H.C.; Chang, C.T.; Cheng, Z.H.; Chen, Y.T. Will an Organic Label Always Increase Food Consumption? It Depends on Food Type and Consumer Differences in Health Locus of Control. *Food Qual. Prefer.* **2018**, *63*, 88–96. [CrossRef]
13. Aharon, A.A.; Nehama, H.; Rishpon, S.; Baron-Epel, O. A Path Analysis Model Suggesting the Association between Health Locus of Control and Compliance with Childhood Vaccinations. *Hum. Vaccin. Immunother.* **2018**, *14*, 1618–1625. [CrossRef]

14. Özdemir, E.Z.; Bektaş, M. The Effects of Self-Efficacy and Locus of Control on Cyberbully/Victim Status in Adolescents. *J. Pediatr. Nurs.* **2021**, *61*, e15–e21. [CrossRef] [PubMed]
15. Octari, T.E.; Suryadi, B.; Sawitri, D.R. The Role of Self-Concept and Health Locus of COntrol on Quality of Life Among Individuals with Diabetes. *J. Psikol.* **2020**, *19*, 80–94. [CrossRef]
16. Levin-Zamir, D.; Baron-Epel, O.B.; Cohen, V.; Elhayany, A. The Association of Health Literacy with Health Behavior, Socioeconomic Indicators, and Self-Assessed Health From a National Adult Survey in Israel. *J. Health Commun.* **2016**, *21*, 61–68. [CrossRef] [PubMed]
17. Segall, M.E.; Wynd, C.A. Health Conception, Health Locus of Control, and Power as Predictors of Smoking Behavior Change. *Am. J. Health Promot.* **1990**, *4*, 338–344. [CrossRef] [PubMed]
18. Bennett, P.; Moore, L.; Norman, P.; Murphy, S.; Tudor-Smith, C. Health Locus of Control and Value for Health in Smokers and Nonsmokers. *Health Psychol.* **1997**, *16*, 179–182. [CrossRef] [PubMed]
19. Kuwahara, A.; Nishino, Y.; Ohkubo, T.; Tsuji, I.; Hisamichi, S.; Hosokawa, T. Reliability and Validity of the Multidimensional Health Locus of Control Scale in Japan: Relationship with Demographic Factors and Health-Related Behavior. *Tohoku J. Exp. Med.* **2004**, *203*, 37–45. [CrossRef] [PubMed]
20. Reitzel, L.R.; Lahoti, S.; Li, Y.; Cao, Y.; Wetter, D.W.; Waters, A.J.; Vidrine, J.I. Neighborhood Vigilance, Health Locus of Control, and Smoking Abstinence. *Am. J. Health Behav.* **2013**, *37*, 334. [CrossRef] [PubMed]
21. Grotz, M.; Hapke, U.; Lampert, T.; Baumeister, H. Health Locus of Control and Health Behaviour: Results from a Nationally Representative Survey. *Psychol. Health Med.* **2011**, *16*, 129–140. [CrossRef]
22. Helmer, S.M.; Krämer, A.; Mikolajczyk, R.T. Health-Related Locus of Control and Health Behaviour among University Students in North Rhine Westphalia, Germany. *BMC Res. Notes* **2012**, *5*, 703. [CrossRef] [PubMed]
23. Mercer, D.A.; Ditto, B.; Lavoie, K.L.; Campbell, T.; Arsenault, A.; Bacon, S.L. Health Locus of Control Is Associated with Physical Activity and Other Health Behaviors in Cardiac Patients. *J. Cardiopulm. Rehabil. Prev.* **2018**, *38*, 394–399. [CrossRef] [PubMed]
24. Clarke, J.H.; MacPherson, B.V.; Holmes, D.R. Cigarette Smoking and External Locus of Control among Young Adolescents. *J. Health Soc. Behav.* **1982**, *23*, 253–259. [CrossRef] [PubMed]
25. Eiser, J.R.; Eiser, C.; Gammage, P.; Morgan, M. Health Locus of Control and Health Beliefs in Relation to Adolescent Smoking. *Br. J. Addict.* **1989**, *84*, 1059–1065. [CrossRef] [PubMed]
26. Lassi, G.; Taylor, A.E.; Mahedy, L.; Heron, J.; Eisen, T.; Munafo, M.R. Locus of Control Is Associated with Tobacco and Alcohol Consumption in Young Adults of the Avon Longitudinal Study of Parents and Children. *R. Soc. Open Sci.* **2019**, *6*, 181133. [CrossRef] [PubMed]
27. Abikoye, G.E.; Fusigboye, A. Gender, Locus of Control and Smoking Habits of Undergraduate Students. *Afr. J. Drug Alcohol Stud.* **2011**, *9*, 71–79. [CrossRef]
28. Kim, Y. Adolescents' Health Behaviours and Its Associations with Psychological Variables. *Cent. Eur. J. Public Health* **2011**, *19*, 205–209. [CrossRef]
29. Booth-Butterfield, M.; Anderson, R.H.; Booth-Butterfield, S. Adolescents' Use of Tobacco, Health Locus of Control, and Self-Monitoring. *Health Commun.* **2009**, *12*, 137–148. [CrossRef] [PubMed]
30. Nutbeam, D. Health Promotion Glossary. *Health Promot. Int.* **1998**, *13*, 349–364. [CrossRef]
31. Sørensen, K.; Pelikan, J.J.M.; Röthlin, F.; Ganahl, K.; Slonska, Z.; Doyle, G.; Fullam, J.; Kondilis, B.; Agrafiotis, D.; Uiters, E.; et al. Health Literacy in Europe: Comparative Results of the European Health Literacy Survey (HLS-EU). *Eur. J. Public Health* **2015**, *25*, 1053–1058. [CrossRef]
32. Berkman, N.D.; Sheridan, S.L.; Donahue, K.E.; Halpern, D.J.; Crotty, K. Low Health Literacy and Health Outcomes: An Updated Systematic Review. *Ann. Intern. Med.* **2011**, *155*, 97–107. [CrossRef]
33. Humphrys, E.; Burt, J.; Rubin, G.; Emery, J.D.; Walter, F.M. The Influence of Health Literacy on the Timely Diagnosis of Symptomatic Cancer: A Systematic Review. *Eur. J. Cancer Care* **2019**, *28*, e12920. [CrossRef] [PubMed]
34. Zaben, K.; Khalil, A. Health Literacy, Self-Care Behavior and Quality of Life in Acute Coronary Syndrome Patients: An Integrative Review. *Open J. Nurs.* **2019**, *9*, 383–395. [CrossRef]
35. Duplaga, M. Determinants and Consequences of Limited Health Literacy in Polish Society. *Int. J. Environ. Res. Public Health* **2020**, *17*, 642. [CrossRef] [PubMed]
36. Clifford, J.S.; Lu, J.; Blondino, C.T.; Do, E.K.; Prom-Wormley, E.C. The Association Between Health Literacy and Tobacco Use: Results from a Nationally Representative Survey. *J. Community Health* **2021**, 1–8. [CrossRef] [PubMed]
37. Lindfors, P.; Kinnunen, J.; Paakkari, L.; Rimpela, A.; Richter, M.; Kuipers, M.; Kunst, A. Adolescent Health Literacy in 3 European Cities and Its Association with Smoking and Smoking Beliefs. *Eur. J. Public Health* **2019**, *29*, ckz186-145. [CrossRef]
38. Zvolensky, M.J.; Mayorga, N.A.; Garey, L. Main and Interactive Effects of E-Cigarette Use Health Literacy and Anxiety Sensitivity in Terms of e-Cigarette Perceptions and Dependence. *Cognit. Ther. Res.* **2019**, *43*, 121–130. [CrossRef]
39. Pelikan, J.M.; Röthlin, F.; Ganahl, K. Measuring Comprehensive Health Literacy in General Populations: Validation of Instrument, Indices and Scales of the HLS-EU Study. In Proceedings of the 6th Annual Health Literacy Research Conference, Bethesda, MD, USA, 13–14 October 2014.
40. Juczyński, Z. Wielowymiarowa Skala Umiejscowienia Kontroli Zdrowia—MHLC. In *NPPPZ–Narzędzia Pomiaru w Promocji i Psychologii Zdrowia*; Pracownia Testów Psychologicznych Polskiego Towarzystwa Psychologicznego: Warszawa, Poland, 2001; pp. 79–86.

41. Duplaga, M.; Grysztar, M. Socio-Economic Determinants of Health Literacy in High School Students: A Cross-Sectional Study. *Int. J. Environ. Res. Public Health* **2021**, *18*, 12231. [CrossRef] [PubMed]
42. Soteriades, S.; Barbouni, A.; Rachiotis, G.; Grevenitou, P.; Mouchtouri, V.; Pinaka, O.; Dadouli, K.; Hadjichristodoulou, C. Prevalence of Electronic Cigarette Use and Its Determinants among 13-to-15-Year-Old Students in Greece: Results from the 2013 Global Youth Tobacco Survey (GYTS). *Int. J. Environ. Res. Public Health* **2020**, *17*, 1671. [CrossRef]
43. Erinoso, O.; Oyapero, A.; Amure, M.; Osoba, M.; Osibogun, O.; Wright, K.; Osibogun, A. Electronic Cigarette Use among Adolescents and Young Adults in Nigeria: Prevalence, Associated Factors and Patterns of Use. *PLoS ONE* **2021**, *16*, e0258850. [CrossRef]
44. Vuolo, M.; Janssen, E.; Le Nézet, O.; Spilka, S. Community- and Individual-Level Risk Factors of Past Month e-Cigarette Use among Adolescents in France. *Drug Alcohol Depend.* **2021**, *226*, 108823. [CrossRef] [PubMed]
45. Cho, M.S. Factors Associated with Cigarette, E-Cigarette, and Dual Use among South Korean Adolescents. *Healthcare* **2021**, *9*, 1252. [CrossRef] [PubMed]
46. Surís, J.C.; Berchtold, A.; Akre, C. Reasons to Use E-Cigarettes and Associations with Other Substances among Adolescents in Switzerland. *Drug Alcohol Depend.* **2015**, *153*, 140–144. [CrossRef] [PubMed]
47. Hrywna, M.; Bover Manderski, M.T.; Delnevo, C.D. Prevalence of Electronic Cigarette Use Among Adolescents in New Jersey and Association With Social Factors. *JAMA Netw. Open* **2020**, *3*, e1920961. [CrossRef]
48. Buu, A.; Hu, Y.H.; Wong, S.W.; Lin, H.C. Internalizing and Externalizing Problems as Risk Factors for Initiation and Progression of E-Cigarette and Combustible Cigarette Use in the US Youth Population. *Int. J. Ment. Health Addict.* **2021**, *19*, 1759–1771. [CrossRef]
49. Lee, A.; Lee, K.S.; Park, H. Association of the Use of a Heated Tobacco Product with Perceived Stress, Physical Activity, and Internet Use in Korean Adolescents: A 2018 National Survey. *Int. J. Environ. Res. Public Health* **2019**, *16*, 965. [CrossRef] [PubMed]
50. Lorenzo-Blanco, E.I.; Unger, J.B.; Thrasher, J. E-Cigarette Use Susceptibility among Youth in Mexico: The Roles of Remote Acculturation, Parenting Behaviors, and Internet Use Frequency. *Addict. Behav.* **2021**, *113*, 106688. [CrossRef] [PubMed]
51. Wiseman, K.P.; Margolis, K.A.; Bernat, J.K.; Grana, R.A. The Association between Perceived E-Cigarette and Nicotine Addictiveness, Information-Seeking, and e-Cigarette Trial among U.S. Adults. *Prev. Med.* **2019**, *118*, 66–72. [CrossRef] [PubMed]
52. Kwon, M.; Park, E. Perceptions and Sentiments About Electronic Cigarettes on Social Media Platforms: Systematic Review. *JMIR Public Health Surveill.* **2020**, *6*, e13673. [CrossRef] [PubMed]
53. Lee, H.Y.; Lin, H.C.; Seo, D.C.; Lohrmann, D.K. Determinants Associated with E-Cigarette Adoption and Use Intention among College Students. *Addict. Behav.* **2017**, *65*, 102–110. [CrossRef]
54. Trucco, E.M.; Fallah-Sohy, N.; Hartmann, S.A.; Cristello, J.V. Electronic Cigarette Use Among Youth: Understanding Unique Risks in a Vulnerable Population. *Curr. Addict. Rep.* **2020**, *7*, 497–508. [CrossRef]

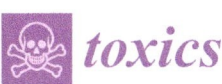

Article

Influence of Electronic Cigarettes on Antioxidant Capacity and Nucleotide Metabolites in Saliva

Dominika Cichońska [1,*], Oliwia Król [2], Ewa M. Słomińska [2], Barbara Kochańska [3], Dariusz Świetlik [4], Jolanta Ochocińska [3] and Aida Kusiak [1]

1. Department of Periodontology and Oral Mucosa Diseases, Medical University of Gdansk, 80-210 Gdansk, Poland; aida.kusiak@gumed.edu.pl
2. Department of Biochemistry, Medical University of Gdansk, 80-210 Gdansk, Poland; oliwia.krol@gumed.edu.pl (O.K.); ewa.slominska@gumed.edu.pl (E.M.S.)
3. Department of Conservative Dentistry, Medical University of Gdansk, 80-210 Gdansk, Poland; barbara.kochanska@gumed.edu.pl (B.K.); jolanta.ochocinska@gumed.edu.pl (J.O.)
4. Department of Biostatistics and Neural Networks, Medical University of Gdansk, 80-210 Gdansk, Poland; dariusz.swietlik@gumed.edu.pl
* Correspondence: dominika.cichonska@gumed.edu.pl

Abstract: The balance between reactive oxygen species production and the activity of antioxidant systems present in saliva is an important element in maintaining oral environment homeostasis. E-cigarettes adversely affect the oral cavity and their cytotoxic effect is related to oxidative stress. The aim of this study was to assess the influence of using electronic cigarettes on antioxidant capacity of saliva. The study involved 110 subjects (35 e-cigarettes users, 33 traditional cigarettes smokers and 42 non-smokers). Laboratory analysis involved quantitation of uric acid, hypoxanthine, xanthine, TAOS (total antioxidant status) and TEAC (Trolox equivalent antioxidant capacity) in saliva. Lower values for TAOS and TEAC were observed among e-cigarettes users and traditional cigarettes smokers in comparison to non-smokers. Uric acid concentration tended to be higher among e-cigarettes users while no differences in hypoxanthine and xanthine saliva concentrations were observed. Electronic cigarettes usage affects antioxidant capacity of saliva to the same extent as traditional cigarettes, when comparing smokers to non-smokers. Further longitudinal studies on a larger study group are needed to assess the effect of changes in antioxidant status on oral health.

Keywords: e-cigarettes; antioxidant capacity; saliva; uric acid

1. Introduction

Homeostasis in oral environment is mainly provided by saliva, produced constantly by large and small salivary glands [1]. Although 99% of saliva consists of water, it contains also inorganic and organic substances which affect its physicochemical properties [2]. Inorganic components such as sodium, potassium, calcium, magnesium, chlorine, fluorine, iodine, bicarbonates and phosphates are present in saliva in ionic form. Organic saliva components include carbohydrates, lipids, hormones, proteins and non-protein nitrogenous substances. [2]. Individual elements occurring in saliva play a strictly defined role in the proper functioning of the whole organism, nourishing and protecting the surrounding tissues. Saliva glycoproteins moisturize the mucosa and provide protection to oral mucosa against mechanical damage. The presence of buffering bicarbonate and phosphate ions enables to neutralize acids derived from food or that are product of bacterial metabolism, which maintains saliva's adequate pH value. Saliva contains also salivary amylase, a protein with enzymatic properties and elements presenting antimicrobial activity such as immunoglobulins A, lysozyme, lactoferrin, histamine and leukocytes [2,3]. Moreover, a variety of antioxidants are also present in saliva [4–7], and the saliva produced by the parotid glands has the highest antioxidant capacity [8].

One of the conditions for maintaining oral environment homeostasis is the balance between ROS (reactive oxygen species) production and the activity of antioxidant systems present in saliva [9]. ROS are mostly generated in cells as a by-product of the mitochondrial electron transport chain, which is dependent on the metabolic status of the cell [10]. Production and effective removal of ROS is crucial in signal transduction, immune defense, matrix remodeling and apoptosis [11]. Low levels of ROS are essential for physiological processes and maintenance of cellular homeostasis [12–14]. However, ROS are also an important effector of cell viability control by inducing a cytostatic effect and modulating cell metabolism and gene expression [11]. The excess of free radicals, especially reactive oxygen species, can lead to oxidative stress, which might become the cause of general and local diseases such as periodontitis, diabetes and rheumatoid arthritis [9,15]. Oxidative stress may lead to the destruction of periodontal structures by the degradation of the extracellular matrix of periodontal tissues, and it promotes inflammatory reactions in periodontitis [16–18]. Human cells and tissues are protected from the toxic effect of free radicals by special mechanisms including antioxidant enzymatic and non-enzymatic systems. Antioxidant enzymatic systems include peroxidase, catalase, superoxide dismutase and myeloperoxidase, whereas antioxidant non-enzymatic systems include uric acid, reduced glutathione, acute phase proteins, cysteine, ascorbic acid, alpha tocopherol, beta-carotene, retinol and methionine [5–7,12,15].

Diverse factors may impact the whole oral environment and composition of saliva is among the most important. Factors that may affect saliva composition include genetic diseases such as Turner syndrome [19], general diseases or tobacco smoking and electronic cigarettes usage [20,21]. Electronic cigarettes are mechanical devices that can be divided into two categories: closed-system and open-system. Closed-system devices tent to resemble traditional cigarettes, are usually disposable and are available in a limited variety of nicotine concentrations and flavors, whereas open-system e-cigarettes are larger in size than traditional cigarettes, can be refilled with e-liquids which are available in a huge variety of flavors and nicotine concentrations and are not disposable after usage [22]. Electronic cigarettes were initially presented as a less harmful substitute for tobacco smoking. However, taking recent research into consideration, this view is controversial [23–27]. It has been proven that electronic cigarettes have a negative effect on oral mucosa leading to death of oral epithelial keratinocytes and periodontal fibroblasts [28–30]. The cytotoxic effect is related to oxidative stress and increased concentration of proinflammatory cytokines [30,31]. Chemical compounds found in tobacco smoke and e-cigarettes liquids can dissolve in saliva, leading to disorders in its biochemical composition [21,32,33].

The aim of this study was to assess the influence of electronic cigarettes usage on the antioxidant capacity of saliva.

2. Materials and Methods

2.1. Patients' Population

This study included 110 patients: 35 patients using e-cigarettes (e-cigarettes users), 33 patients smoking traditional cigarettes and 42 non-smoking patients (non-smokers). They were students at the Medical University of Gdansk and young patients, who volunteered for a periodontal examination in the Department of Periodontology and Oral Mucosa Diseases. All participants were generally healthy people aged 20 to 30. Patients with periodontitis and diseases which might interfere condition of oral mucosa like diabetes, disorders of salivary secretion, oral mucosa diseases and people taking medications permanently and treated with antibiotics or steroid preparations in the last 6 months and patients consuming alcoholic beverages were excluded from the research. E-cigarettes users had been using open-system electronic cigarettes with a small nicotine concentration for at least 6 months. Traditional cigarettes smokers were smoking at least 10 cigarettes per day for at least 6 months. People smoking both traditional and electronic cigarettes were not included in this research. The study was conducted in 2018–2019. The study protocol has been approved by the Ethics Committee of Medical University of Gdansk,

Poland (NKBBN/161/2014). Ethical aspects of the research followed the World Medical Association Declaration of Helsinki.

2.2. Saliva Collection

Mixed unstimulated saliva was collected into a sterile silicon Corning-type test-tube from all patients who participated in this study. Saliva was collected in morning hours, two hours after the last intake of food or drink. Unstimulated salivary samples were obtained by expectoration in absence of chewing movements.

The samples were clarified by centrifugation (2000× g; 10 min) and immediately stored for the subsequent determination of uric acid, hypoxanthine, xanthine, TAOS (total antioxidant status) and TEAC (Trolox equivalent antioxidant capacity).

2.3. Analysis of Saliva

The whole mixed unstimulated saliva was analyzed in the biochemical laboratory of Conservative Dentistry Medical University of Gdansk and Department of Biochemistry, Medical University of Gdansk, Poland.

To determine nucleotide metabolite concentration, saliva samples were extracted with 1.3 M $HClO_4$ (1:1 volume ratio) and centrifuged (20,800× g/10 min/4 °C). The supernatants were accumulated and brought to pH 6.0–6.5 using 3 M K_3PO_4 solution. After 15-min incubation on ice, samples were centrifuged at (20,800× g/10 min/4 °C), and the supernatants were analyzed using high-performance liquid chromatography (HPLC) as we have described previously in detail.

Determination of sixteen nucleotides, nucleosides and bases was carried out using high-performance liquid chromatography and its application to the study of purine metabolism in hearts for transplantation [34].

Liquid chromatographic evaluation of purine production in the donor human heart during transplantation was performed [35].

The total antioxidant status (TAOS) in saliva was measured by the 2,2′-azino-bis(3-ethylbenzothiazoline-6-sulphonic acid; ABTS) assay, which was based on the capacity of saliva to scavenge the ABTS+ radical. The relative inhibition of ABTS+ formation, after the saliva addition, is proportional to the antioxidant capacity of the sample 1. For the measurement of the total antioxidant status in saliva, 15 µL of saliva was diluted with 180 µL phosphate buffer (0.076 M NaH_2PO_4 + 0.23 M Na_2HPO_4 in pure water), and then, it was incubated for 10 min at room temperature in a 96-well plate with a 5 µL reaction mixture containing 7 mM ABTS and 2.45 mM potassium persulfate (solved in phosphate buffer: 0.22 M NaH_2PO_4 + 0.37 M Na_2HPO_4) solved in pure water, pH 7.2. Prior to testing, the reaction mixture was incubated overnight, placing it in the dark at room temperature. The absorbance in the test and control samples (15 µL saline instead of saliva) was read at 630 nm, using a BioTek microplate reader. Results expressed as a percentage inhibition of the reaction were calculated as follows: TAOS [%] = 100 × (Ac−At)/Ac, where Ac is the absorbance of the control sample absorbance and At is the test sample absorbance.

To calculate Trolox equivalent antioxidant capacity (TEAC), a calibration curve for Trolox standard solutions was prepared. Volumes of 15 µL of 30, 100, 500 and 1000 µM Trolox standards were diluted and incubated with reaction mixture in the same manner as in saliva. Antioxidant concentration, as mM Trolox equivalents (TEAC value), in the saliva samples were calculated on the basis of a linear regression equation obtained from the plotted Trolox calibration curve [36].

2.4. Statistical Analysis

The statistical analyses have been performed using the statistical suite StatSoft. Inc. (Tulsa, OK, USA) (2014), STATISTICA (data analysis software system) version 12.0. (2014) from www.statsoft.com and Excel. The significance of the difference between more than two groups was assessed with the one-way analysis of variance (ANOVA Kruskal–Wallis). In the case of statistically significant differences between two groups, post hoc tests were utilized. Correlations were assessed with Pearson and Spearman tests. In all the calculations, the statistical significance level of $p < 0.001$ and $p < 0.0001$ has been used.

3. Results

Table 1 presents the value of uric acid, hypoxanthine, xanthine, uric acid + xanthine, TAOS and TEAC levels on unstimulated saliva among e-cigarette users, cigarette smokers and non-smokers.

Table 1. Mean values of uric acid, hypoxanthine, xanthine, uric acid + xanthine, TAOS and TEAC on unstimulated saliva among e-cigarette users, cigarette smokers and non-smokers.

Groups	UA [µmol/L]	Hx [µmol/L]	X [µmol/L]	UA + X [µmol/L]	TAOS [%]	TEAC [mM]
	X̄ (SEM)	X̄ (SEM)	X̄ (SEM)	X̄ (SEM)	X̄ (SEM)	X̄ (SEM)
E-cigarettes users	193.3 (14.1) n = 35	7.7 (0.9) n = 35	8.3 (1.8) n = 35	201.6 (14.5) n = 35	68.9 (1.7) [a] n = 35	1.3 (0.04) [c] n = 35
Cigarettes smokers	172.4 (16.8) n = 33	8.3 (1) n = 33	6.1 (1.1) n = 33	178.5 (16.8) n = 33	63.6 (2.4) [b] n = 31	1.2 (0.05) [d] n = 31
Non-smokers	158.9 (10.3) n = 42	9.5 (1.2) n = 42	9.3 (1.3) n = 42	168.2 (10.6) n = 42	78.1 (1.1) [a,b] n = 38	1.5 (0.03) [c,d] n = 38

Legend: UA—uric acid, Hx—hypoxanthine, X—xanthine, TAOS—total antioxidant status, TEAC—Trolox equivalent antioxidant capacity, mean values, SEM—standard error of mean; a,b,c,d—testify to statistically significant values; [a-a, b-b, c-c, d-d]—groups with statistical significance, $p < 0.001$ for [a-a, b-b], $p < 0.0001$ for [c-c, d-d].

The concentration of uric acid among e-cigarettes users was 193.3 µmol/L (14.1); the result in the group of traditional cigarette smokers was 172.4 µmol/L (16.8) and in the group of non-smokers was 158.9 µmol/L (10.3). The concentration of uric acid in group of e-cigarettes users was higher than among traditional cigarettes smokers and non-smokers; however, no statistically significant differences were observed. Saliva concentrations of uric acid are presented in Figure 1.

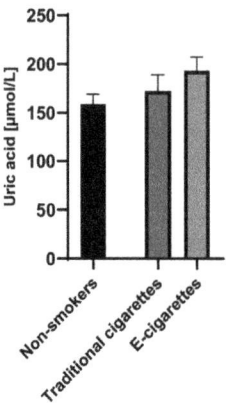

Figure 1. Concentration of uric acid in groups of e-cigarettes users, traditional cigarettes smokers and non-smokers.

The concentration of hypoxanthine in the group of e-cigarettes users was 7.7 µmol/L (0.9), among traditional cigarettes smokers was 8.3 µmol/L (1) and in non-smokers group was 9.5 µmol/L (1.2). Although the concentrations of hypoxanthine among e-cigarettes users were lower than values in the non-smokers group and among traditional cigarettes smokers, no statistically significant differences were observed. Saliva concentrations of hypoxanthine are presented in Figure 2.

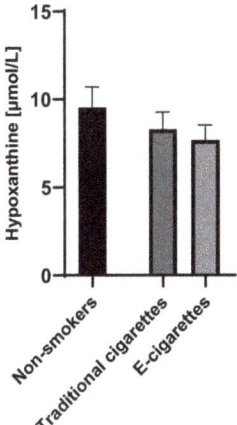

Figure 2. Concentration of hypoxanthine in groups of e-cigarettes users, traditional cigarettes smokers and non-smokers.

The concentration of xanthine in the group of e-cigarettes users was 8.3 µmol/L (1.8), in the group of traditional cigarettes smokers was 6.1 µmol/L (1.1) and among non-smokers was 9.3 µmol/L (1.3). The concentrations of hypoxanthine among e-cigarettes users were higher than the values among traditional cigarettes smokers and lower than the values in the group of non-smokers; therefore, no statistically significant differences were observed. Saliva concentrations of xanthine are presented in Figure 3.

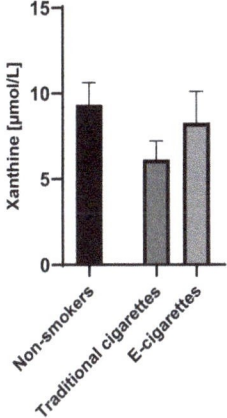

Figure 3. Concentration of xanthine in groups of e-cigarettes users, traditional cigarettes smokers and non-smokers.

The combined concentration of uric acid and xanthine among e-cigarettes users was 201.6 µmol/L (14.5), among traditional cigarettes smokers was 178.5 µmol/L (16.8) and among non-smokers was 168.2 µmol/L (10.6). Although the combined concentrations of uric acid and xanthine in the group of e-cigarettes users were higher than among traditional cigarettes smokers and non-smokers, no statistically significant differences were observed. Combined saliva concentrations of uric acid and xanthine are presented in Figure 4.

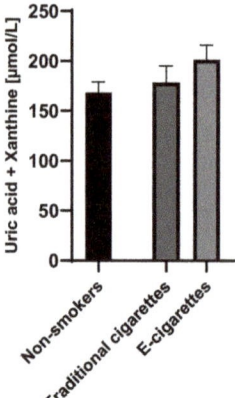

Figure 4. Combined concentrations of uric acid and xanthine in groups of e-cigarettes users, traditional cigarettes smokers and non-smokers.

The values of TAOS in the group of e-cigarettes users was 68.9% (1.7), among traditional cigarettes smokers was 63.6% (2.4) and among non-smokers was 78.1% (1.1). The values of TAOS in the groups of e-cigarettes users and traditional cigarettes smokers were lower than among non-smokers. Statistically significant differences on the level of $p < 0.001$ were observed among e-cigarettes users in comparison to non-smokers and on the level of $p < 0.0001$ among traditional cigarettes smokers in comparison to non-smokers. Values of TAOS are presented in Figure 5.

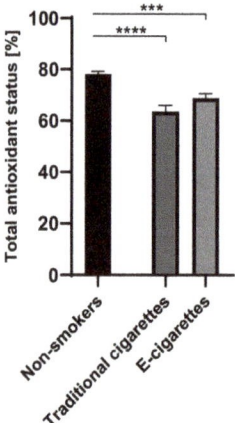

Figure 5. Values of TAOS (total antioxidant status) in groups of e-cigarettes users, traditional cigarettes smokers and non-smokers. *** $p < 0.001$; **** $p < 0.0001$.

The value of TEAC in the group of e-cigarettes users was 1.3 mM (0.04), in the group of traditional cigarettes users was 1.2 mM (0.05) and among non-smokers was 1.5 mM (0.03). The values of TEAC among e-cigarettes users and traditional cigarettes smokers were lower than in the non-smokers group. Statistically significant differences on the level of $p < 0.001$ were observed in the group of e-cigarettes users compared to the non-smokers and on the level of $p < 0001$ between traditional cigarettes smokers and non-smokers. Values of TEAC are presented in Figure 6.

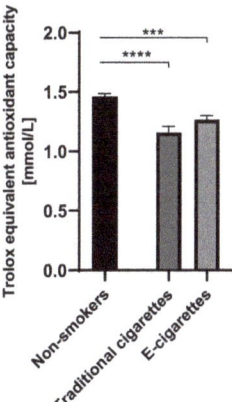

Figure 6. Values of TEAC (Trolox equivalent antioxidant capacity) in groups of e-cigarettes users, traditional cigarettes smokers and non-smokers. *** $p < 0.001$; **** $p < 0.0001$.

Statistically significant correlations between values of TAOS on level of $p < 0.0003$ in the group of e-cigarette users and on the level of $p < 0.0001$ in the group of traditional cigarettes smokers were also observed and are presented in Figures 7–10.

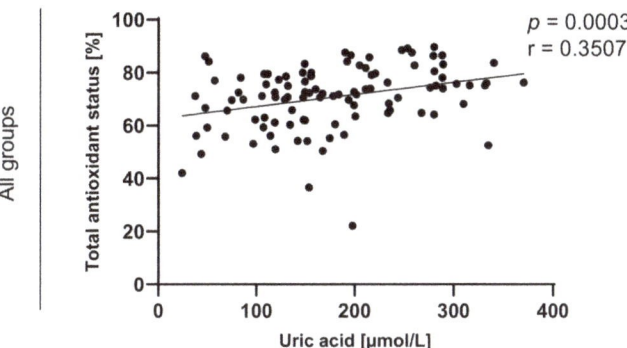

Figure 7. Correlation between uric acid and TAOS (total antioxidant status) among e-cigarettes users, traditional cigarettes smokers and non-smokers.

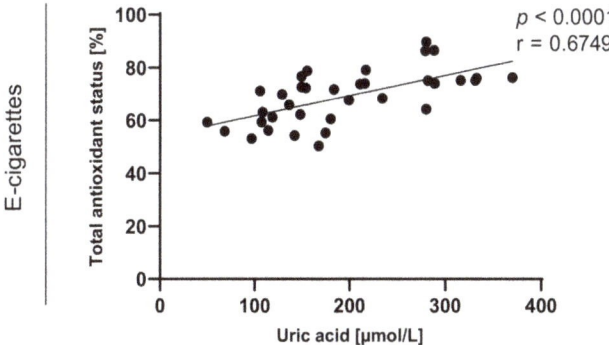

Figure 8. Correlation between uric acid and TAOS (total antioxidant status) among e-cigarettes users.

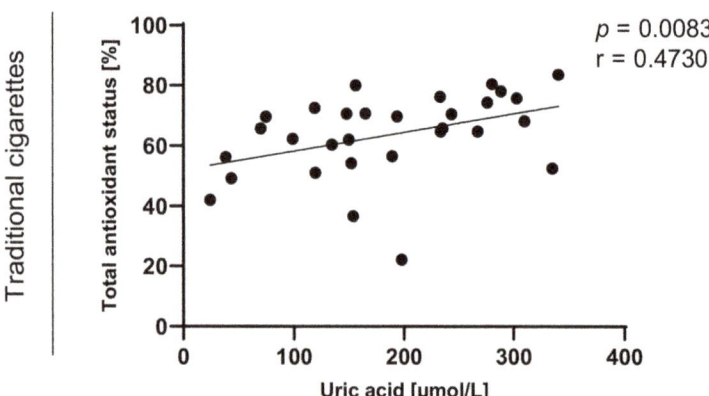

Figure 9. Correlation between uric acid and TAOS (total antioxidant status) among traditional cigarettes smokers.

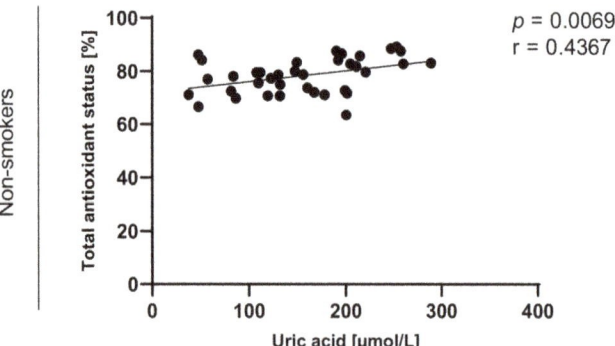

Figure 10. Correlation between uric acid and TAOS (total antioxidant status) among non-smokers.

4. Discussion

The most important finding of this study was determining that the oxidant status of saliva is reduced by use of electronic cigarettes to the same extent as it is by traditional cigarettes smoking. This highlights the important risk of the adverse effects of electronic cigarettes, in contrast to the common view of their limited toxicity.

Saliva is the first body fluid that has a direct contact with both tobacco smoke and electronic cigarettes vapor and is in the first line in antioxidant defense [5]. Tobacco smoke is a complex mixture of chemical compounds, which are a source of free radicals and oxidants causing adverse side effects in the oral cavity [37,38]. Tobacco smoking might be the reason for an adaptive response, consequently leading to an increase in the antioxidant levels in saliva or to a decrease in saliva antioxidant defenses [39]. Liquids used in electronic cigarettes mainly consist of propylene glycol, glycerin, nicotine and flavor additives [23–25]. However, e-liquids heated to high temperatures might become a source of detectable levels of potentially harmful chemicals as formaldehyde, acrolein, heavy metals and acetaldehyde carbonyls [40,41]. Oxidants or reactive oxygen species are also generated by vaporizing e-liquids, which are influenced by the heating element of the electronic cigarette and associated with e-liquid flavor. The aerosol generated by electronic cigarettes might pose an impact on levels of oxidative stress [42]; however, it has not been proven yet which electronic cigarettes' factors might be related to oxidative stress generation [43].

Uric acid (UA) is the most important non-enzymatic antioxidant present in saliva. This is a plasma born antioxidant that facilitates removal of hydroxyl radical and superoxide anion [6,44]. Increased concentration of uric acid in saliva might reflect a response to oxidative stress and be related to periodontitis or cancer [44–46]. Our results indicate that uric acid concentration in the saliva of e-cigarettes users tended to be higher than among traditional cigarettes smokers and non-smokers. Studies conducted by Kodakova et al. [39] and Zappacosta et al. [4] indicated no differences in the level of uric acid in saliva between traditional cigarettes smokers and non-smokers. On the contrary, Greabu et al. [47], Ahmadi-Motamayel [48] and Abdolsamadi et al. [49] observed the decreased uric acid levels in the saliva of traditional cigarettes smokers compared to non-smokers. Our results show little effect of traditional cigarette smoking on uric acid concentration in saliva. The trend towards an increase in uric acid concentration in e-cigarettes users may indicate facilitated transport of uric acid from blood into saliva, and this effect is worth further investigation.

Hypoxanthine and xanthine are products of purine metabolism. Adenine nucleotides could be converted in several steps into hypoxanthine, which is then transformed to xanthine and then to uric acid [50]. Our results indicated that saliva concentration of hypoxanthine and xanthine in electronic cigarettes users and traditional cigarettes smokers tended to be lower than among non-smokers. Concentrations of hypoxanthine among traditional cigarettes were higher and that of xanthine lower in comparison to e-cigarettes users. Such pattern together with uric acid concentration changes highlights a shift towards uric acid concentration either by accelerated breakdown of hypoxanthine or xanthine or due to increased transport of uric acid. Our study is the first analysis of the impact of e-cigarettes usage and of smoking traditional cigarettes on the levels of hypoxanthine and xanthine in saliva.

Total antioxidant status (TAOS) is the sum of all antioxidants present in saliva, and uric acid makes up to 85% of the TAOS [5]. Measurement of TAOS value reflects the current efficiency of antioxidant mechanisms. Initially, during exposure to oxygen free radicals, an adaptive increase in TAOS value was observed, while sustained exposure to oxygen free radicals led to a decrease in the concentration of antioxidants, which resulted in a decrease in the TAOS value [51]. In our research TAOS in the saliva of e-cigarettes users and traditional cigarettes smokers was lower than among non-smokers. Hamo Mahmood et al. also observed the decrease of TAOS among traditional cigarettes smokers in comparison to non-smokers [52]. Research conducted by Bakhtiari et al., on the TAOS in the saliva of traditional cigarettes smokers also demonstrated lower values than among non-smokers [53]. Kodakova et al. [39] and and Zappacosta et al. [4] reported no differences in levels of TAOS in saliva between traditional cigarettes smokers and non-smokers. However, Greabu et al. [47], Ahmadi-Motamayel [48] and Nagler [54] observed the increase of TAOS in the saliva of traditional cigarettes smokers compared to non-smokers. According to Hamo Mahmood et al., the reduction of TAOS among traditional cigarettes smokers might be related to the exhaustion of saliva antioxidants caused by the presence of high amounts of free radicals in cigarette smoke, which may lead to an oxidative stress [52].

Trolox equivalent antioxidant capacity (TEAC) enables to measure total antioxidant capacity of saliva by assessing the capacity of a compound to scavenge ABTS radicals [55,56]. In our research, the values of TEAC among e-cigarettes users and traditional cigarettes smokers were lower than in non-smokers group. Statistically significant differences were observed between both e-cigarettes users compared to non-smokers and traditional cigarettes smokers compared to non-smokers. Research on the impact of e-cigarettes and traditional cigarettes on TEAC has not been published yet.

The salivary antioxidant system is relevant when considering saliva's anti-cancer capacity and protection from development of periodontal diseases [9,46,56]. Among patients with periodontitis, a decreased efficiency of antioxidant mechanisms has been observed [9]. Konopka et al., demonstrated lower values of TAOS in saliva among patients with periodontitis as compared to control group [9]. The decreased values of TAOS in saliva might be related to the depletion of antioxidants as a result of a chronic inflammation. The connection between periodontitis and the antioxidant potential of saliva is also confirmed by a positive correlation between the concentration of uric acid in saliva and the parameters of periodontal tissues inflammation [9]. Disorders of antioxidant potential are also strictly related to the risk of oral cancer development. Free radicals and ROS can induce DNA damage, which may lead to cancerous transformation. Those negative effects of ROS are counteracted by antioxidants [57].

5. Conclusions

Electronic cigarettes usage adversely affects the antioxidant capacity of saliva, in comparison to non-smokers, to the same extent as smoking traditional cigarettes. This might present an important clinical risk of oral cavity disorders. Further longitudinal studies on a larger group should be conducted in order to assess how the changes observed in the antioxidant capacity of saliva translate to oral health.

Author Contributions: Conceptualization, D.C. and A.K.; methodology, D.C., A.K., E.M.S., B.K., O.K. and J.O.; formal analysis, A.K. and E.M.S.; investigation, D.C., A.K., O.K. and J.O.; data curation, D.C., A.K., E.M.S., O.K. and J.O.; writing—original draft preparation, D.C., A.K. and E.M.S.; writing—review and editing, D.C., A.K. and E.M.S. visualization, D.C. and O.K.; statistical analysis, O.K. and D.Ś.; supervision, A.K., E.M.S. and B.K. All authors have read and agreed to the published version of the manuscript.

Funding: This research received no external funding.

Institutional Review Board Statement: The study was conducted according to the guidelines of the Declaration of Helsinki and approved by the Ethics Committee of Medical University of Gdansk, Poland (NKBBN/161-386/2017, approval date: 11.09.2017).

Informed Consent Statement: Informed consent was obtained from all subjects involved in the study.

Conflicts of Interest: The authors declare no conflict of interest.

References

1. Pink, R.; Simek, J.; Vondrakova, J. Saliva as a diagnostic medium. *Biomed. Pap. Med. Fac. Univ. Palacky Olomouc Czech Republ.* **2009**, *153*, 103–110. [CrossRef]
2. Lynge Pedersen, A.M.; Belstrøm, D. The role of natural salivary defences in maintaining a healthy oral microbiota. *J. Dent.* **2019**, *80*, 3–12. [CrossRef] [PubMed]
3. Dyba, J.; Lenkowski, M.; Surdacka, A. Evaluating the diagnostic potential of saliva in respect of periodontal disease as well as changes occurring within the endothelium. *Dent. Forum* **2017**, *1*, 21–25.
4. Zappacosta, B.; Persichilli, S.; De Sole, P.; Mordente, A.; Giardia, B. Effect of smoking one cigarette on antioxidant metabolites in the saliva of healthy smoker. *Arch. Oral Biol.* **1999**, *44*, 485–488. [CrossRef]
5. Battino, M.; Ferreiro, M.S.; Gallardo, I.; Newman, H.N.; Bullon, P. The antioxidant capacity of saliva. *J. Clin. Periodontal.* **2002**, *29*, 189–194. [CrossRef]
6. Nagler, R.M.; Klein, I.; Zarzhersky, N.; Drigues, N.; Reznick, A.Z. Characterization of the differentiated antioxidant profile of human saliva. *Free Radic. Biol. Med.* **2002**, *32*, 268–277. [CrossRef]
7. Mandel, I.D. The role of saliva in maintaining oral homeostasis. *J. Am. Dent. Assoc.* **1989**, *119*, 298–304. [CrossRef] [PubMed]
8. Roblegg, E.; Coughran, A.; Sirjani, D. Saliva: An all-rounder of our body. *Eur. J. Pharm. Biopharm.* **2019**, *142*, 133–141. [CrossRef]
9. Konopka, T.; Gmyrek-Marciniak, A.; Kozłowski, Z.; Kaczmarek, U.; Wnukiewicz, J. Potencjał antyoksydacyjny śliny u pacjentów z zapaleniem przyzębia i rakiem płaskonabłonkowym dna jamy ustnej. *Dent. Med. Probl.* **2006**, *43*, 354–362.
10. Venditti, P.; Di Stefano, L.; Di Meo, S. Mitochondrial metabolism of reactive oxygen species. *Mitochondrion* **2013**, *13*, 71–82. [CrossRef] [PubMed]
11. Betteridge, D.J. What is oxidative stress? *Metabolism* **2000**, *49*, 3–8. [CrossRef]
12. Valko, M.; Leibfritz, D.; Moncol, J.; Cronin, M.T.D.; Mazur, M.; Teser, J. Free radicals and antioxidants in normal physiological functions and human disease. *Int. J. Biochem. Cell Biol.* **2006**, *39*, 44–84. [CrossRef]
13. Becker, L.B. New concepts in reactive oxygen species and cardiovascular reperfusion physiology. *Cardiovasc. Res.* **2004**, *61*, 461–470. [CrossRef] [PubMed]
14. Valko, M.; Leibfritz, D.; Moncol, J.; Cronin, M.T.D.; Mazur, M. Free radicals, metals and antioxidants in oxidative-stress included cancer. *Chem. Biol. Interact.* **2006**, *160*, 1–40. [CrossRef] [PubMed]
15. Dąbrowska, Z.N.; Bijowska, K.; Dąbrowska, E.; Pietuska, M. Effect of oxidants and antioxidants on oral health. *Med. Ogólna Nauki Zdrowiu* **2020**, *26*, 87–93. [CrossRef]

16. Kimura, S.; Yonemura, T.; Kaya, H. Increased oxidative product formation by peripheral blood polymofronuclear leukocytes in human periodontal disease. *J. Periodontal. Res.* **1993**, *28*, 197–203. [CrossRef]
17. Knaś, M.; Maciejczyk, M.; Waszkiel, D.; Zalewska, A. Oxidative stress and salivary antioxidants. *Dent. Med. Probl.* **2013**, *50*, 461–466.
18. Wang, Y.; Andrukhov, O.; Rausch-Fan, X. Oxidative stress and antioxidant system in periodontotitis. *Front. Physiol.* **2017**, *8*, 910. [CrossRef]
19. Kusiak, A.; Kochańska, B.; Limon, J.; Ochocińska, J. The physico-chemical properties of saliva in Turner's syndrome. *Dent. Forum* **2011**, *39*, 19–23.
20. Weiner, D.; Levy, Y.; Khankin, E.V.; Reznick, A.Z. Inhibition of salivary amylase activity by cigarette smoke aldehydes. *J. Physiol. Pharmacol.* **2008**, *59*, 727–737.
21. Cichońska, D.; Kusiak, A.; Kochańska, B.; Ochocińska, J.; Świetlik, D. Influence of electronic cigarettes on selected antibacterial properties of saliva. *Int. J. Environ. Res. Public Health* **2019**, *16*, 4433. [CrossRef]
22. Chen, C.; Zhuang, Y.L.; Zhu, S.H. E-Cigarette design preference and smoking cessation: A U.S. population study. *Am. J. Prev. Med.* **2016**, *51*, 356–363. [CrossRef]
23. Bertholon, J.F.; Becquemin, M.H.; Annesi-Maesano, I.; Dautzenberg, B. Electronic cigarettes: A short review. *Respiration* **2013**, *86*, 433–438. [CrossRef] [PubMed]
24. McNeill, A.; Brose, L.S.; Calde, R.R.; Hitchman, S.C.; Hajek, P.; McRobbie, H. E-cigarettes: An evidence update. A report commissioned by Public Health England. *Public Health Engl.* **2015**, *11*, 14–15.
25. Brown, C.J.; Cheng, J.M. Electronic cigarettes: Product characterization and design considerations. *Tob. Control* **2014**, *23*, 4–10. [CrossRef] [PubMed]
26. Chen, M.S.; Hall, M.G.; Parada, H.; Peebles, K.; Brodar, K.E.; Brewer, N.T. Symptoms during adolescents' first use of cigarettes and e-cigarettes: A pilot study. *Int. J. Environ. Res. Public Health* **2017**, *14*, 1260. [CrossRef]
27. Pisinger, C.; Dossing, M. A systematic review of health effects of electronic cigarettes. *Prev. Med.* **2014**, *69*, 248–260. [CrossRef]
28. Yu, V.; Rahimy, M.; Korrapati, A. Electronic cigarettes induce DNA stand breaks and cell death independently of nicotine in cell lines. *Oral Oncol.* **2016**, *52*, 58–65. [CrossRef] [PubMed]
29. Semlali, A.; Chakir, J.; Goulet, J.P.; Chmielewski, W.; Rouabhia, M. Whole cigarette smoke promotes human gingival epithelial cell apoptosis and inhibits cell repair processes. *J. Periodontal. Res.* **2011**, *46*, 533–541. [CrossRef]
30. Sundar, I.K.; Javed, F.; Romanos, G.E.; Rahman, I. E-cigarettes and flavorings induce inflammatory and pro-senescence responses in oral epithelial cells and periodontal fibroblasts. *Oncotarget* **2016**, *7*, 77196–77204. [CrossRef] [PubMed]
31. Holliday, R.; Kist, R.; Bauld, L. E-cigarette vapour is not inert and exposure can lead to cell damage. *Evid. Based Dent.* **2016**, *17*, 2–3. [CrossRef] [PubMed]
32. Salaspuro, V.; Salaspuro, M. Synergistic effect of alcohol drinking and smoking on in vitro acetaldehyde concentration in saliva. *Int. J. Cancer* **2004**, *111*, 480–483. [CrossRef] [PubMed]
33. Alqahtani, S.; Cooper, B.; Spears, C.A.; Wright, C.; Shannahan, J. Electronic nicotine delivery system-induced alterations in oral health via saliva assessment. *Exp. Biol. Med.* **2020**, *245*, 1319–1325. [CrossRef] [PubMed]
34. Smolenski, R.T.; Lachno, D.R.; Ledingham, S.J.; Yacoub, M.H. Determination of sixteen nucleotides, nucleosides and bases using high-performance liquid chromatography and its application to the study of purine metabolism in hearts for transplantation. *J. Chromatogr.* **1990**, *18*, 414–420. [CrossRef]
35. Smolenski, R.T.; Yacoub, M.H. Liquid chromatographic evaluation of purine production in the donor human heart during transplantation. *Biomed. Chromatogr.* **1993**, *7*, 189–195. [CrossRef] [PubMed]
36. Miller, N.J.; Rice-Evans, C.; Davies, M.J.; Gopinathan, V.; Milner, A. A novel method for measuring antioxidant capacity and its application to monitoring the antioxidant status in premature neonates. *Clin. Sci.* **1993**, *84*, 407–412. [CrossRef]
37. Nagler, R.M.; Reznick, A.Z. Cigarette smoke effects on salivary antioxidants and oral cancer-novel concepts. *IMAJ* **2004**, *6*, 691–694.
38. Nagler, R.; Lischinsky, S.; Diamond, E.; Drigues, N.; Klein, I.; Reznick, A.Z. Effect of cigarette smoke on salivary proteins and enzyme activities. *Arch. Biochem. Biophys.* **2000**, *15*, 229–236. [CrossRef]
39. Kondakova, I.; Lissi, E.A.; Pizarro, M. Total reactive antioxidant potential in human saliva of smokers and non-smokers. *Biochem. Mol. Biol. Int.* **1999**, *47*, 911–920. [CrossRef]
40. Kosmider, L.; Sobczak, A.; Fik, M.; Knysak, J.; Zaciera, M.; Kurek, J.; Goniewicz, M.L. Carbonyl compounds in electronic cigarette vapors: Effects of nicotine solvent and battery output voltage. *Nicotine Tob. Res.* **2014**, *16*, 1319–1326. [CrossRef]
41. Goniewicz, M.L.; Knysak, J.; Gawron, M.; Kosmider, L.; Sobczak, A.; Kurek, J.; Prokopowicz, A.; Jablonska-Czapla, M.; Rosik-Dulewska, C.; Havel, C.; et al. Levels of selected carcinogens and toxicants in vapour from electronic cigarettes. *Tob. Control* **2014**, *23*, 133–139. [CrossRef]
42. Derruau, S.; Robinet, J.; Untereiner, V.; Piot, O.; Sockalingum, G.D.; Lorimier, S. Vibrational spectroscopy saliva profiling as biometric tool for disease diagnostics: A systematic literature. *Molecules* **2020**, *25*, 4142. [CrossRef]
43. Lerner, C.A.; Sundar, I.K.; Yao, H.; Gerloff, J.; Ossip, D.J.; McIntosh, S.; Robinson, R.; Rahman, I. Vapors produced by electronic cigarettes and e-juices with flavorings induce toxicity, oxidative stress, and inflammatory response in lung epithelial cells and in mouse lung. *PLoS ONE* **2015**, *6*, e0116732. [CrossRef]

44. Gawron-Skarbek, A.; Prymont-Przymińska, A.; Sobczak, A.; Guligowska, A.; Kostka, T.; Nowak, D.; Szatko, F. A comparison of native and non-urate total antioxidant capacity of fasting plasma and saliva among middle-aged and older subjects. *Redox Rep.* **2018**, *23*, 7–62. [CrossRef]
45. Almadori, G.; Bussu, F.; Galli, J.; Limongelli, A.; Persichilli, S.; Zappacosta, B.; Minucci, A.; Paludetti, G.; Giardina, B. Salivary glutathione and uric acid levels in patients with head and neck squamous cell carcinoma. *Head Neck* **2007**, *29*, 648–654. [CrossRef] [PubMed]
46. Moore, S.; Calder, K.A.C.; Miller, N.J.; Rice-Evans, C.A. Antioxidant activity of saliva and periodontal disease. *Free Radic. Res.* **1994**, *21*, 417–425. [CrossRef] [PubMed]
47. Greabu, M.; Battino, M.; Totan, A.; Mohora, M.; Mitrea, N.; Totan, C.; Spinu, T.; Didilescu, A. Effect of gas phase and particulate phase of cigarette smoke on salivary antioxidants. What can be the role of vitamin C and pyridoxine? *Pharmacol. Rep.* **2007**, *59*, 613–618. [PubMed]
48. Ahmadi-Motamayel, F.; Falsafi, P.; Abolsamadi, H.; Goodarzi, M.T.; Poorolajal, J. Evaluation of salivary antioxidants and oxidative stress markers in male smokers. *Comb. Chem. High Throughput Screen* **2019**, *22*, 496–501. [CrossRef]
49. Abdolsamadi, H.R.; Goodarzi, M.T.; Mortazavi, H.; Robati, M.; Ahmadi-Motemaye, F. Comparison of salivary antioxidants in healthy smoking and non-smoking men. *Chang. Gung Med. J.* **2011**, *34*, 607–611.
50. Xiang, L.W.; Li, J.; Lin, J.M.; Li, H.F. Determination of gouty arthritis' biomarkers in human urine using reversed-phase high-performance liquid chromatography. *J. Pharm. Anal.* **2014**, *4*, 153–158. [CrossRef] [PubMed]
51. Prior, R.L.; Cao, G. In vivo total antioxidant capacity: Comparison of different analytical methods. *Free Radic. Biol. Med.* **1999**, *27*, 1173–1181. [CrossRef]
52. Hamo Mahmood, I.; Abdullah, K.S.; Othman, S.H. The total antioxidant status in cigarette smoking individuals. *MJBU* **2007**, *25*, 45–50. [CrossRef]
53. Bakhtiari, S.; Azimi, S.; Mehdipour, M.; Amini, S.; Elmi, Z.; Namazi, Z. Effect of cigarette smoke on salivary total antioxidant capacity. *J. Dent. Res. Dent. Clin. Dent. Prospects* **2015**, *9*, 281–284. [CrossRef]
54. Nagler, R.M. Altered salivary profile in heavy smokers and its possible connection to oral cancer. *Int. J. Biol. Mark.* **2007**, *22*, 274–280. [CrossRef]
55. Van den Berg, R.; Haenen, G.R.M.M.; van den Berg, H.; Bast, A. Applicability of an improved TEAC assay for evaluation of antioxidant capacity measurements of mixtures. *Food Chem.* **1999**, *66*, 511–517. [CrossRef]
56. Rao, R.K.; Thomas, D.W.; Pepperl, S.; Porreca, F. Salivary epidermal growth factor plays a role in protection of ileal mucosal integrity. *Dig. Dis. Sci.* **1997**, *42*, 2175–2181. [CrossRef]
57. Valko, M.; Izakovic, M.; Mazur, M.; Rhodes, C.J.; Telser, J. Role of oxygen radicals in DNA damage and cancer incidence. *Mol. Cell Biochem.* **2004**, *266*, 37–56. [CrossRef] [PubMed]

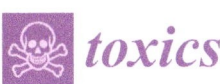

Article

Comparative Reactive Oxygen Species (ROS) Content among Various Flavored Disposable Vape Bars, including Cool (Iced) Flavored Bars

Shaiesh Yogeswaran, Thivanka Muthumalage and Irfan Rahman *

Department of Environmental Medicine, University of Rochester Medical Center, Box 850, 601 Elmwood Avenue, Rochester, NY 14642, USA; Shaiesh_Yogeswaran@urmc.rochester.edu (S.Y.); Thivanka_Muthumalage@urmc.rochester.edu (T.M.)
* Correspondence: Irfan_Rahman@urmc.rochester.edu; Tel.: +1-(585)-275-6911

Citation: Yogeswaran, S.; Muthumalage, T.; Rahman, I. Comparative Reactive Oxygen Species (ROS) Content among Various Flavored Disposable Vape Bars, including Cool (Iced) Flavored Bars. *Toxics* 2021, 9, 235. https://doi.org/10.3390/toxics9100235

Academic Editors: Andrzej Sobczak and Leon Kośmider

Received: 3 August 2021
Accepted: 16 September 2021
Published: 25 September 2021

Publisher's Note: MDPI stays neutral with regard to jurisdictional claims in published maps and institutional affiliations.

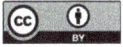

Copyright: © 2021 by the authors. Licensee MDPI, Basel, Switzerland. This article is an open access article distributed under the terms and conditions of the Creative Commons Attribution (CC BY) license (https://creativecommons.org/licenses/by/4.0/).

Abstract: Studies have shown that aerosols generated from flavored e-cigarettes contain Reactive Oxygen Species (ROS), promoting oxidative stress-induced damage within pulmonary cells. Our lab investigated the ROS content of e-cigarette vapor generated from disposable flavored e-cigarettes (vape bars) with and without nicotine. Specifically, we analyzed vape bars belonging to multiple flavor categories (Tobacco, Minty Fruit, Fruity, Minty/Cool (Iced), Desserts, and Drinks/Beverages) manufactured by various vendors and of different nicotine concentrations (0–6.8%). Aerosols from these vape bars were generated via a single puff aerosol generator; these aerosols were then individually bubbled through a fluorogenic solution to semi-quantify ROS generated by these bars in H_2O_2 equivalents. We compared the ROS levels generated by each vape bar as an indirect determinant of their potential to induce oxidative stress. Our results showed that ROS concentration (μM) within aerosols produced from these vape bars varied significantly among different flavored vape bars and identically flavored vape bars with varying nicotine concentrations. Furthermore, our results suggest that flavoring chemicals and nicotine play a differential role in generating ROS production in vape bar aerosols. Our study provides insight into the differential health effects of flavored vape bars, in particular cool (iced) flavors, and the need for their regulation.

Keywords: vaping; ENDS; disposable e-cigarettes; vape bars; flavoring; flavoring chemicals; reactive oxygen species (ROS); disposables; oxidative stress

1. Introduction

Despite the significant decline in youth e-cigarette usage since the Federal Drug Enforcement Agency's (FDA) flavored e-cigarette enforcement policy which was enacted in February 2020, youth e-cigarette use within the United States remains significantly high [1]. Moreover, according to a cross-sectional study conducted by the Centers for Disease Control and Prevention (CDC), in 2020, 4.7% of middle school students (550,000) and 19.6% of high school students (3.02 million) reported current e-cigarette use [1]. The prevalence of e-cigarette usage in the United States, especially amongst its youth, is partly due to the switch many cartridge-based e-cigarette users made to using disposable e-cigarettes; the FDA's 2020 e-cigarette flavoring enforcement policy prompted this action [1]. Further, the FDA's flavoring enforcement policy only applies to flavoring for cartridge-based Electronic Nicotine Delivery System (ENDS) products; these products include cartridge-based e-cigarettes and pre-filled pod devices [1]. More specifically, the FDA's February 6th, 2020 e-cigarette enforcement policy for cartridge-based ENDS products applies to all flavors with nicotine, excluding menthol and tobacco [1]. Moreover, the FDA's enforcement policy involves requiring all manufacturers and retailers in the United States to remove all flavored cartridge-based ENDS products with nicotine from the market except tobacco-flavored and menthol-flavored cartridge-based ENDS products [1]. All flavored products without nicotine (zero nicotine) are still available in the market. Furthermore, products exempt from the previously mentioned enforcement policy include disposable e-cigarettes with or without nicotine in certain states within the United States. A disposable e-cigarette is a type of ENDS product which can be discarded or thrown away once it runs out of e-liquid or charge. According to the 2020 National Youth Tobacco Survey (NYTS) conducted by the CDC, the use of disposable e-cigarettes (e-cigs) by high-school students who were already e-cig users had increased significantly from 2.4% in 2019 to 26.5% in 2020. Additionally, according to the 2020 NYTS, the number of middle-school e-cig users who specifically used disposable e-cigs increased from 3.3% in 2019 to 15.2% in 2020 [1]. One aspect of disposable e-cigs which is attractive to youth e-cigarette users is the convenience at which they can be used; they do not require recharging or refilling with e-liquids like cartridge-based products. Additionally, disposable devices are much cheaper and practical to use than their refillable counterparts.

With the substantial rise in the availability of different e-liquid flavors in recent years, investigating the role that e-liquid flavoring chemicals have in inducing pulmonary pathophysiological effects has become more complicated [2]. Further, the long-term effects of e-cigarette vapor exposure on human health require further investigation. However, studies so far have shown that e-cigarette aerosol production involves generating reactive oxygen species (ROS) [3]. ROS can be generated either intracellularly (via mitochondrial oxidative phosphorylation) or may arise from exogenous sources (cigarette smoke, e-cigarette aerosols, and environmental pollution,) [4]. Specific ROS include hydrogen peroxide (H_2O_2), hydroxyl radical ($^{\bullet}OH$), and superoxide radical ($O_2^{\bullet -}$) [5]. ROS plays a crucial role in modulating the immune-inflammatory system and activating different signal transduction pathways and cell signaling processes for inflammatory responses [6].

The normal physiological balance between ROS and antioxidants can be disturbed through the inhalation of exogenous sources of ROS, thus leading to the damage of cellular structures. Further, an excess in intracellular ROS levels causes oxidative damage to the cellular membrane, intracellular lipids, intracellular enzymes, and intracellular DNA (iDNA). Moreover, excess ROS can also induce a vicious cycle of chronic inflammation in the lungs due to excessive ROS leading to the activation of specific immune cells, polymorphonuclear neutrophils (PMNs); activated PMNs can, in turn, generate more ROS in pulmonary cells [7]. This subsequent chronic inflammation leads to airways becoming more thickened and prone to mucus secretion, also known as airway modeling, this later resulting in lung dysfunction [8]. Regarding exogenous ROS sources, studies in the past have shown that tobacco smoke-generated ROS can induce DNA damage within lung epithelial cells and premature pulmonary cell death, leading to the development of lung cancer and COPD/emphysema, respectively [9]. Additionally, one study had shown that through activating the heating element of an e-cigarette and then aerosolizing its e-liquid component, ROS is produced; which can be drawn from the device into the lungs, directly causing inflammatory response [10].

Despite the well-known adverse health effects of conventional cigarette smoking, one of the main factors driving both youth and adult appeal for e-cigarettes is the availability of many different flavors. These flavors add to the allure many have for e-cigarettes by creating sensory perceptions of palatable tastes, which conceal the bitter taste of nicotine [11]. Further, one survey found that the availability of fruit and candy e-liquid flavors significantly contributes to the prevalence of youth e-cigarette usage in the United States; adults seem to prefer more traditional flavors, such as tobacco [11]. Likewise, according to a Morbidity and Mortality Weekly Report by the CDC conducted in September 2020, among current users of flavored disposable e-cigarettes, the most commonly used flavor type was those under the fruit classification (82.7%; 650,000 [1]). Additionally, according to the same Morbidity and Mortality Weekly Report by the CDC, the following three most widely used vape bar flavors were those falling under the mint classification (51.9%; 410,000), those falling under the sweet categorizations (candy, desserts, etc.) (41.7%; 330,000), and those falling under the menthol (cool/iced) classification (23.3%; 180,000), respectively [1].

Accordingly, with the recent surge in flavored disposable e-cig use during this past year, more research should be conducted which investigates how ROS content within aerosols generated from disposable e-cigarettes are modulated by flavoring chemicals.

In addition to flavor, another factor contributing to the prevalence of disposable e-cigarette usage in this country is the range of nicotine concentrations which are available for these devices. Nicotine is a highly addictive alkaloid present within the aerosol generated by e-cigarettes as well as within the smoke generated from conventional cigarettes [12]. For disposable e-cigarettes sold within the United States, nicotine content ranges from 0 mg/mL (0%, nicotine-free option) to 68 mg/mL (6.8%). Furthermore, nicotine is extremely addictive and can harm the neural development of those under the age of 25, which is most troubling given the prevalence of e-cigarette use among adolescents in this country [13]. Exposure to nicotine through inhaling e-cigarette generated aerosols has contributed to prolonging e-cigarette usage amongst a significant portion of the country, especially those under the age of 25 [14]. Despite youth e-cigarette usage continuing to be a rising health concern in the U.S, studies investigating how exogenous ROS generation varies as a function of nicotine concentration in ENDS products are lacking. Additionally, with the recent surge in flavored disposable e-cig use and the wide range of nicotine content available for these products, research should be conducted to determine how ROS or free radical generation among disposable e-cigarettes varies as a function of nicotine concentration. Consequently, in our study, we hypothesize that ROS levels within the aerosols generated from disposable e-cigarettes will vary with different flavors as well with different nicotine concentrations. Furthermore, disposable e-cigarettes with a wide range of salt nicotine concentrations (0–6.8%) and within six main flavor categories (Tobacco, Minty Fruit, Fruity, Minty/Cool (Iced), Desserts, and Drinks/Beverages) from different vendors were analyzed. Additionally, we analyzed vape bars of identical flavors manufactured from the same company, but with varying concentrations of nicotine. The company (vendor) that produced these bars that we subsequently analyzed were Bolt, Flair Plus, and SMOQ. Bolt and Flair Plus disposable bars, which contain a solution comprising Propylene Glycol (PG) and Vegetable Glycerin (VG) mixed in a 1:1 ratio; likewise, these bars use a 1.6 and 1.8 Ohm coil, respectively, to aerosolize their component e-liquid. Accordingly, our subsequent comparative acellular ROS analyses included semi-quantified ROS content within aerosols produced from our PG:VG controls heated using 1.6 and 1.8 Ohm coils; the controls were made using a 1:1 (i.e., 50:50 ratio) ratio of PG and VG in this pilot/preliminary screening study.

2. Materials and Methods

2.1. Vape Bar Procurement

Vape bars were purchased from various locations and manufacturers locally within Rochester, NY and from various online websites/vendors. The disposable e-cigarettes used in this experiment contained a wide range of salt nicotine concentrations (0–6.8%) and were categorized into six main flavor categories (Tobacco, Minty Fruit, Fruity, Minty/Cool (Iced), Desserts, and Drinks/Beverages). The commercial manufacturers of the disposable vape bars used were Blu, Bolt, Cyclone, Eonsmoke, Flair Plus, Fling, Fliq, FreshBar, Hyde, Hyppe Bar, Jolly, Lit, NJOY, Phantom, Puff Bar, SMOQ, SOL, Tsunami Twin, Vice, Zaero, and Zero Disposable.

2.2. Generation of Vape Bar Aerosols

A fluorogenic dye was made using 0.01N NaOH, $2'7'$ dichlorofluorescein diacetate (H_2DCF-DA) (EMD Biosciences, San Diego, CA, USA) (Cat # 287810), phosphate (PO_4) buffer, and horseradish peroxidase (Thermo Fisher Scientific, Waltham, MA, USA) (Cat# 31491). The PO_4 buffer was made using dibasic sodium phosphate (Sigma-Aldrich, St. Louis, MO, USA) (Cat# S0876) and sodium phosphate monobasic (JT Baker, Phillipsburg, NJ, USA) (Cat # 02-004-215). Afterward, i.e., upon bubbling, the resulting fluorogenic dye was analyzed via fluorescence spectroscopy with a maximum excitation and emission spectra of 475 and 535 nm, respectively. The standards used in this experiment ranged from 0 to 50 µM, each made from 1.25 mM H_2O_2 solution, which was prepared from 30% H_2O_2 (H_2O_2) (Thermo Fischer Scientific, Waltham, MA, USA) (Cat# H323-500) and double-distilled water (ddH_2O). To enumerate, 1.25 mM H_2O_2 was diluted to 0.90 mM H_2O_2 using ddH_2O, and that resulting 0.90 mM hydrogen peroxide solution was used in preparing the previously mentioned standards. Further, to ensure the desired concentration of H_2O_2 had been prepared using the 30% H_2O_2 solution (1.25 mM), Ultraviolet/Visible (UV/Vis) spectroscopy was used. To further explain, after adding 113 µL of 30% H_2O_2 to 999.887 mL of ddH_2O, 1 mL of the resulting solution was added to a quartz cuvette (Sigma-Aldrich, St. Louis, MO, USA) (Cat # C-9542). The quartz cuvette, which has a 10 mm light path, was then inserted into a UV/Vis Spectrophotometer (Beckman Colter, Brea, CA, USA) (Cat# DU 250) and exposed to 240 nm light. Afterward, the absorbance was read and divided by 0.0436 (the extinction coefficient); the extinction coefficient was determined through previous H_2O_2 standardization tests and calibration curves generated. The resulting calculation should produce 1.25 mM; this signifying the correct concentration of H_2O_2 was produced using double distilled water and 30% H_2O_2. Further, before adding 1 mL of the resulting H_2O_2 solution into a quartz cuvette to then be inserted into the UV/Vis Spectrophotometer, ddH_2O was pipetted into the same quartz cuvette and used as a blank.

Regarding the puff generation protocol itself, using a standard lab vacuum and a Buxco Individual Cigarette Puff Generator (Data Sciences International (DSI), St. Paul, MN, USA) (Cat#601-2055-001), the aerosol generated from each vape bar was individually bubbled through 10 mL of H_2DCF-DA solution within a 50 mL conical tube, at 1.5 L/min (Figure 1). Moreover, two lime glass Pasteur pipettes (VWR, Radnor, PA, USA) (Cat # 14672-380) were inserted into the fluorogenic dye within a 50 mL conical tube via a two-hole stopper. Regarding the two Pasteur pipettes inserted into the respective 50 mL conical tube, the fine tip of one of the pipettes was manually broken (or shortened) before being inserted into the two-hole stopper; the fine tip of this pipette did not touch the fluorogenic dye. Next, the end of the same Pasteur pipette, the end usually attached to a rubber bulb, was connected to a vacuum using rubber tubing. Regarding the second Pasteur pipette inserted into the two-hole stopper on the 50 mL conical tube containing the dye, its fine tip was also shortened (via manual breaking), but not as much as the previously mentioned pipette ("shorter" Pasteur pipette). Moreover, the "longer" Pasteur pipette had its fine tip immersed within the fluorogenic dye inside the conical tube. Subsequently, the "shorter" Pasteur pipette was connected to a Fume Hood vacuum, and the "longer" Pasteur pipette was connected to the Puff Generator machine; specifically, rubber tubing was used for connecting the pipettes to the vacuum and Puff Generator. To be more specific, the ends of each pipette (the ends of lime glass Pasteur pipettes which are usually connected to a rubber bulb) were connected to the rubber tubing. Furthermore, the entirety of the puffing protocol for each vape bar and control was conducted in a fume hood; additionally, surrounding lights were turned off to reduce exposure of the fluorogenic dye to light. Furthermore, each 50 mL conical tube containing 10 mL of fluorogenic dye was wrapped with aluminum foil to minimize the dye's exposure to light. A red light was used to see whether the vape bar generated aerosols were indeed being bubbled through the fluorogenic dye; this is due to H_2DCF-DA not absorbing red light.

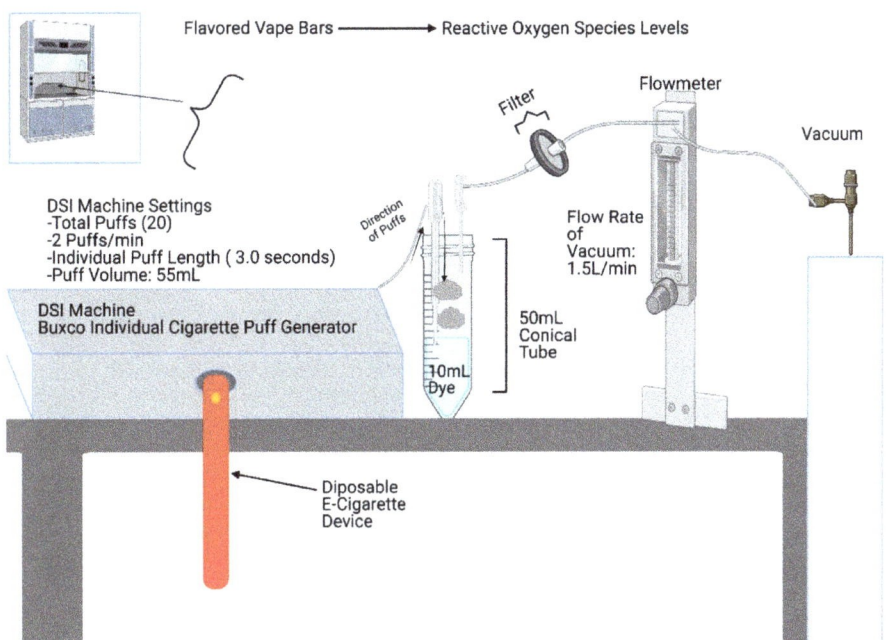

Figure 1. Disposable E-cigarette exposure generation system. This schematic shows the apparatus used to bubble the 10 mL fluorogenic dye within each 50 mL conical tube using the aerosol emitted from the vape bar inserted into the DSI Puff Generator machine. Using a standard lab vacuum, the fluorogenic dye was bubbled at 1.5 L/min, and "puffs" were generated from each vape bar using the DSI Machine above. The DSI machine provided a total of 20 puffs, each puff lasting three seconds and having a volume of 55.0 mL. Each conical tube was wrapped in aluminum foil to protect the fluorogenic dye from light. The entirety of the "bubbling" process using the DSI machine and vacuum apparatus was performed inside a chemical fume hood.

In conjunction with the aforementioned puff generation set-up, once a vape bar was inserted into the Buxco Puff Generator, aerosol was generated and bubbled into the fluorogenic dye under a specific puff profile regiment. Under the particular puff regiment used in the study, a total of 20 puffs was generated through the Puff Generator apparatus; the puffing frequency was two puffs/min, and each puff had a volume of 55 mL and lasted 3.0 s. Different components making up the interior of the Puff Generator (the artificial lung, inhalation actuator, and exhalation actuator) worked together simultaneously to smoke the vape bar to the puff regiment inputted by the user. Further, the Puff Generator smoked each vape bar for ten minutes; the resulting aerosols then traveled from the tubing attached to the Puff Generator to the Pasteur pipette inserted into the 50 mL conical tube. Moreover, once ten minutes of a specific puff regiment had passed for one particular vape bar, the 50 mL conical tube containing the dye which had just been bubbled through with the aerosol of that specific vape bar was inverted several times and then put in ice. Additionally, tubing which connected the Puff Generator to the 10 mL fluorogenic dye within a respective 50 mL conical tube was rinsed with 70% Ethanol and then sterile ddH$_2$O in between replicates for a bar of a specific flavor, vendor, and nicotine concentration and in between puffing regiments for different vape bars. After bubbling all vape bars in duplicates, each resulting fluorogenic dye sample was given 15 min to react within a 37 °C degree water bath (VWR 1228 Digital Water Bath); the resulting solution was then immediately analyzed via fluorescence spectroscopy.

2.3. Generation of Aerosols from Propylene Glycol: Vegetable Glycerin (PG:VG) Solutions, Negative Controls, and Positive Controls

The same puff generator device and puffing regiment used for bubbling the aerosols generated from the vape bars analyzed were used when bubbling solutions consisting of Propylene Glycol (PG) (Sigma-Aldrich, St. Louis, MO, USA) (Cat # P4347) and Vegetable Glycerin (VG) (Sigma-Aldrich, St. Louis, MO, USA) (Cat # G5516). In other words, a PG:VG control (humectant control) was used in conjunction with our vape bar analyses. To further explain, a PG:VG solution was prepared in a 15 mL conical tube; PG and VG were added together in a 1:1 ratio. Subsequently, the prepared PG:VG solution was vortexed for one minute, inverted several times, and then left on a laboratory shaker (Labnet, Edison, NJ, USA) (Mo: Gyrotwister GX-1000) at ten revolutions per minute (10 rpm) overnight before being used in an acellular ROS assay the following day. On the day of the acellular ROS analysis, 700µL of the PG:VG solution was pipetted into a new empty refillable JUUL pod with a 1.8 Ohm cotton wick atomizer (OVNStech, Shenzen, GD, China) (Mo: WO1 JUUL Pods). Subsequently, the PG:VG solution was allowed to sit in the pod for three to five minutes before being inserted into a rechargeable e-cigarette device (JUUL Labs Inc., Washington, DC, USA) (Mo: Rechargeable JUUL Device w/USB charger). Next, the JUUL device was inserted into the Puff Generator and was smoked under the same puff regiment as the disposable vape bars which were analyzed. Similar to the 1.8 Ohm coil PG:VG control described, the same process was used with a refillable cartridge using a 1.6 Ohm coil; in this case, Eleaf Elven pod cartridges (Eleaf Elven, Shenzen, GD, China) (Mo: Eleaf Elven Pod Cartridge) were used and inserted into a different rechargeable e-cigarette device (Eleaf Elven, Shenzen, GD, China) (Mo: Eleaf Elven Pod System).

For our negative control, air was bubbled through the fluorogenic dye; this was achieved by using the Puff Generator under the same puffing regiment as before but without inserting a disposable vape bar into the machine. For our positive control, cigarette smoke generated through burning conventional research cigarettes (Kentucky Tobacco Research & Development Center in the University of Kentucky, Lexington, KY, USA) (Mo: 3R4F) was bubbled through the fluorogenic dye. Also, the fluorogenic dye through which the 3R4F research cigarette smoke was bubbled through was diluted four-fold with freshly made dye. Each control (PG:VG heated with a 1.6 Ohm coil, PG:VG heated with a 1.8 Ohm coil, air, and the 3R4F cigarette) was run in duplicates.

2.4. Fluorescence Spectroscopy and ROS Quantification

After bubbling aerosols from every vape bar during a specific day in which an acellular ROS assay was conducted, 100 µL of each prepared standard and each bubbled dye solution was added to 3.0 mL of fluorogenic dye.Further, 3.0 mL of dye was first added to a 16 × 100 mm Durex Borosilicate Glass culture tube (VWR) (Cat #: 47729-576), and then 100 µL of the bubbled dye solution and each standard was individually added to these culture tubes. Next, each culture tube was vortexed gently. Subsequently, each culture tube was placed within a 37 °C water bath for 15 min. Further, during the 15-min incubation period, surrounding lights were turned off, and only red lights were used. Afterward, standards were measured on a spectrofluorometer (Thermo Fisher Scientific, Waltham, MA, USA) (Mo. FM109535) in fluorescence intensity units (FIU); the same was carried out with the fluorogenic dye samples through which vape bar aerosols were bubbled; all of which was performed using the previously mentioned culture tubes. Additionally, readings displayed on the fluorometer (concentration in µM) were based on the generated hydrogen peroxide standard curve and measured as hydrogen peroxide, H_2O_2 equivalents.

2.5. Statistical Analysis

Statistical analyses of significance were calculated using one-way ANOVA as well as Tukey's post-hoc test for multiple pair-wise comparisons by GraphPad Prism Software version 8.1.1. Samples were run in duplicates and experiments were repeated until consistent data were obtained. The results are shown as mean ± SEM with duplicates analyses. Data were considered to be statistically significant for p values < 0.05.

3. Results

3.1. Total ROS Concentration within Aerosols Generated from Vape Bars Vary by Flavor

Our data show that aerosols generated from disposable flavored vape bars produced differential H_2O_2 equivalents. The aerosols generated from different flavored vape bars contained significantly different total ROS concentrations (μM H_2O_2) (Figures 2–7). The disposable vape bars with the highest ROS content within each of the six previously mentioned flavor categories (Tobacco, Minty Fruit, Minty/Cool (Iced), Fruity, Drinks/Beverages, and Desserts) were Hyde American Tobacco (5% nicotine), Hyppe Bar: Cool Melon (5% nicotine), NJOY: Cool Menthol (6% nicotine), Puff Bar: Blue Razz (5% nicotine), SMOQ: Pink Lemonade (5% nicotine), and Strawberries and Cream (5% nicotine), respectively (Figures 2–7). The aerosol produced by the 5% nicotine Hyde American Tobacco flavored bar contained 10.43–10.72 μM H_2O_2 (Figure 2), the aerosol produced by the 5% nicotine Hyppe Bar Cool Melon bar was 9.44–9.76 μM H_2O_2 (Figure 3), and the aerosol generated from the 5% Puff Bar Blue Razz contained a ROS content of 8.15–9.11 μM H_2O_2 (Figure 5). Moreover, the ROS content within the aerosols generated by SOL: Spearmint (5% nicotine), SMOQ: Pink Lemonade (5% nicotine), Strawberries and Cream (5% nicotine), was 8.78–9.25 μM H_2O_2, 15.32–15.63 μM H_2O_2, and 8.11–8.39 μM H_2O_2, respectively (Figures 4, 6 and 7, respectively). Among the fruity-flavored vape bars analyzed, ROS levels generated from the 0 and 5% nicotine-containing Blue Razz bars were the highest among every 0% nicotine-containing fruity-flavored bar (5.68–5.82 μM H_2O_2) and every nicotine-containing fruity-flavored bar (8.15–9.11 μM H_2O_2), respectively (Figure 5). Additionally, the highest ROS content among all vape bars analyzed in this experiment was found within the aerosol generated by the 5% nicotine-containing SMOQ: Pink Lemonade vape bar (15.32–15.63 μM H_2O_2) under the "Drinks/Beverages" flavor category (Figure 6).

Among the 0% nicotine vape bars analyzed, bars which generated aerosols containing the highest ROS content within the Tobacco, Minty Fruit, and Minty/Cool (Iced) flavor categories were Cyclone's Bold Tobacco flavored-bar (0% nicotine), Bolt's Lychee Ice flavored-bar (0% nicotine), and Flair Plus's Cool Mint flavored-bar (0% nicotine), respectively (Figures 2–4). Additionally, the 0% nicotine bars which generated aerosols containing the highest ROS content within the Fruity, Drink, and Dessert flavor categories were Zaero's Blue Razz flavored bar (0% nicotine), Bolt's Orange Pop flavored bar (0% nicotine), and Fling's Vanilla flavored bar (0% nicotine) (Figures 5–7).

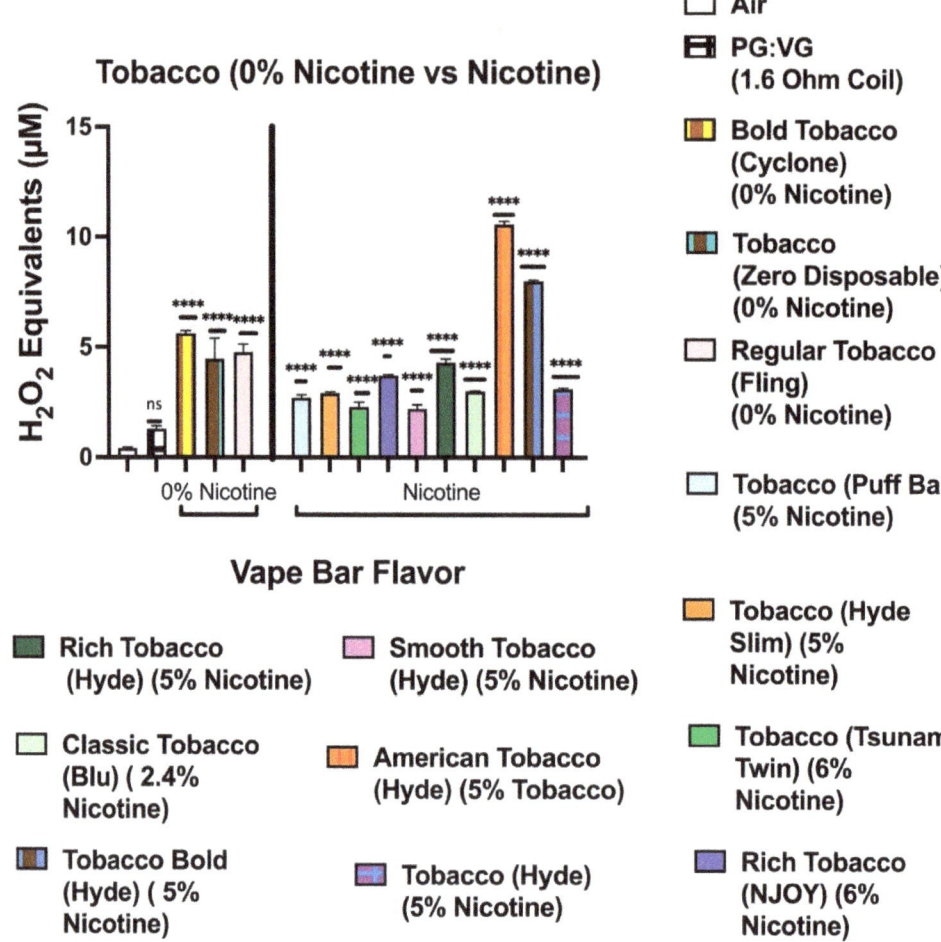

Figure 2. Generation of ROS by different tobacco-based flavors from various vendors. Acellular ROS was measured using a hydrogen peroxide standard within aerosols generated from various tobacco flavored disposable e-cigarette devices. Acellular ROS was also measured from the 1:1 ratio PG:VG control used. Each tobacco-based vape bar's flavor, brand, and nicotine concentration are listed and color-coded. The resistance of the coil used to heat and aerosolize the PG:VG solution is also listed. All flavors and PG:VG controls listed on the graph above were compared to the control value of air. Data are represented as mean ± SEM, and significance was determined by one-way ANOVA. **** $p < 0.0001$ versus air controls. ns is abbreviated for "Non-Significant" versus air-controls ($p > 0.05$).

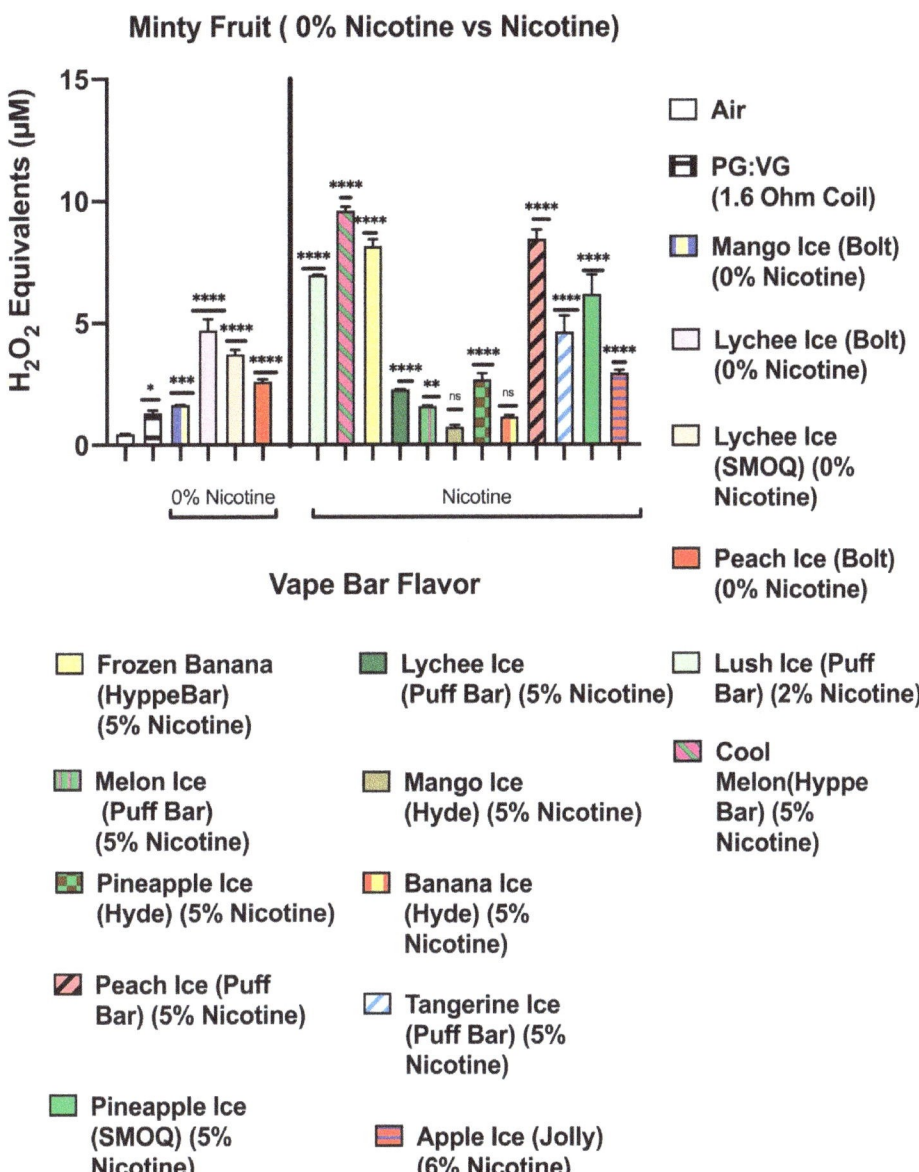

Figure 3. Generation of ROS by different minty fruit flavors from various vendors. Acellular ROS was measured from aerosols generated from various different minty fruit flavored disposable e-cigarette devices using a hydrogen peroxide standard. Acellular ROS was also measured from the 1:1 ratio PG:VG control used. Each minty fruit-based vape bar's flavor, brand, and nicotine concentration are listed and color-coded. The resistance of the coil used to heat and aerosolize the PG:VG solution is also is also listed. All flavors and PG:VG controls listed on the graph above were compared to the control value of air. Data are represented as mean ± SEM, and significance was determined by one-way ANOVA. * $p < 0.05$, ** $p < 0.01$, *** $p < 0.001$, and **** $p < 0.0001$ versus air controls. ns is abbreviated for "Non-Significant" versus air controls ($p > 0.05$).

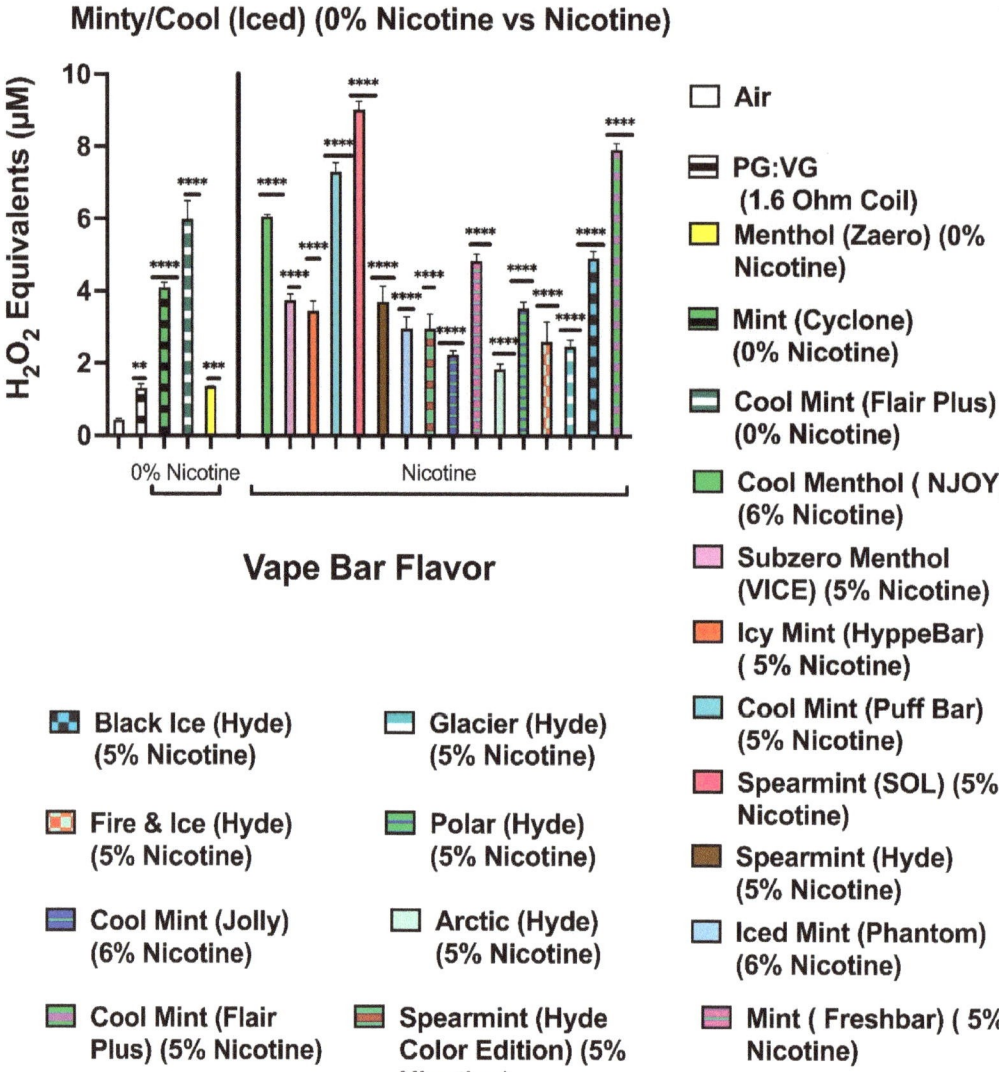

Figure 4. Generation of ROS by different Minty/Cool (Iced) flavors from various vendors. Acellular ROS was measured from aerosols generated from various different minty/cool (iced)-flavored disposable e-cigarette devices using a hydrogen peroxide standard. Acellular ROS was also measured from the 1:1 ratio PG:VG control used. Each Minty/Cool (Iced)-based vape bar's flavor, brand, and nicotine concentration are listed and color-coded. The resistance of the coil used to heat and aerosolize the PG:VG solution is also listed. All flavors and PG:VG controls listed on the graph above were compared to the control value of air. Data are represented as mean ± SEM, and significance was determined by one-way ANOVA. Data are represented as mean ± SEM, and significance was determined by one-way ANOVA. ** $p < 0.01$, *** $p < 0.001$, and **** $p < 0.0001$ versus air controls. ns is abbreviated for "Non-Significant" versus air controls ($p > 0.05$).

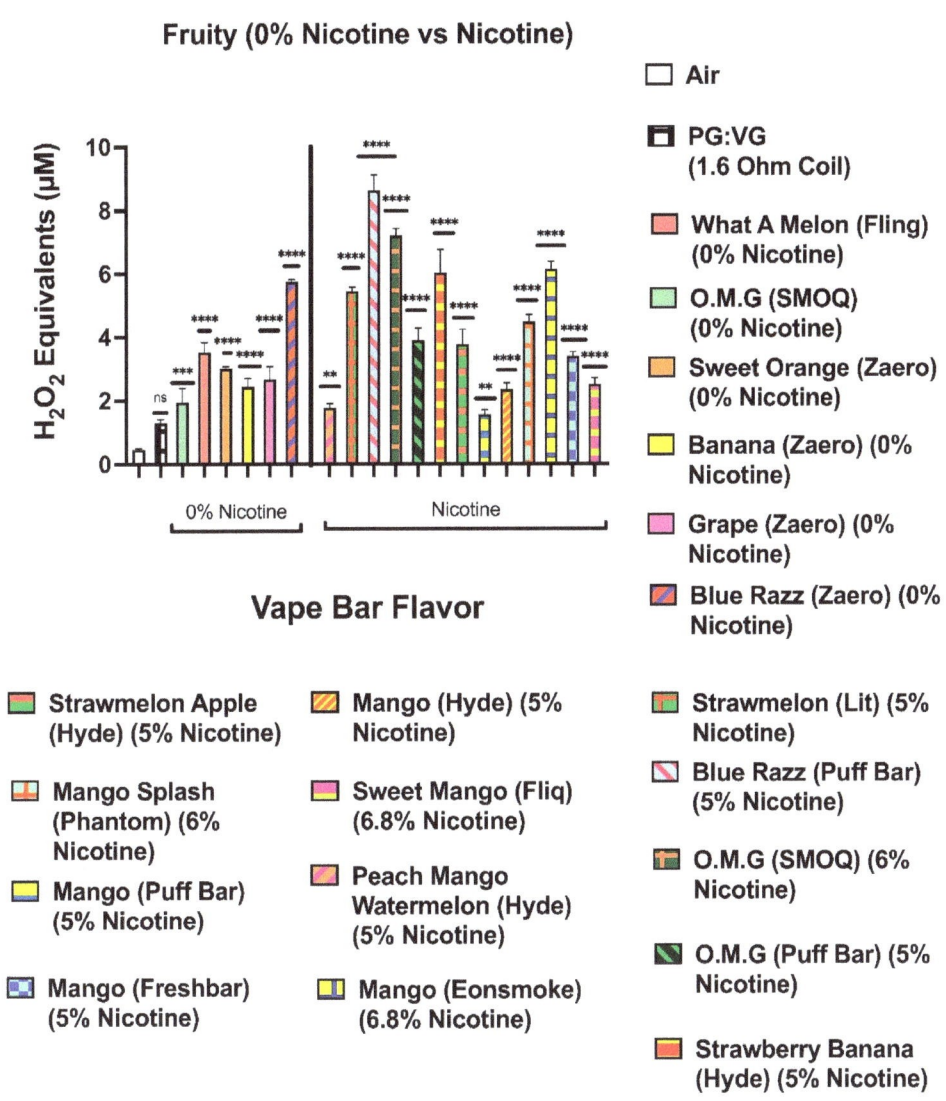

Figure 5. Generation of ROS by different fruity flavors from various vendors. Acellular ROS was measured from aerosols generated from various fruit-flavored disposable e-cigarette devices using a hydrogen peroxide standard. Acellular ROS was also measured from the 1:1 ratio PG:VG control used. Each fruity-based vape bar's flavor, brand, and nicotine concentration are listed and color-coded. The resistance of the coil used to heat and aerosolize the PG:VG solution is also listed. All flavors and PG:VG controls listed on the graph above were compared to the control value of air. Data are represented as mean ± SEM, and significance was determined by one-way ANOVA.** $p < 0.01$ *** $p < 0.001$, and **** $p < 0.0001$ versus air controls. ns is abbreviated for "Non-Significant" versus air controls ($p > 0.05$).

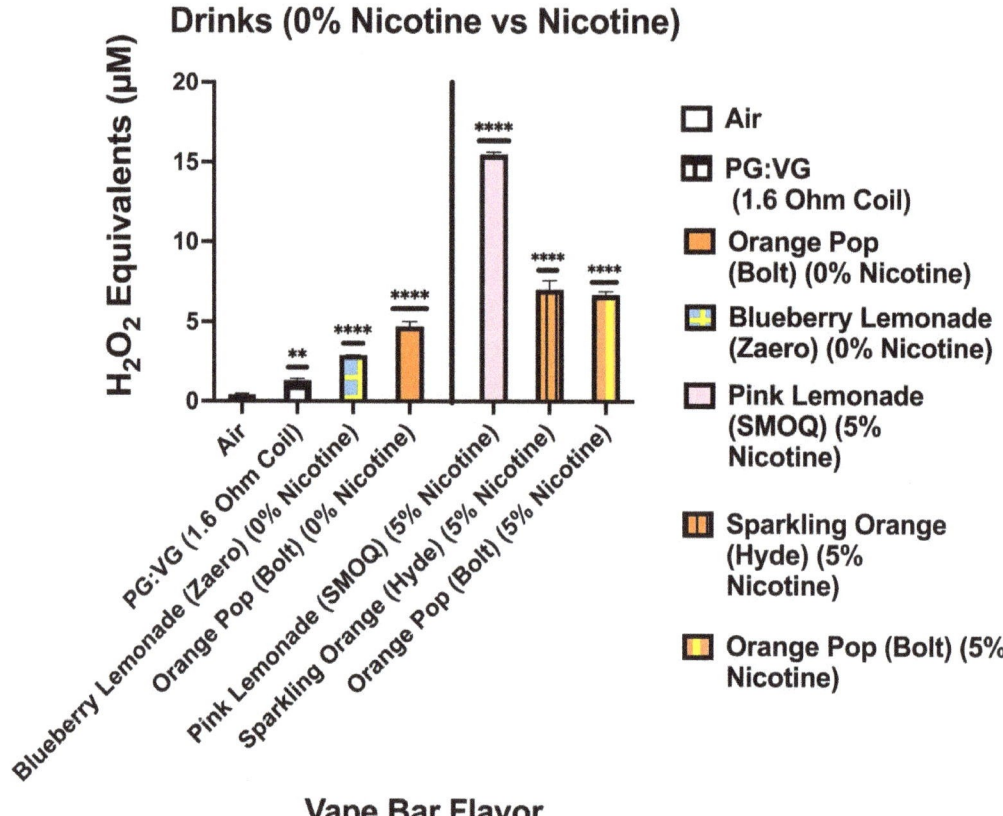

Figure 6. Generation of ROS by different drink flavors from various vendors. Acellular ROS was measured from aerosols generated from various drink flavored disposable e-cigarette devices using a hydrogen peroxide standard. Acellular ROS was also measured from the 1:1 ratio PG:VG control used. Each drink-based vape bar's flavor, brand, and nicotine concentration are listed and color-coded. The resistance of the coil used to heat and aerosolize the PG:VG solution is also listed. All flavors and PG:VG controls listed on the graph above were compared to the control value of air. Data are represented as mean ± SEM, and significance was determined by one-way ANOVA. ** $p < 0.01$ and **** $p < 0.0001$ versus air controls. ns is abbreviated for "Non-Significant" versus air controls ($p > 0.05$).

3.2. Total ROS Concentration in Aerosols Generated by Identical Flavored Vape Bars Vary with Nicotine Concentration

Comparatively, we observed significant variations in generated ROS levels among identically flavored disposable vape bars of varying nicotine concentrations. The variations in ROS levels among identically flavored vape bars with different nicotine concentrations were observed for eight specific flavors (Blue Razz, Mango Ice, Peach Ice, Lychee Ice, Cool Mint, Orange Pop, Melon Ice Cream, and O.M.G (Orange, Mango, and Guava)) (Figures 8–12). When analyzing ROS content produced from aerosols generated by Blue Razz flavored vape bars, we found that the aerosol generated by the nicotine-containing bar (5% nicotine) had significantly higher ROS than the respective non-nicotine-containing bar (0% nicotine) (Figure 8a). Likewise, we found that the aerosol generated by the nicotine-containing (5% nicotine) Peach Ice bar contained a significantly higher ROS content than that produced from a non-nicotine-containing Peach Ice bar (0% nicotine) (Figure 8b). In contrast, for both the Mango Ice and Lychee Ice flavors, we found that the aerosol generated from the non-nicotine-containing bar generated a significantly higher level of ROS than its respective nicotine-containing counterpart (Figure 9).

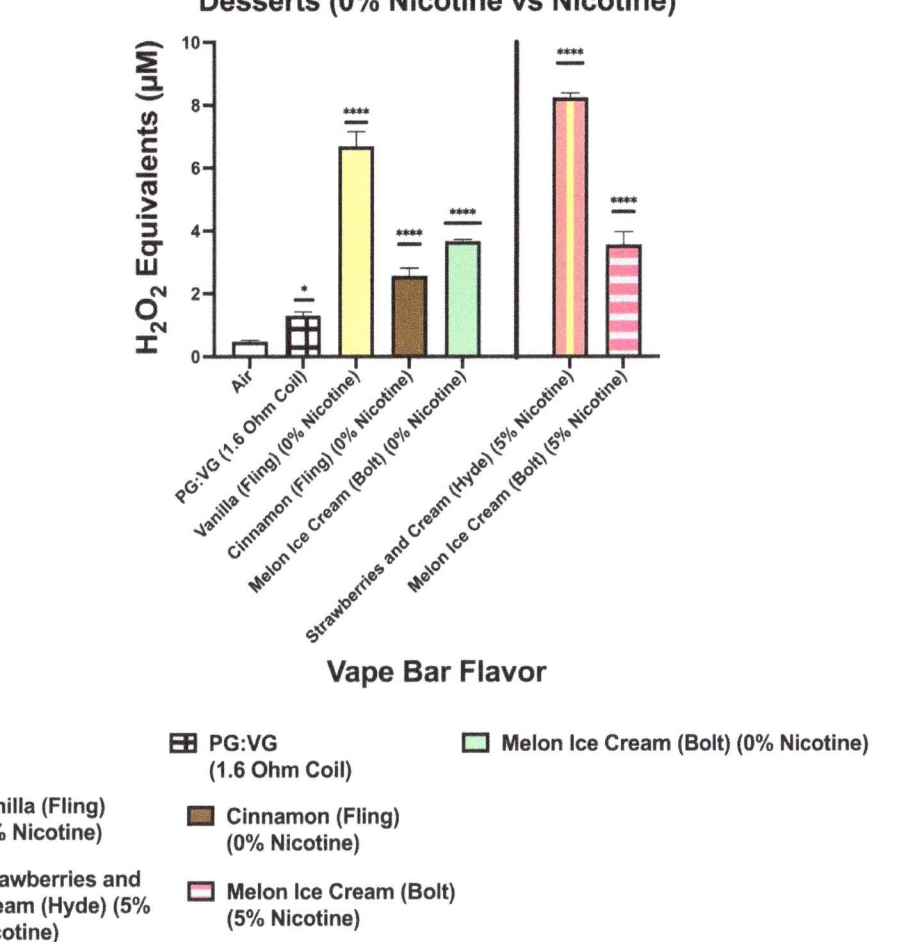

Figure 7. Generation of ROS by different dessert flavors from various vendors. Acellular ROS was measured from aerosols generated from various dessert flavored disposable e-cigarette devices using a hydrogen peroxide standard. Acellular ROS was also measured from the PG:VG control used. Acellular ROS was also measured from the 1:1 ratio PG:VG control which was used. Each dessert-based vape bar's flavor, brand, and nicotine concentration are listed and color-coded. The resistance of the coil used to heat and aerosolize the PG:VG solution is also listed. All flavors and PG:VG controls listed on the graph above were compared to the control value of air. Data are represented as mean ± SEM, and significance was determined by one-way ANOVA. * $p < 0.05$ and **** $p < 0.0001$ versus air controls. ns is abbreviated for "Non-Significant" versus air controls ($p > 0.05$).

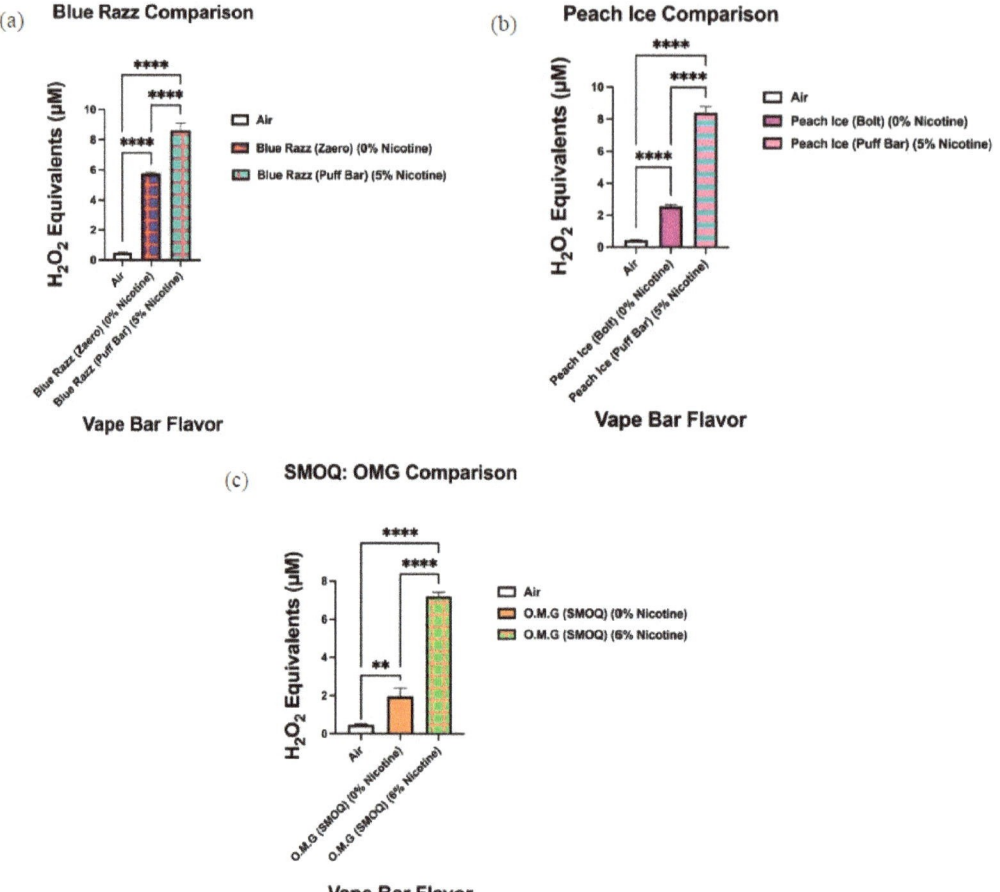

Figure 8. Direct relationship between ROS generation and nicotine concentration within aerosols generated from Blue Razz (**a**), Peach Ice (**b**), and O.M.G (**c**) flavored vape bars. Acellular ROS was measured within aerosols generated from disposable e-cigarettes of the same flavor but different nicotine concentrations using a hydrogen peroxide standard. The disposable vape bars that are shown above within each graph (**a**,**b**) are of the same specific flavor, but each bar was manufactured from a different vendor; these flavors are Blue Razz (**a**) and Peach Ice (**b**). The O.M.G flavored vape bars of differing nicotine concentrations which were analyzed were manufactured from the same vendor (SMOQ) (**c**). Names of each vape bar's flavor, its brand, and its respective nicotine concentration are listed on the side of each respective graph. Pairwise comparisons consisted of those between ROS generated from vape bars and those of other vape bars as well as with the air control. Data are represented as mean ± SEM, and significance was determined using a one-way ANOVA. ** $p < 0.01$ and **** $p < 0.0001$ versus air controls and for specific pairwise comparisons.

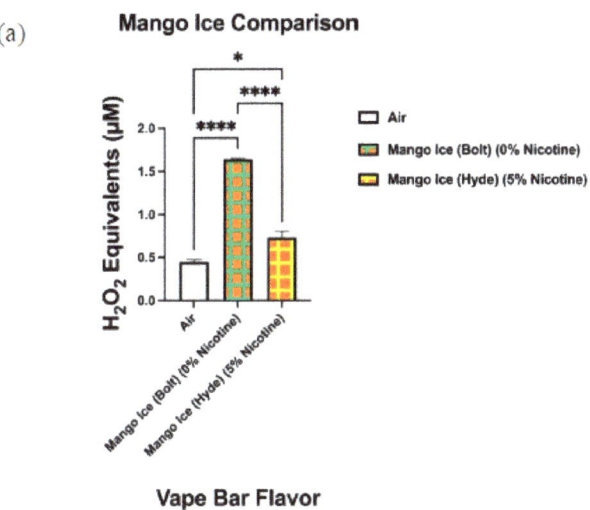
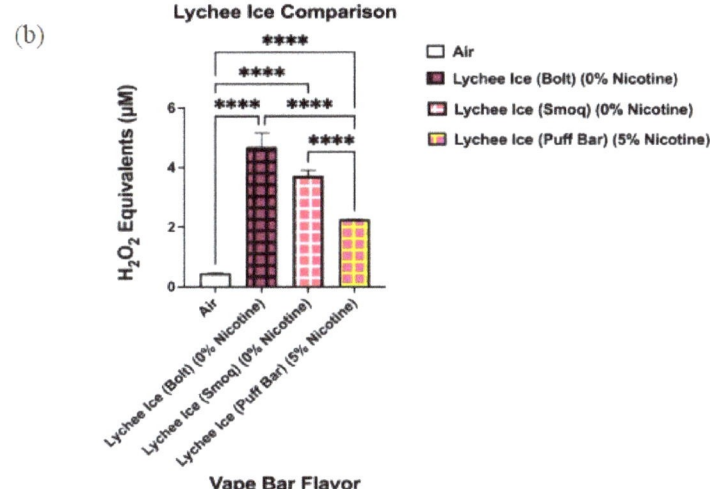

Figure 9. Inverse relationship between ROS generation and nicotine concentration in aerosols generated from Mango Ice (**a**) and Lychee Ice (**b**) flavored disposable e-cigarettes. Acellular ROS was measured using a hydrogen peroxide standard within aerosols generated from disposable e-cigarettes of the same flavor but different nicotine concentrations. Regarding disposable vape bars that were of the same specific flavor (Mango Ice (**a**) and Lychee Ice (**b**)), each vape bar was manufactured from a different vendor. The names of each vape bar's flavor, its brand, and its respective nicotine concentration are listed on the side of each respective graph. Pairwise comparisons consisted of those between aerosols generated from vape bars and other vape bars as well as with air. All flavors were compared to the control value of air and to other flavors. Data are represented as mean ± SEM, and significance was determined by one-way ANOVA. * $p < 0.05$ and **** $p < 0.0001$ for specific pairwise comparisons.

(a)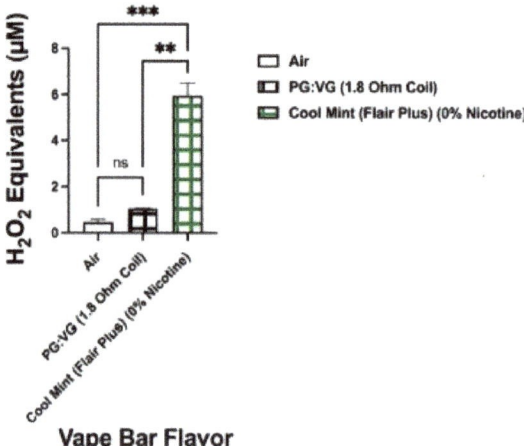

(b)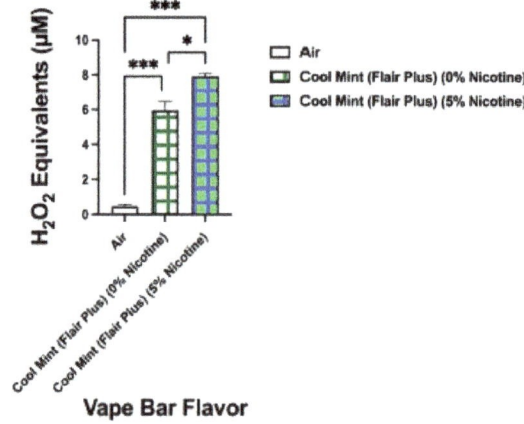

Figure 10. Differential ROS levels among aerosols produced from Cool Mint flavored vape bars of varying nicotine concentrations manufactured by Flair Plus. Acellular ROS was measured using a hydrogen peroxide standard within aerosols generated from vape bars of varying concentrations of nicotine (0 and 5%) of the same flavor and vendor (Flair Plus and Cool Mint), respectively. The corresponding 0% nicotine-containing bar was compared to a PG:VG control; this PG:VG control contained the same PG:VG ratio and was heated using a coil of the same resistance as the vape bar shown above (**a**). Another comparison in ROS concentration was made between the aerosols generated from the 0% nicotine containing Flair Plus: Cool Mint bar and the 5% nicotine-containing Flair Plus: Cool Mint bar (**b**). The name of each vape bar's flavor, its brand, and its respective nicotine concentration are listed on the side of each respective graph; the same labeling method was used for the PG:VG control analyzed. Data are represented as mean ± SEM, and significance was determined using a one-way ANOVA. * $p < 0.05$, ** $p < 0.01$, and *** $p < 0.001$ for specific pairwise comparisons shown above. ns is abbreviated for "Non-Significant" versus air controls ($p > 0.05$).

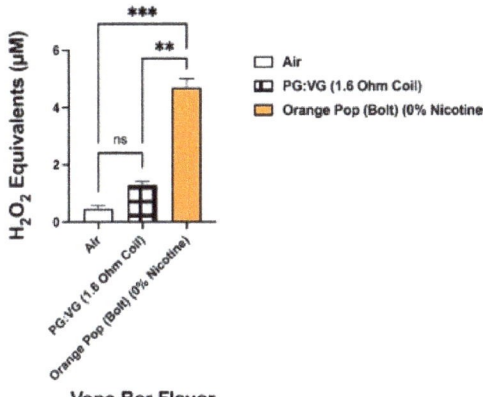

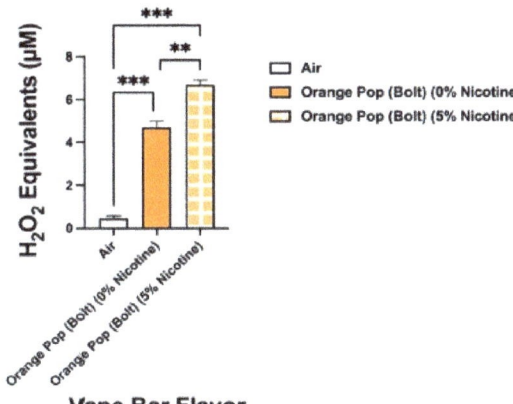

Figure 11. Differential ROS levels among aerosols produced from Orange Pop flavored vape bars of varying nicotine concentrations manufactured by Bolt. Acellular ROS was measured using a hydrogen peroxide standard within aerosols generated from vape bars of varying nicotine concentrations which were of the same flavor and vendor (Orange Pop and Bolt, respectively). The corresponding 0% nicotine-containing bar was compared to a PG:VG control; this PG:VG control contained the same PG:VG ratio and was heated using a coil of the same resistance as the vape bar shown above (**a**). Another comparison in ROS concentration was made between the aerosols generated from the 0% nicotine-containing Bolt: Orange Pop bar and the 5% nicotine-containing Bolt: Orange Pop (**b**). The name of each vape bar's flavor, its brand, and its respective nicotine concentration are listed on the side of each respective graph; the same labeling method was used for the PG:VG control analyzed. Data are represented as mean ± SEM, and significance was determined using a one-way ANOVA. ** $p < 0.01$ and *** $p < 0.001$ for specific pairwise comparisons shown above. ns is abbreviated for "Non-Significant" versus air controls ($p > 0.05$).

(a) **Bolt: Melon Ice Cream Comparison (0% Nicotine vs PG:VG)**

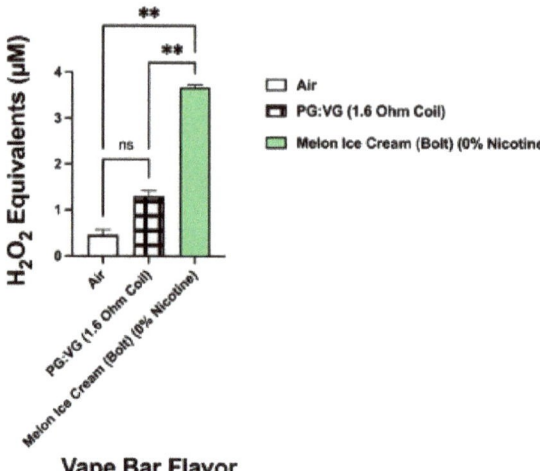

(b) **Bolt: Melon Ice Cream Comparison (0% Nicotine vs 5% Nicotine)**

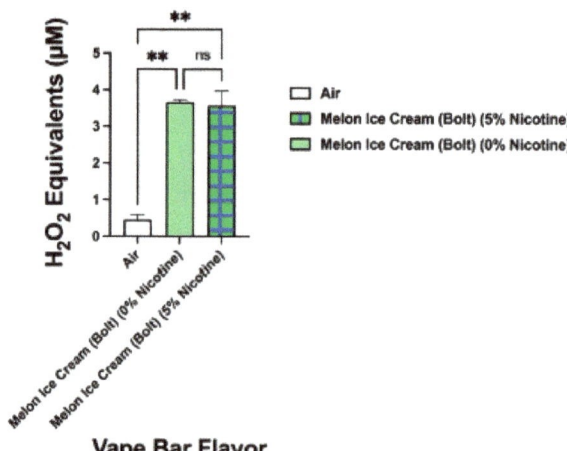

Figure 12. Differential ROS levels among aerosols generated from Melon Ice Cream flavored vape bars of varying nicotine concentrations manufactured by Bolt. Acellular ROS was measured using a hydrogen peroxide standard within aerosols generated from vape bars of various nicotine concentrations (0 and 5%) of the same flavor and vendor (Melon Ice Cream and Bolt, respectively). The corresponding 0% nicotine-containing bar was compared to a PG:VG control; this PG: VG control contained the same PG:VG ratio and was heated using a coil of the same resistance as the vape bar shown above (**a**). Another comparison in ROS concentration was made between the aerosols generated from the 0% nicotine-containing Bolt: Melon Ice Cream bar and the 5% nicotine-containing Bolt: Melon Ice Cream (**b**). The name of each vape bar's flavor, its brand, and its respective nicotine concentration are listed on the side of each respective graph; the same labeling method was used for the PG:VG control analyzed. Data are represented as mean ± SEM, and significance was determined using a one-way ANOVA. ** $p < 0.01$ for specific pairwise comparisons shown above. ns is abbreviated for "Non-Significant" versus air controls ($p > 0.05$).

When analyzing the ROS content within aerosols produced by vape bars of the same flavor and vendor (Bolt, Flair Plus, and SMOQ, etc.), we observed significant variations in ROS levels among bars of varying nicotine concentrations (Figures 10–12). Further, the ROS concentration within aerosol generated from the 0% nicotine Cool Mint bar from Flair Plus, 5.40–6.50 μM H_2O_2, was significantly lower than that within the aerosol generated from its corresponding 5% nicotine bar, 7.73–8.11 μM H_2O_2 (Figure 10b). Regarding the two Orange Pop vape bars made by Bolt, which we analyzed, aerosol within the corresponding 0% nicotine bar contained a ROS concentration of 4.39–5.00 μM H_2O_2, which is significantly lower than the ROS concentration within the aerosol generated from its respective 5% nicotine bar, 6.48–6.90 μM H_2O_2 (Figure 11b). Similarly, like Orange Pop, Melon Ice Cream is another flavor manufactured by Bolt at both 0% nicotine and 5% nicotine. Regarding the semi-quantification of ROS within the aerosols produced by the Melon Ice Cream flavored bar from Bolt, the ROS concentration within Bolt's 0% nicotine Melon Ice Cream bar is 3.61–3.73 μM H_2O_2 (Figure 12b). Likewise, 3.61–3.73 μM H_2O_2 is not significantly different from the ROS concentration within the aerosol generated from the corresponding 5% nicotine bar, 3.16–3.97 μM H_2O_2 (Figure 12b). Regarding other comparisons of semi-quantified ROS levels within aerosols generated from vape bars of varying nicotine concentrations of the same flavor and vendor, SMOQ's O.M.G bars were also analyzed (Figure 8c). The ROS concentration within the aerosol generated from SMOQ's 6% nicotine O.M.G bar (6.96–7.43 μM H_2O_2) was significantly higher than that within the aerosol generated from the corresponding 0% nicotine bar (1.5–2.4 μM H_2O_2) (Figure 8c).

Regarding the non-nicotine-containing Flair Plus: Cool Mint bar (0% nicotine), the non-nicotine-containing Bolt: Orange Pop bar (0% nicotine), and the non-nicotine-containing Bolt: Melon Ice Cream bar (0% nicotine), there were significant differences between ROS levels within each aerosol generated from each of the three bars and the ROS levels within their respective aerosolized PG:VG controls. To further explain, the ROS content within the aerosol generated from Flair Plus's 0% nicotine Cool Mint bar (5.40–6.50 μM H_2O_2) was significantly higher than that within the aerosol generated from PG:VG solution aerosolized (1.03–1.06 μM H_2O_2). To clarify, this specific PG:VG control aerosolized contains the same PG:VG ratio (1:1) and was heated using a coil of the same resistance as that used in the Flair Plus: Cool Mint bar (0% nicotine), 1.8 Ohms (Figure 10a).

Likewise, the ROS concentration within aerosol generated from the 0% nicotine Bolt: Orange Pop bar (4.39–5.00 μM H_2O_2) was significantly higher than that within the aerosol generated from the PG:VG solution vaporized using a 1.6 Ohm coil (1.18–1.42 μM H_2O_2) (Figure 11a). The resistance of the coil used in all Bolt disposable bars is 1.6 Ohms. Similarly, the respective PG:VG control used in the subsequent pairwise comparison with the 0% nicotine Bolt: Orange Pop bar (Figure 11a) had the same ratio of PG and VG as the respective bar (1:1). Regarding the non-nicotine-containing Bolt: Melon Ice Cream bar, the ROS concentration within the aerosolized 0% nicotine bar (3.61–3.73 μM H_2O_2) was significantly higher than that generated from the PG:VG control (1.18–1.42 μM H_2O_2) (Figure 12a). Again, to clarify, this specific PG:VG control, used in the aforementioned pairwise comparison, contains the same PG:VG ratio (1:1) and was heated using a coil of the same resistance as that used in the Bolt: Melon Ice Cream bar (0% nicotine), 1.6 Ohms.

4. Discussion

When analyzing the ROS content emitted by vape bars within each flavor category (Tobacco, Fruity, Minty Fruit, Minty/Cool (Iced), Drinks/Beverages, and Desserts), we observed differential ROS production among the different flavored bars. In addition, within each of the six flavor categories analyzed, different flavored disposable vape bars with the same nicotine content produced variable levels of ROS relative to the respective air control. The Tobacco, Fruity, Minty Fruit, Minty/Cool (Iced), Drinks/Beverages, and Dessert flavor categories with and without nicotine were selected for our analyses due to the popularity of these flavor categories among e-cigarette users, especially among e-cigarette users in middle and high school, after the FDA's 2020 e-cigarette flavoring enforcement policy [1]. Furthermore, the FDA's 2020 flavoring enforcement policy prohibits companies from selling cartridge-based e-cigarettes with dessert, candy, fruit, mint flavors with nicotine, as well as any flavor excluding tobacco or menthol [1]. Any flavors without nicotine (zero nicotine) are still sold in the United States without any regulations, which are used in the present study.

Vape bars under the Minty Fruit flavor category were analyzed due to their recent rise in popularity among youth e-cigarette users. Further, around the same time that disposable e-cigarette sales surged following the FDA's flavored e-cigarette enforcement policy on nicotine in 2020, a significantly high number of minty fruit e-cigarette flavors had entered marketplaces [15]. Further, the increased usage of minty (cool/iced) fruit flavors among e-cigarette users in the country necessitated us to analyze these flavors because of their potential to make further regulatory action more complicated due to Iced Fruit flavors not fitting into existing flavor categorizations [15]. Research investigating how flavoring chemicals affect ROS generation in e-cigarette generated aerosols has been explored minimally; however, a few recent studies have delved into the dependence that ROS generation from e-cigarettes may have on flavoring chemicals. Our study found that ROS levels generated from cigar/cigarillo smoke varied among different flavors [16]. Regarding studies conducted with e-cigarettes, another study found that ROS generation within the aerosols generated from cartridge-based e-cigarette devices was highly dependent on the vendor, puffing pattern, voltage, and the flavor of the cartridge-based e-cigarette device used [3]. Moreover, our lab's previous study found that the flavorings used in e-liquids can induce an inflammatory response in monocytes; the study further found that this response is mediated through ROS production [17].

Additionally, we show that ROS content in aerosols generated in vape bars of identical flavors (Blue Razz, Peach Ice, Lychee Ice, Mango Ice, Orange Pop, Melon Ice Cream, Cool Mint, and O.M.G) varied among identically flavored bars of different nicotine content. However, only five out of eight flavors mentioned showed the corresponding nicotine-containing bar generating significantly higher ROS levels than its respective 0% nicotine-containing bar. Here, our data showed that the nicotine-containing Mango Ice and Lychee Ice bars contained significantly lower ROS levels than their corresponding 0% nicotine-containing bar. These results observed among the Mango Ice and Lychee Ice bars of differing nicotine content may have occurred because the pairwise comparisons between these identically flavored bars did not control for the vendor. In the pairwise comparisons between the 0% nicotine-containing Mango Ice bar and the 5% nicotine Mango Ice bar, each bar was made by a different manufacturer. Additionally, because each Mango Ice bar was manufactured by a different vendor, the PG:VG content within each bar may have also been different between the identically flavored bars. Previous studies have shown that the ratio of PG and VG used within an e-liquid led to significant alterations in ROS levels within generated aerosols. Similarly, when analyzing and comparing ROS content among the aerosols generated from the different Lychee Ice bars (0% nicotine and 5% nicotine-containing bars), each bar was made by a different vendor. Further, this means that among the Lychee Ice, Peach Ice, Mango Ice, and Blue Razz bars analyzed, pairwise comparisons between the 0% nicotine-containing bar and the 5% nicotine-containing bar did not control for the vendor. Similarly, this may explain the reason for a consistent relationship between increasing nicotine content and ROS generation is not seen among the Lychee Ice, Mango Ice, Peach Ice, and Blue Razz flavored bars. The ROS generated from the nicotine-containing Mango Ice and Lychee Ice bars was significantly lower than that within the aerosols generated from the corresponding 0% nicotine bar. In contrast, our data analyzing the Blue Razz and Peach Ice bars showed a direct relationship between increasing nicotine content and ROS production.

Consequently, to control for the vendor in determining how nicotine affects ROS generation, one could analyze the ROS content within aerosols generated by vape bars of the same flavor and vendor but of differing nicotine content. Correspondingly, we did this by determining the ROS concentration within aerosols generated from the Flair Plus: Cool Mint, Bolt: Orange Pop, Bolt: Melon Ice Cream, and SMOQ: O.M.G bars.

Further, among three of the four vendor-specific flavors, we found that the aerosol from the respective nicotine-containing bar contained a significantly higher level of ROS than the corresponding 0% nicotine-containing bar. For instance, the 5% nicotine Flair Plus: Cool Mint bar generated an aerosol that contained a significantly higher level of ROS than that within its respective 0% nicotine bar; this suggests that nicotine contributes to this significant difference in ROS levels. Similar results were also observed when comparing the 0 and 5% nicotine-containing Orange Pop bars manufactured by Bolt and the O.M.G flavored bars (0 and 6% nicotine) manufactured by SMOQ. Further, we realized that to better elucidate the role nicotine in affecting ROS generated from flavored vape bars, more comparative acellular ROS analyses are needed between bars of the same specific flavor and vendor, but different nicotine concentrations. Further work is required to analyze more vape bars with differing nicotine concentrations made from the same vendor and of the same specific flavor.

Previous studies have shown that nicotine and the other constituents of e-liquids (flavoring agents, propylene glycol (PG), and vegetable glycerin (VG)) contribute to ROS production [5,18]. Similarly, Haddad et al. have shown that the ROS emission from aerosolized e-liquids was significantly affected by the PG:VG ratio of the e-liquid [19]. Propylene Glycol (PG) and Vegetable Glycerol (VG) are humectants, substances used to maintain moisture. Furthermore, PG and VG's ability to attract and retain moisture allows e-cigarette users to feel what is known as a "throat hit". A "Throat hit" refer to the sensation one who uses ENDS products feels in their throat caused by nicotine inhalation. Regarding one of the specific findings from Haddad Et al., the study found that increasing the percentage of VG within the base PG:VG liquid component of an e-liquid used within a rechargeable e-cigarette significantly increased ROS flux [19]. Similarly, another study by Bitzer et al. found increases in the PG content of an e-liquid used in rechargeable e-cigarettes led to heavy increases in free-radical production within the resulting aerosolized e-liquid [18].

These previous studies compelled us to determine the ROS concentration with the PG:VG base solution used within the vape bars analyzed in our study. We reasoned that by semi-quantifying the ROS content within the aerosols produced from the PG:VG component of vape bars we analyzed, the role flavoring chemicals and nicotine have in contributing to ROS production during e-liquid heating and aerosolization can be further elucidated. However, out of every vape bar analyzed in our study, the only two companies which provided the PG:VG content online were Bolt and Flair Plus; for both companies, the e-liquid component of the vape-bar contained a 1:1 ratio PG:VG solution. Accordingly, we prepared a 1:1 ratio PG:VG solution to be smoked and aerosolized using the Puff Generator in tandem with the other analyzed vape bars. Additionally, when looking into other specifications of the Flair Plus and Bolt bars analyzed, we saw that each vendor used a coil of a different resistance: 1.6 and 1.8 Ohms, respectively. Accordingly, we analyzed the ROS content within a 1:1 ratio PG:VG solution aerosolized using a 1.6 Ohm coil (via Eleaf Elven cartridges) and a 1.8 Ohm coil (via OVN: W01 JUUL cartridges).

Regarding how flavoring chemicals used in vape bars contribute to ROS emissions from vape bar-generated aerosols, research delving into how the interactions between different components of e-liquids contribute to ROS generation is lacking. However, a study by Son, Yeongkwon et al. found that the flavoring chemicals within flavoring agents (those including maltol, benzyl acetate, and anethole, etc.) may undergo redox cycling with transition metal ions found with e-liquids and produce •OH [5]. Additionally, a previous study from our lab (Lerner et. al.) found that the oxidative nature of non-vaporized e-liquids is dependent on the flavoring additives used in an e-liquid [10]. For example, e-liquids containing fruity or sweet flavors were stronger oxidizing agents than corresponding tobacco flavored e-liquids [10]. Together, Lerner et al. findings and the present study suggest that flavoring chemicals themselves influence ROS production during e-liquid aerosolization. Our results comparing the ROS content within aerosols generated from different bars within each of the six major flavor categories (Tobacco, Minty Fruit, Minty/Cool (Iced), Fruity, Drinks/Beverages, and Desserts) suggest that ROS generation varies among different flavored bars. However, comparative acellular ROS analyses between a 0% nicotine-containing flavored vape bar and the PG:VG solution making up that same vape bar are needed to further investigate the role of flavoring agents in ROS production within vape bars. To further explain, a PG:VG solution heated and aerosolized using a coil of the same resistance as the flavored vape bars of interest is needed. By comparing the ROS generated between a 0% nicotine-containing flavored vape bar and an accurate PG:VG control, one can see whether the flavoring agents themselves play a role in changing the ROS levels generated upon a vape bar aerosolization.

Consequently, we conducted pairwise comparisons between ROS levels produced from three 0% nicotine-containing bars and their respective PG:VG controls. These three aforementioned 0% nicotine bars were manufactured by Flair Plus and Bolt; two of which were manufactured by Bolt and one of which was manufactured by Flair Plus. Next, when comparing the ROS content within the aerosol generated from the 0% nicotine Flair Plus: Cool Mint bar with that within the aerosol produced from its respective PG:VG control, the ROS content generated from the 0% nicotine bar was significantly higher than that within aerosolized PG:VG control. Moreover, the PG:VG ratio and the coil's resistance used in the PG:VG control were the same as that used in the 0% nicotine-containing Flair Plus: Cool Mint bar; this specific pairwise comparison minimized PG:VG content and coil resistance as potential confounding influences. Accordingly, the previously mentioned results suggest that flavoring chemicals themselves (in particular the ones used to make the Cool Mint flavor) significantly contribute to ROS generation upon e-liquid heating and subsequent aerosolization.

Similarly, pairwise comparisons between the 0% nicotine Bolt: Orange Pop bar and its respective PG:VG control and between the 0% nicotine Bolt: Melon Ice Cream bar and its PG:VG control also suggest the same conclusion we reached upon our analysis of the 0% nicotine-containing Cool Mint bar from Flair Plus and its PG:VG control. To clarify Bolt disposable bars have a PG:VG ratio of 1:1 and use a 1.6 Ohm coil to heat their e-liquid component. Consequently, the PG:VG control used in the pairwise comparisons with the aforementioned Bolt 0% nicotine bars contained a PG:VG ratio of 1:1 and was aerosolized using a 1.6 Ohm coil. Subsequently, our data showed that both 0% Bolt bars (Orange Pop and Melon Ice Cream) contain a significantly higher ROS content than their corresponding PG:VG controls. These results further suggest that flavoring agents (in this case, the ones used to make Orange Pop and Melon Ice Cream flavors) significantly contribute to ROS generation by flavored vape bars.

Regarding a limitation of our study, the only PG:VG controls we used were those with a 1:1 ratio composition of both PG and VG. These were heated using 1.6- and 1.8-Ohm coils. PG:VG controls utilizing this specific ratio of PG and VG (1:1) and which were heated using 1.6- and 1.8-Ohm coils. This was used because the PG:VG ratio and the resistance of the coils used in the Flair Plus and Bolt bars we had analyzed. Flair Plus and Bolt were the only two commercial manufacturers of the disposable vape bars used in this study that provided information on their PG: VG content, coil resistance, and that manufactured both non-nicotine-containing and nicotine-containing bars. Further, we could not find the resistance of the coils used in many of the other vape bars we analyzed, nor could we find the PG:VG ratio used within those bars. Consequently, our PG:VG controls were modeled after the specifications of the Flair Plus and Bolt bars analyzed. Additionally, in our data comparing the ROS generated from every single vape bar within each of the six major flavor categories analyzed, we only included the PG:VG control heated using a 1.6 Ohm coil. We did this because information on the resistance of the coils used in many of the other vape bars included in this study was not provided by the respective vendors of those bars. Secondly, we realized that out of all the vape bars we analyzed whose vendors provided information on their coil resistance, the highest number of bars used a 1.6 Ohm coil. Consequently, to maintain consistency among the first six graphs provided in the paper, we only included the 1.6 Ohm PG:VG control within each of those six graphs. However, acellular ROS assays and comparative analyses between different flavored vape bars in future studies should only be conducted once the resistance of coils used in the vape bars one plans to analyze is known. This is because coil resistance is a key part of the heating and aerosolization process within ENDS [20], and possibly in vape bars. Accordingly, future related studies must include PG:VG controls that are aerosolized using coils of the same resistance of each vape bars analyzed in the respective study.

Similarly, regarding another limitation of this study, the only two commercial manufacturers of the vape bars we analyzed in our study that provided information on PG:VG ratios used in component e-liquids were Flair Plus and Bolt. Consequently, the PG:VG controls we used consisted only of a 1:1 ratio of PG:VG as these were the PG and VG ratios used in bars from Bolt and Flair Plus. The other commercial manufacturers of the vape bars we analyzed in our study did not provide information on the ratio of PG and VG contained in their vape bars. Consequently, we could not semi-quantify the ROS within aerosols produced from solutions of the same PG:VG ratio as those used in many of the vape bars we analyzed in this study. For these reasons, when producing graphs and including pairwise comparisons between the Blue Razz, Peach Ice, Mango Ice, and Lychee Ice bars of differing nicotine content, we did not include the ROS generated from our PG:VG controls. Our reasoning for this was because we did not know the ratio of the PG:VG used within the Blue Razz, Peach Ice, Mango Ice, and Lychee Ice bars; consequently, conducting pairwise comparisons between the PG:VG controls we used and each of the Blue Razz, Peach Ice, Mango Ice, and Lychee Ice bars of varying nicotine content would not have been scientifically sound. Furthermore, NMR spectroscopy using the e-liquids isolated from all the vape-bar we analyzed will determine each bar's specific PG:VG ratio. In the future, when conducting acellular ROS analyses of flavored vape bars, we will use NMR spectroscopy to determine each bar's PG:VG ratio to make an accurate PG:VG control for subsequent acellular ROS assays (both for bars whose manufactures provide information of PG:VG ratios and those which do not).

Moreover, assessing the ROS generation due to 'cooling agents' in ENDS is vital in determining the toxicity of vape bars with dual and multi flavors. Studies have found variations in the levels of synthetic cooling agents, such as WS-3 and WS-23, in cool (iced) flavors among e-cigarettes manufactured by various companies [21,22]. These cooling agents induce cytotoxicity in BEAS-2B lung epithelial cells, suggesting their adverse toxic effects upon inhalation [21]. Furthermore, future studies assessing the acellular ROS generation by cooling agents should consider the confounding factors, such as flavor category and nicotine concentration, as these constituents form secondary reactive species upon heating. Further, these future acellular ROS analyses must include a fruity-flavored vape bar (e.g., apple), its respective cool (iced) flavor (e.g., apple ice), an appropriate PG:VG control, and an appropriate salt nicotine control (using a PG:VG solvent) [23]. Additionally, acellular ROS assays conducted to investigate the effects cooling agents have in ROS generation from vape bars must include fruity flavored and respective cool (iced) flavored vape bars manufactured by various vendors. This may include flavored bars with or without nicotine (tobacco and mint/menthol flavors) [24].

Overall, our results suggest that different flavoring chemicals used in vape bars contribute to variations in the breakdown of the chemical bonds holding together the components of the e-liquid within a vape bar during thermal degradation, leading to differential ROS levels in generated aerosols. Additionally, our pairwise comparisons made between vape bars with different nicotine concentrations but the same specific flavor and vendor suggest nicotine itself has a role in influencing ROS generation within aerosolizing vape bars. In general, cool (iced) flavors generated differential ROS than their counterpart non-cool (iced) flavors. However, further assays are needed to elucidate how both the flavor of a vape bar and its corresponding nicotine concentration affect ROS generation within vape bars, and immune-inflammatory responses in mouse model as seen previously [25]. Future studies can use Gas Chromatography–Mass Spectrometry (GC–MS) to analyze the compounds within flavoring agents within flavored vape bars. For example, using GC-MS to analyze the e-liquids extracted from minty and cool (iced) vape bars can provide more insight on the cooling agents used within these specific flavored vape bars. In addition, Electron Paramagnetic Resonance (EPR) Spectroscopy can analyze the relative proportions of specific ROS (H_2O_2, $O_2^{\bullet-}$, and $^{\bullet}OH$) and free radicals within the aerosol generated from vape bars.

Future studies involving acellular ROS analyses using different flavored vape bars should also include a PG:VG control which includes nicotine (either free-base or nicotine benzoate). Further, when analyzing the ROS generated from vape bars of the same flavor and vendor but different nicotine concentrations, in addition to making a PG:VG control made up of the same ratio of PG and VG and heated using a coil of the same resistance as that used in the vape bars of interest, one can also make another control consisting of PG:VG and nicotine. Further, one can make a PG:VG control which includes the same percentage of nicotine salt used in the e-liquid component of their bars of interest. Subsequently, acellular ROS analyses among bars of the same flavor and vendor but different nicotine concentrations, a PG:VG control and PG:VG control with nicotine may show whether or not ROS generated from vape bars varies as a function of nicotine content. However, due limitations in our inventory, we could not produce a PG:VG w/nicotine control and aerosolize it to semi-quantify its ROS content.

5. Conclusions

Overall, our results concur with our initial hypothesis that ROS generated from disposable e-cigarette bars varies among different flavors and flavors of different nicotine content. The breakdown of chemical bonds holding together an e-liquid via thermal degradation leads to ROS production in generated aerosols. Further, any alterations in ROS production from e-liquids must arise due to changes in the breakdown of these chemical bonds during thermal degradation (in frequency, timing, etc.). Accordingly, our results seem to suggest that both flavoring agents and nicotine in some way alter the breakdown of chemical bonds holding together a vape bar's component e-liquid.

Future studies are required to analyze a much higher number of flavored vape bars to better understand the relationship between nicotine and ROS generation and between flavoring chemicals and ROS generation within disposable e-cigarettes. Furthermore, in addition to analyzing a greater number of vape bars, more acellular ROS comparisons should be performed between vape bars that control for the vendor in multiple emerging flavors/vendors which are present in the market, thereby reducing the confounding influence a specific vendor may have on ROS generation. Additionally, for future studies analyzing the ROS generated by bars of the same specific flavor and vendor, corresponding PG:VG and PG:VG w/nicotine controls should be used for every vape bar analyzed.

Furthermore, the chemical constituents of a vape bar's flavoring agents with differential cool (iced) flavors, and the quantities of specific free radicals within its generated aerosols can be determined through GC–MS and EPR Spectroscopy, respectively. These assays can be used to understand how the physicochemical interactions inside an e-liquid undergoing thermal degradation contribute to differential ROS generation among different flavors. Further, in conjunction with the recommended future studies, the results of our preliminary study can generate evidence used in favor of public health and regulatory policies that lead to the regulation of products, such as vape bars and other flavored/non-flavored ENDS.

Author Contributions: Conceptualization, T.M. and I.R.; methodology, T.M.; assay performance: S.Y. software, S.Y.; validation, S.Y., T.M. and I.R.; formal analysis, S.Y.; investigation, S.Y.; resources, I.R.; data curation, S.Y.; writing—original draft preparation, S.Y.; writing—review and editing, S.Y., T.M. and I.R.; visualization, S.Y.; supervision, I.R.; project administration, I.R.; funding acquisition, I.R. All authors have read and agreed to the published version of the manuscript.

Funding: This research was supported by our TCORS Grant: CRoFT 1 U54 CA228110-01.

Institutional Review Board Statement: All experiments performed in this study were approved and in accordance with the University of Rochester Institutional Biosafety Committee. Additionally all protocols, procedures, and data analysis in this study followed the NIH guidelines and standards of reproducibility and scientific rigor by an unbiased approach. (Biosafety Study approval

#Rahman/102054/09-167/07-186; identification code: 07-186; date of approval: 01/05/2019). No animals or human subjects were used.

Informed Consent Statement: Not applicable as study did not involve humans.

Data Availability Statement: We declare that we have provided all the data in figures.

Acknowledgments: Figure 1 and the Graphical Abstract were made using BioRender; each image (except the colored e-cigarette bars) was created from scratch using an original design concept. Regarding the images of the colored e-cigarette bars used in the Graphical Abstract and Figure 1, those were created using Adobe Illustrator from scratch using an original design concept. All stock images used in Figure 1 and the Graphical Abstract were stock images directly from BioRender, with the exception of the "Minty leaves" stock image used in the graphical abstract. The "Minty leaves" image used in the graphical abstract was an Adobe Stock image which was purchased and subsequently downloaded (purchased with a standard license which includes using the stock image in a publication).

Conflicts of Interest: The authors declare no conflict of interest.

References

1. Wang, T.W.; Neff, L.J.; Park-Lee, E.; Ren, C.; Cullen, K.A.; King, B.A. E-Cigarette Use Among Middle and High School Students—United States. *Mmwr-Morb. Mortal. Wkly. Rep.* **2020**, *69*, 1310–1312. [CrossRef] [PubMed]
2. Rehan, H.S.; Maini, J.; Hungin, A.P.S. Vaping versus Smoking: A Quest for Efficacy and Safety of E-cigarette. *Curr. Drug Saf.* **2018**, *13*, 92–101. [CrossRef]
3. Zhao, J.; Zhang, Y.; Sisler, J.D.; Shaffer, J.; Leonard, S.S.; Morris, A.M.; Qian, Y.; Bello, D.; Demokritou, P. Assessment of Reactive Oxygen Species Generated By Electronic Cigarettes Using Acellular and Cellular Approaches. *J. Hazard. Mater.* **2018**, *344*, 549–557. [CrossRef] [PubMed]
4. Yao, H.; Rahman, I. Current concepts on oxidative/carbonyl stress, inflammation and epigenetics in pathogenesis of chronic obstructive pulmonary disease. *Toxicol. Appl. Pharmacol.* **2011**, *254*, 72–85. [CrossRef] [PubMed]
5. Son, Y.; Mishin, V.; Laskin, J.D.; Mainelis, G.; Wackowski, O.A.; Delnevo, C.; Schwander, S.; Khlystov, A.; Samburova, V.; Meng, Q. Hydroxyl Radicals in E-Cigarette Vapor and E-Vapor Oxidative Potentials under Different Vaping Patterns. *Chem. Res. Toxicol.* **2019**, *32*, 1087–1095. [CrossRef] [PubMed]
6. Schieber, M.; Chandel, N.S. ROS Function in Redox Signaling and Oxidative Stress. *Curr. Biol.* **2014**, *24*, R453–R462. [CrossRef]
7. Mittal, M.; Siddiqui, M.R.; Tran, K.; Reddy, S.P.; Malik, A.B. Reactive Oxygen Species in Inflammation and Tissue Injury. *Antioxid. Redox. Signal.* **2014**, *20*, 1126–1167. [CrossRef] [PubMed]
8. Goldkorn, T.; Filosto, S.; Chung, S. Lung Injury and Lung Cancer Caused by Cigarette Smoke-Induced Oxidative Stress: Molecular Mechanisms and Therapeutic Opportunities Involving the ceramide-Generating Machinery and epidermal Growth Factor Receptor. *Antioxid. Redox. Signal.* **2014**, *21*, 2149–2174. [CrossRef]
9. Sundar, I.K.; Mullapudi, N.; Yao, H.; Spivack, S.D.; Rahman, I. Lung cancer and its association with chronic obstructive pulmonary disease: Update on nexus of epigenetics. *Curr. Opin. Pulm. Med.* **2011**, *17*, 279–285. [CrossRef]
10. Lerner, C.A.; Sundar, I.K.; Yao, H.; Gerloff, J.; Ossip, D.J.; McIntosh, S.; Robinson, R.; Rahman, I. Vapors Produced by Electronic Cigarettes and E-Juices with flavorings Induce Toxicity, Oxidative Stress, and Inflammatory Response in Lung Epithelial Cells and in Mouse Lung. *PLoS ONE* **2015**, *10*, e0116732. [CrossRef]
11. Soneji, S.; Bond, T.; Mason, P. Association between Initial Use of e-Cigarettes and Subsequent Cigarette Smoking among Adolescents and Young Adults: A Systematic Review and Meta-analysis. *JAMA Pediatr.* **2017**, *171*, 788–797. [CrossRef] [PubMed]
12. Djordjevic, M.V.; Doran, K.A. Nicotine Content and Delivery across Tobacco Products. *Handb. Exp. Pharmacol.* **2009**, *4*, 61–82.
13. Grant, J.E.; Lust, K.; Fridberg, D.J.; King, A.C.; Chamberlain, S.R. E-Cigarette Use (Vaping) is Associated with Illicit Drug Use, Mental Health Problems, and Impulsivity in University Students. *Ann. Clin. Psychiatry.* **2019**, *31*, 27–35.
14. Jankowski, M.; Krzystanek, M.; Zejda, J.E.; Majek, P.; Lubanski, J.; Lawson, J.A.; Brozek, G. E-Cigarettes are More Addictive than Traditional Cigarettes-A Study in Highly Educated Young People. *Int. J. Environ. Res. Public. Health* **2019**, *16*, 2279. [CrossRef] [PubMed]
15. Leventhal, A.; Dai, H.; Barrington-Trimis, J.; Sussman, S. 'Ice' flavoured e-cigarette use among young adults. *Tob. Control.* **2021**. [CrossRef] [PubMed]
16. Lawyer, G.R.; Jackson, M.; Prinz, M.; Lamb, T.; Wang, Q.; Muthumalage, T.; Rahman, I. Classification of Flavors in Cigarillos and Little Cigars and Their Variable Cellular and Acellular Oxidative and Cytotoxic Responses. *PLoS ONE* **2019**, *14*, e0226066. [CrossRef] [PubMed]
17. Muthumalage, T.; Prinz, M.; Ansah, K.O.; Gerloff, J.; Sundar, I.K.; Rahman, I. Inflammatory and Oxidative Responses Induced by Exposure to Commonly Used e-Cigarette Flavoring Chemicals and Flavored e-Liquids without Nicotine. *Front. Physiol.* **2017**, *8*, 1130. [CrossRef] [PubMed]
18. Bitzer, Z.T.; Goel, R.; Reilly, S.M.; Foulds, J.; Muscat, J.; Elias, R.J.; Richie, J.P., Jr. Effects of Solvent and Temperature on Free Radical Formation in Electronic Cigarette Aerosols. *Chem. Res. Toxicol.* **2018**, *31*, 4–12. [CrossRef]

19. Haddad, C.; Salman, R.; El-Hellani, A.; Talih, S.; Shihadeh, A.; Saliba, N.A. Reactive Oxygen Species Emissions from Supra- and Sub-Ohm Electronic Cigarettes. *J. Anal. Toxicol.* **2019**, *43*, 45–50. [CrossRef]
20. Hiler, M.; Karaoghlanian, N.; Talih, S.; Maloney, S.; Breland, A.; Shihadeh, A.; Eissenberg, T. Effects of Electronic Cigarette Heating Coil Resistance and Liquid Nicotine Concentration on User Nicotine Delivery, Heart Rate, Subjective Effects, Puff Topography, and Liquid Consumption. *Exp. Clin. Psychopharmacol.* **2020**, *28*, 527–539. [CrossRef]
21. Omaiye, E.E.; Luo, W.; McWhirter, K.J.; Pankow, J.F. Flavour chemicals, synthetic coolants and pulegone in popular mint-flavoured and menthol-flavoured e-cigarettes. *Tob. Control* **2021**, 1–7. [CrossRef]
22. Jabba, S.V.; Erythropel, H.C.; Torres, D.G.; Delgado, L.A.; Anastas, P.T.; Zimmerman, J.B.; Jordt, S.-E. Synthetic Cooling Agents in US-marketed E-cigarette Refill Liquids and Disposable E-cigarettes: Chemical Analysis and Risk Assessment. *bioRxiv* **2021**. [CrossRef]
23. Kaur, G.; Muthumalage, T.; Rahman, I. Mechanisms of toxicity and biomarkers of flavoring and flavor enhancing chemicals in emerging tobacco and non-tobacco products. *Toxicol. Lett.* **2018**, *288*, 143–155. [CrossRef]
24. Kaur, G.; Gaurav, A.; Lamb, T.; Perkins, M.; Muthumalage, T.; Rahman, I. Current Perspectives on Characteristics, Compositions, and Toxicological Effects of E-Cigarettes Containing Tobacco and Menthol/Mint Flavors. *Front. Physiol.* **2020**, *11*, 613948. [CrossRef]
25. Szafran, B.N.; Pinkston, R.; Perveen, Z.; Ross, M.K.; Morgan, T.; Paulsen, D.B.; Penn, A.L.; Kaplan, B.L.F.; Noël, A. Electronic-Cigarette Vehicles and Flavoring Affect Lung Function and Immune Responses in a Murine Model. *Int. J. Mol. Sci.* **2020**, *21*, 6022. [CrossRef] [PubMed]

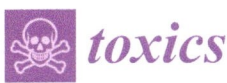

Article

Cross-Sectional Associations of Smoking and E-cigarette Use with Self-Reported Diagnosed Hypertension: Findings from Wave 3 of the Population Assessment of Tobacco and Health Study

Connor R. Miller [1,*], Hangchuan Shi [2,3], Dongmei Li [2] and Maciej L. Goniewicz [1]

1. Roswell Park Comprehensive Cancer Center, Department of Health Behavior, Buffalo, NY 14263, USA; maciej.goniewicz@roswellpark.org
2. Department of Clinical & Translational Research, University of Rochester Medical Center, Rochester, NY 14627, USA; hangchuan_shi@urmc.rochester.edu (H.S.); dongmei_li@urmc.rochester.edu (D.L.)
3. Department of Public Health Sciences, University of Rochester Medical Center, Rochester, NY 14627, USA
* Correspondence: connor.miller@roswellpark.org

Citation: Miller, C.R.; Shi, H.; Li, D.; Goniewicz, M.L. Cross-Sectional Associations of Smoking and E-cigarette Use with Self-Reported Diagnosed Hypertension: Findings from Wave 3 of the Population Assessment of Tobacco and Health Study. *Toxics* **2021**, *9*, 52. https://doi.org/10.3390/toxics9030052

Academic Editor: Peter Franklin

Received: 3 December 2020
Accepted: 5 March 2021
Published: 9 March 2021

Publisher's Note: MDPI stays neutral with regard to jurisdictional claims in published maps and institutional affiliations.

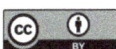

Copyright: © 2021 by the authors. Licensee MDPI, Basel, Switzerland. This article is an open access article distributed under the terms and conditions of the Creative Commons Attribution (CC BY) license (https://creativecommons.org/licenses/by/4.0/).

Abstract: Following their introduction a decade ago, electronic cigarettes (e-cigarettes) have grown in popularity. Given their novelty, knowledge of the health consequences of e-cigarette use remains limited. Epidemiologic studies have not comprehensively explored associations between e-cigarette use and hypertension, a highly prevalent health condition and major contributor to cardiovascular disease burden. In this study, cross-sectional associations of cigarette smoking and e-cigarette use (vaping) with self-reported diagnosed hypertension were evaluated among 19,147 18–55 year old respondents in Wave 3 (2015–2016) of the Population Assessment of Tobacco and Health Study. Multivariable analyses first modeled smoking and vaping as separate 2-category variables, then as a 6-category composite variable accounting for former smoking. After adjusting for potential confounders, current vaping (aOR = 1.31; 95%CI: 1.05–1.63) and current smoking (aOR = 1.27; 95%CI: 1.10–1.47) were both associated with higher odds of hypertension. In analyses modeling smoking and vaping compositely, respondents who were concurrently smoking and vaping had the highest odds of hypertension (aOR = 1.77; 95%CI: 1.32–2.39 [referent: never smokers]). These results differ somewhat from prior epidemiologic studies of vaping and respiratory outcomes, which consistently report smaller point estimates for current vaping than for current smoking. Our findings reinforce the uncertainty surrounding long-term health consequences of vaping, as well as highlight important distinctions between respiratory and cardiovascular outcomes when considering the harm reduction potential of e-cigarettes.

Keywords: tobacco; e-cigarettes; smoking; hypertension; epidemiology

1. Introduction

Tobacco's status as a leading cause of preventable disease and premature mortality spans many decades [1]. While intense focus from researchers and policy makers has contributed substantially to recent decreases in use [2], tobacco remains a major public health concern: in 2017, an estimated 7.1 million deaths and the loss of 182 million disability-adjusted life years were attributed to tobacco use across the globe [3]. Notably, the vast majority of tobacco-related death and morbidity are caused by smoke from combusted tobacco products [4], which contains numerous cardiovascular toxicants [5]. A seminal 2005 publication estimated that 1 in 10 deaths from cardiovascular disease (CVD) could be attributed to tobacco smoking in the year 2000 [6], reinforcing the importance of smoking as a modifiable risk factor in efforts to reduce global burden of CVD.

In light of the detriment caused by smoking tobacco, electronic cigarettes (e-cigarettes) were developed as alternatives to combusted cigarettes in the late 2000s. E-cigarettes encompass a range of devices which heat and aerosolize a solution that typically contains nicotine and a mixture of propylene glycol, glycerin and various flavoring additives. Laboratory studies have shown that the amount and concentration of toxicants in e-cigarette aerosol are substantially lower than in cigarette smoke [7–9]. As such, e-cigarettes are often promoted as potentially-modified risk products compared with cigarettes, and the majority of adult e-cigarette users (vapers) are current or former cigarette smokers, many of whom reference 'quitting smoking' as a primary reason for initiating use [10].

The potential public health implications of smokers fully transitioning away from cigarettes in favor of vaping are still not well understood. Knowledge regarding associations between vaping and a multitude of clinical health outcomes, including cardiovascular conditions, is currently limited. A handful of published studies have examined cross-sectional associations between CVD and vaping in large free-living samples of the US adult population [11–14]. Conflicting results have been reported, and the topic has incurred contentious debate, particularly surrounding methodological decisions regarding confounding of the association by history of cigarette smoking among adult e-cigarette users.

Notably, epidemiological studies have yet to examine associations between vaping and important clinical risk factors of CVD (i.e., diabetes mellitus, hypertension, hyperlipidemia), most of which are known to be adversely associated with smoking cigarettes. Of particular interest is hypertension, as it remains the leading risk factor for CVD worldwide, and for which an estimated 10.4 million deaths and 218 million disability-adjusted life years were attributed in 2017 [3]. Transient increases in systolic blood pressure have been observed following an acute bout of vaping in humans [15], while accelerated aortic stiffness and abnormal vascular inflammation have been reported after substantial exposure to e-cigarette aerosols in mice and in vitro studies, respectively [16,17], both of which could contribute to the development of hypertension if confirmed in humans [18]. Likewise, cigarette smoking causes a short-term spike in blood pressure [19], while its adverse impact on endothelial function, vascular injury, and arterial compliance suggest a potential role in hypertension pathogenesis [20]. However, epidemiological studies of associations between smoking and chronic blood pressure alterations have reported mixed findings, with some publications observing a higher and others a lower risk of hypertension among habitual cigarette smokers compared to never smokers [21].

Given the equivocal state of evidence for cigarette smoking and a lack of evidence for vaping, the present study evaluated cross-sectional associations of vaping and cigarette smoking with self-reported hypertension in a nationally representative sample of US adults, with a focus on young and middle-aged adults. Multiple statistical modeling approaches were employed in an attempt to scrutinize the association between vaping and hypertension independently from cigarette smoking, as well as approximating cumulative exposure to both products together.

2. Materials and Methods

2.1. Study Population

The present study analyzed data from the Wave 3 Population Assessment of Tobacco and Health (PATH) Study public use files (available at: https://www.icpsr.umich.edu/web/NAHDAP/studies/36498/datadocumentation (accessed on 8 March 2021)). The PATH Study is a nationally representative prospective cohort study evaluating tobacco use behaviors, perceptions, and tobacco-related health outcomes among youth and adults in the United States [22]. The PATH Study utilized a four-stage stratified area probability sampling method to assemble the baseline cohort, with a two-phase design for sampling adults at the final stage. Additional information regarding study design and methodology has been published [23].

Initial data collection for Wave 1 occurred between September 2013 and December 2014. The Wave 1 weighted recruitment rate was 54.0%, of which 74.0% completed the survey, resulting in a baseline cohort containing 32,320 adult respondents (age 18+ years). Subsequent waves of data were collected from October 2014 to October 2015 (Wave 2;

n = 28,362 adults) and again from October 2015 to October 2016 (Wave 3; n = 28,148 adults). The weighted response rates at Wave 2 and Wave 3 were 83.2% and 78.4%, respectively.

Compared to older adults, (a) hypertension is less widespread and (b) survival bias and reverse causality are less likely to influence associations of interest in this study. Therefore, our primary analyses focused on young and middle-aged adults (18–54 years) at Wave 3 (n excluded for being 55+ years = 6095). In primary analyses, we further excluded respondents who were current-established users (i.e., had ever used a specified product fairly regularly and currently use every day or some days) of 'other' tobacco products: traditional cigars, hookah, cigarillos, filtered cigars, pipes, snus, or smokeless tobacco (additional n excluded = 2906). This left an analytic sample of n = 19,147.

2.2. Assessment of Hypertension

The outcome of interest for this analysis was self-reported diagnosed hypertension. At Wave 1, PATH respondents were asked "Has a doctor, nurse or other health professional ever told you that you had high blood pressure?", and at Waves 2 and 3 they were asked "In the past 12 months, has a doctor, nurse or other health professional told you that you had high blood pressure?". Wave 3 respondents who reported ever being diagnosed with high blood pressure were subsequently asked "In the past 12 months, has your high blood pressure been under control?". Those who selected *yes* or *no* to this question were classified as having hypertension, while those who selected *never had high blood pressure* were re-classified as not having hypertension (See Figure S1 for additional details).

2.3. Assessment of Smoking and Vaping Status

Separate binary variables were defined for current smoking and current vaping. Current vapers had ever used e-cigarettes, ever used them fairly regularly, and currently used them every day or some days. Current smokers had smoked at least 100 cigarettes in a lifetime, and currently smoked every day or some days. Furthermore, integrating the category of former smokers (smoked 100 cigarettes in their lifetime, but did not currently smoke on an everyday or someday basis at time of survey), we derived a composite smoking and vaping variable with six categories: (1) exclusive vapers who were never smokers, (2) exclusive vapers who were former smokers, (3) dual users, (4) exclusive smokers, (5) former smokers and (6) never smokers.

2.4. Assessment of Covariates

To control for potential confounding, the following variables were adjusted for in all primary multivariable analyses: age, sex, race-ethnicity, education, annual household income, insurance status, marital status, leisure-time physical activity, body mass index (BMI), heavy alcohol use, hypercholesterolemia, and diabetes mellitus. Leisure-time physical activity categories were defined according to the question "in a typical week, how many days do you do any physical activity or exercise of at least moderate intensity, such as brisk walking, bicycling or swimming at a regular pace?" (0 days/week, 1–3 days/week, ≥4 days/week). Heavy alcohol use was defined as having 5 or more alcoholic drinks in one day on 5 or more days in the past month. Hypercholesterolemia and diabetes mellitus were classified according to similar case-finding questions as the outcome variable (hypercholesterolemia: [a] "[Have you ever been told by/ In the past 12 months, has] . . . a doctor, nurse or other health professional told you that you had high cholesterol?", [b] "In the past 12 months, have you taken any medications to reduce cholesterol?"; diabetes: [a] "[Have you ever been told by/ In the past 12 months, has] . . . a doctor, nurse or other health professional that you have diabetes, sugar diabetes, high blood sugar, or borderline diabetes?" [b] "What type of diabetes do you have?"). All adjusted covariates were employed as categorical variables.

2.5. Statistical Analysis

Analyses were conducted using survey analysis procedures (i.e., *proc surveylogistic*) in SAS v9.4 (SAS Institute Inc., Cary, NC, USA), with a significance level for two-sided tests set at 0.05. The balanced repeated replication (BRR) method was used to form replicate weights in variance estimation to account for the complex sampling design in the cross-sectional PATH Wave 3 data. We used weighted frequency distributions and the Rao-Scott modified likelihood ratio test to examine weighted bivariate associations between covariates and current vaping and smoking status. Multivariable weighted logistic regression models estimated adjusted odds ratios (aORs) and 95% confidence intervals (CIs) for associations of vaping and smoking with hypertension. Two sets of primary multivariable analyses were conducted: first, modeling smoking and vaping as separate 2-category variables, then modeling smoking and vaping as a 6-category composite variable.

In sensitivity analyses (see supplement files), current users of 'other' tobacco products were re-introduced to the analytic sample. Two additional binary covariates controlling for current combusted (traditional cigars, hookah, cigarillos, filtered cigars, or pipes) and smokeless (snus or smokeless) tobacco use were incorporated into these multivariable logistic regression models. Missing data were handled as listwise deletions in multivariable models (details provided in Tables S2 and S3).

3. Results

Among the 19,147 PATH Wave 3 respondents included in the analytic sample, there were 1100 (3.7% [3.4–4.0]) current vapers and 5654 (19.5% [18.7–20.3]) current smokers (Table 1). Most current vapers were current or former smokers. Aside from insurance status, history of hypercholesterolemia, and history of diabetes mellitus, all other Table 1 characteristics were significantly associated with current vaping status (χ^2 $p < 0.05$). All Table 1 characteristics except BMI and history of diabetes mellitus were significantly associated with current smoking status (χ^2 $p < 0.05$). Table S1 shows descriptive statistics according to the six-category composite smoking and vaping variable. Over three-quarters of current exclusive vapers who never smoked were 18–24 years old, and almost half had a BMI <25 kg/m^2. The four categories comprised of current or former smokers were predominantly 35 years and older, while a clear majority had BMI >25 kg/m^2.

Overall, 17.3% (16.4–18.1) of respondents had self-reported hypertension in 2015–2016 (Table 1). Self-reported hypertension was higher among current vapers than those who were not current vapers, as well as among current smokers than those who were not current smokers. The prevalence of self-reported hypertension across composite smoking and vaping categories are presented in Figure 1. In pairwise comparisons, prevalence among never smokers and current exclusive vapers who had never smoked each differed from the other four categories.

Table 1. Descriptive statistics for the analytic sample overall, stratified by current vaping status, and stratified by current smoking status.

Characteristic	Overall Sample (n = 19,147)		Current Vaping Status				Current Smoking Status			
			No (n = 18,013)		Yes (n = 1100)		No (n = 13,481)		Yes (n = 5654)	
	n	% (95% CI)	n	% (95% CI)	n	% (95% CI)	n	% (95% CI)	n	% (95% CI)
Hypertension *†										
No	16,267	82.7 (81.9–83.6)	15,344	82.9 (82.0–83.7)	897	78.7 (75.8–81.3)	11,851	84.0 (83.0–84.9)	4404	77.4 (76.0–78.8)
Yes	2859	17.3 (16.4–18.1)	2650	17.1 (16.3–18.0)	201	21.3 (18.7–24.2)	1618	16.0 (15.1–17.0)	1241	22.6 (21.2–24.0)
Vaping status †										
Never vaper	16,040	91.3 (90.8–91.8)	—	—	—	—	11,968	95.6 (95.2–95.9)	4064	73.8 (72.2–75.4)
Former vaper	1565	5.0 (4.6–5.3)	—	—	—	—	618	2.3 (2.1–2.6)	946	15.9 (14.7–17.1)
Current vaper	1100	3.7 (3.4–4.0)	—	—	—	—	517	2.1 (1.8–2.4)	581	10.3 (9.4–11.3)
Smoking status *										
Never smoker	2832	16.2 (15.3–17.1)	10,227	66.3 (65.0–67.6)	184	12.9 (10.8–15.5)	—	—	—	—
Former smoker	10,426	64.3 (63.0–65.6)	2498	15.6 (14.7–16.5)	333	32.7 (29.4–36.2)	—	—	—	—
Current smoker	5654	19.5 (18.7–20.3)	5056	18.1 (17.4–18.9)	581	54.4 (50.4–58.2)	—	—	—	—
Age *†										
18–24 years	7238	18.7 (18.2–19.3)	6838	18.5 (17.9–19.1)	389	25.1 (22.5–28.0)	6154	20.2 (19.5–20.9)	1082	12.6 (11.7–13.5)
25–34 years	4985	27.3 (26.4–28.3)	4695	27.3 (26.3–28.3)	282	29.4 (26.6–32.3)	3265	26.6 (25.4–27.8)	1718	30.5 (28.9–32.1)
35–44 years	3549	26.0 (25.0–27.1)	3300	26.0 (25.0–27.1)	239	24.9 (22.3–27.7)	2133	25.5 (24.2–26.7)	1412	28.3 (26.8–29.9)
45–54 years	3375	27.9 (27.0–28.9)	3180	28.2 (27.3–29.1)	190	20.6 (17.9–23.7)	1929	27.7 (26.7–28.8)	1442	28.6 (27.3–30.1)
Sex *†										
Female	10,505	53.8 (53.1–54.5)	9951	54.1 (53.4–54.8)	538	44.9 (41.3–48.5)	7419	54.8 (53.9–55.6)	3081	49.7 (48.2–51.1)
Male	8626	46.2 (45.5–46.9)	8046	45.9 (45.2–46.6)	562	55.1 (51.5–58.7)	6048	45.2 (44.4–46.1)	2571	50.3 (48.9–51.8)
Race-ethnicity *†										
Non-Hispanic White	10,428	59.4 (58.7–60.1)	9627	58.8 (58.1–59.6)	786	76.0 (72.7–79.0)	6792	57.3 (56.4–58.1)	3632	68.7 (67.0–70.3)
Non-Hispanic Black	2674	11.6 (11.1–12.1)	2613	11.8 (11.3–12.4)	57	5.3 (4.0–7.0)	1968	11.6 (11.0–12.2)	703	11.7 (10.7–12.9)
Hispanic	4256	19.8 (19.2–20.4)	4083	20.1 (19.5–20.7)	161	11.5 (9.4–14.0)	3432	21.2 (20.5–22.0)	820	13.6 (12.6–14.6)
Non-Hispanic Other	1580	9.2 (8.6–9.7)	1485	9.3 (8.7–9.8)	94	7.2 (5.4–9.4)	1162	9.9 (9.3–10.6)	417	6.0 (5.3–6.8)
Annual household income *†										
≥USD 50,000	6793	48.3 (47.0–49.5)	6449	48.7 (47.5–50.0)	340	37.1 (33.8–40.6)	5402	52.8 (51.5–54.2)	1388	29.7 (27.8–31.5)
<USD 50,000	11,045	51.7 (50.5–53.0)	10,331	51.3 (50.0–52.5)	689	62.9 (59.4–66.2)	7043	47.2 (45.8–48.5)	3994	70.3 (68.5–72.2)
Education status *†										
Bachelors and beyond	4085	30.9 (30.2–31.5)	3949	31.5 (30.8–32.2)	133	14.4 (11.9–17.3)	3514	35.4 (34.6–36.2)	570	11.8 (10.6–13.3)
Some college	6812	33.0 (32.2–33.8)	6309	32.6 (31.8–33.4)	496	45.5 (42.1–48.9)	4792	32.5 (31.6–33.4)	2019	35.3 (33.8–36.9)
High school or less	8166	36.1 (35.4–36.8)	7681	35.9 (35.2–36.7)	463	40.1 (36.6–43.7)	5122	32.1 (31.2–33.1)	3035	52.8 (51.1–54.5)
Leisure-time physical activity *†										
≥4 days/week	7638	38.2 (37.0–39.3)	7191	38.1 (37.0–39.3)	439	39.1 (35.8–42.5)	5477	38.1 (36.7–39.5)	2156	38.3 (36.7–40.0)
1–3 days/week	8427	46.5 (45.4–47.6)	7953	46.6 (45.5–47.7)	457	42.2 (38.8–45.7)	6191	48.2 (46.9–49.4)	2233	39.5 (38.0–41.0)
0 days/week	3015	15.3 (14.6–16.1)	2808	15.2 (14.5–16.0)	199	18.6 (15.9–21.7)	1773	13.7 (12.8–14.6)	1239	22.2 (20.9–23.4)
Body mass index *										
<18.5 kg/m^2	528	2.2 (2.0–2.5)	494	2.2 (2.0–2.4)	32	2.6 (1.7–3.9)	381	2.2 (1.9–2.5)	146	2.4 (2.0–2.8)
18.5–24.9 kg/m^2	6975	33.5 (32.4–34.6)	6559	33.4 (32.4–34.6)	409	35.1 (31.7–38.7)	5086	33.6 (32.3–34.8)	1888	33.2 (31.8–34.6)
25.0–29.9 kg/m^2	5469	31.9 (30.8–33.1)	5183	32.2 (31.0–33.3)	273	26.1 (23.3–29.0)	3828	32.0 (30.7–33.4)	1638	31.5 (30.1–33.0)
≥30 kg/m^2	5636	32.4 (31.2–33.5)	5259	32.2 (31.0–33.4)	367	36.2 (32.8–39.8)	3810	32.2 (30.9–33.6)	1824	32.9 (31.3–34.4)
Heavy alcohol use *†										
No	17,920	95.3 (94.8–95.7)	16,901	95.5 (95.0–95.9)	990	90.9 (88.8–92.6)	12,922	96.8 (96.4–97.2)	4988	88.8 (87.7–89.9)
Yes	1111	4.7 (4.3–5.2)	1008	4.5 (4.1–5.0)	98	9.1 (7.4–11.2)	510	3.2 (2.8–3.6)	600	11.2 (10.1–12.3)
Insurance status †										
Insured	15,495	85.0 (84.2–85.8)	14,587	85.1 (84.2–85.9)	889	83.0 (80.2–85.5)	11230	87.2 (86.3–88.1)	4260	75.9 (74.3–77.4)
Uninsured	3452	15.0 (14.2–15.8)	3240	14.9 (14.1–15.8)	199	17.0 (14.5–19.8)	2100	12.8 (11.9–13.7)	1345	24.1 (22.6–25.7)
Marital status *†										
Married	6393	49.9 (48.8–51.1)	6034	50.5 (49.3–51.6)	346	34.6 (31.4–38.0)	4561	53.4 (52.1–54.6)	1830	35.6 (33.6–37.6)
Widowed, divorced or separated	2378	13.4 (12.7–14.2)	2196	13.2 (12.4–14.1)	176	18.9 (16.4–21.7)	1086	10.8 (10.0–11.6)	1289	24.6 (23.1–26.1)
Never married	10,150	36.6 (35.7–37.6)	9570	36.3 (35.3–37.3)	566	46.5 (43.0–50.0)	7692	35.9 (34.8–37.0)	2451	39.8 (37.9–41.8)
Hyperlipidemia †										
No	16,867	84.3 (83.4–85.1)	15,891	84.2 (83.4–85.0)	947	85.3 (82.9–87.5)	12,089	84.5 (83.6–85.5)	4768	83.1 (82.0–84.1)
Yes	2277	15.7 (14.9–16.6)	2120	15.8 (15.0–16.6)	152	14.7 (12.5–17.1)	1390	15.5 (14.5–16.4)	885	16.9 (15.9–18.0)
Diabetes mellitus										
No	17,784	91.5 (90.8–92.1)	16,750	91.5 (90.8–92.2)	1005	91.1 (88.7–93.0)	12,655	91.6 (90.8–92.4)	5119	90.9 (90.0–91.7)
Yes	1336	8.5 (7.9–9.2)	1240	8.5 (7.8–9.2)	91	8.9 (7.0–11.3)	815	8.4 (7.6–9.2)	519	9.1 (8.3–10.0)

Reported statistics (other than frequencies) represent weighted values according to PATH Study specifications. Due to some missing data points, subgroup frequencies do not all add up to the full analytic sample (n = 19,147). Details provided in supplement file. * Indicates Rao-Scott χ^2 test $p < 0.05$ comparing current vaper v. never/former vaper. † Indicates Rao-Scott χ^2 test $p < 0.05$ comparing current smoker v. never/former smoker. CI = confidence interval.

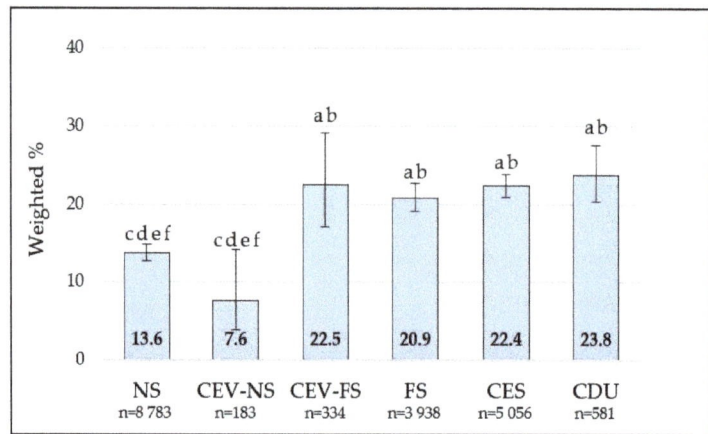

Figure 1. Prevalence of self-reported hypertension according to smoking and vaping status. NS = never smoker; CEV-NS = current exclusive vaper who never smoked; CEV-FS = current exclusive vaper who formerly smoked; FS = former smoker; CES = current exclusive smoker; CDU = current dual user. Superscript letters indicate significant differences during Bonferroni-adjusted pairwise comparisons: a = NS; b = CEV-NS; c = CEV-FS; d = FS; e = CES; f = CDU.

Table 2 displays multivariable results for weighted logistic regression modeling smoking and vaping as separate risk factors. Following adjustment for relevant sociodemographic factors, health behaviors, and clinical variables, current smokers had 27% higher odds of hypertension than those who were not, and current vapers had 31% higher odds of hypertension than those who were not. Relationships between established risk factors for hypertension were as expected, with particularly strong associations seen for age, BMI, hyperlipidemia and diabetes mellitus.

Table 2. Prevalence of hypertension and multivariable odds for hypertension among the analytic sample, modeling current smoking and vaping as separate variables.

Variable		Prevalence of Hypertension		Multivariable Odds of Hypertension
	n	Cases	% (95% CI)	aOR (95% CI)
Current vaper				
No	18,013	2650	17.1 (16.3–18.0)	REF
Yes	1100	201	21.3 (18.7–24.2)	1.31 (1.05–1.63)
Current smoker				
No	13,481	1618	16.0 (15.1–17.0)	REF
Yes	5654	1241	22.6 (21.2–24.0)	1.27 (1.10–1.47)
Age				
18–24 years	7238	310	4.5 (3.8–5.1)	REF
25–34 years	4985	573	10.9 (9.7–12.2)	2.33 (1.82–2.99)
35–44 years	3549	798	18.3 (16.8–19.9)	3.58 (2.82–4.55)
45–54 years	3375	1178	31.1 (29.2–33.0)	6.19 (4.90–7.83)
Sex				
Female	10,505	1465	15.2 (14.1–16.4)	REF
Male	8626	1393	19.7 (18.4–20.9)	1.60 (1.39–1.85)
Race-ethnicity				
Non-Hispanic White	10,428	1538	17.6 (16.4–18.8)	REF
Non-Hispanic Black	2674	581	26.1 (24.0–28.4)	1.56 (1.32–1.84)
Hispanic	4256	452	12.8 (11.4–14.3)	0.67 (0.54–0.82)
Non-Hispanic Other	1580	230	12.4 (10.1–15.0)	0.95 (0.72–1.24)

Table 2. Cont.

Variable		Prevalence of Hypertension		Multivariable Odds of Hypertension
	n	Cases	% (95% CI)	aOR (95% CI)
Annual household income				
≥USD 50,000	6793	927	15.7 (14.3–17.3)	REF
<USD 50,000	11,045	1801	19.2 (18.1–20.5)	1.32 (1.09–1.60)
Education status				
Bachelors and beyond	4085	557	13.9 (12.4–15.7)	REF
Some college	6812	1069	18.1 (16.9–19.5)	1.10 (0.92–1.32)
High school or less	8166	1223	19.3 (18.1–20.5)	1.08 (0.89–1.33)
Insurance status				
Insured	15,495	2437	18.0 (17.0–19.0)	REF
Uninsured	3452	400	13.4 (12.0–15.0)	0.70 (0.58–0.85)
Marital status				
Married	6393	1208	18.0 (16.8–19.3)	REF
Widowed, divorced or separated	2378	648	26.0 (23.6–28.6)	1.26 (1.01–1.57)
Never married	10,150	960	12.9 (11.9–13.9)	1.23 (1.04–1.45)
Leisure-time physical activity				
≥4 days/week	7638	953	15.3 (14.1–16.5)	REF
1–3 days/week	8427	1244	16.5 (15.5–17.6)	0.92 (0.80–1.07)
0 days/week	3015	651	24.3 (22.2–26.5)	1.18 (0.98–1.42)
Body mass index				
<18.5 kg/m^2	528	26	5.9 (3.3–10.2)	REF
18.5–24.9 kg/m^2	6975	420	6.6 (5.8–7.5)	1.10 (0.52–2.34)
25.0–29.9 kg/m^2	5469	790	15.4 (14.2–16.7)	1.98 (0.95–4.13)
≥30 kg/m^2	5636	1527	30.5 (28.9–32.2)	4.11 (1.98–8.55)
Heavy alcohol use				
No	17,920	2629	17.0 (16.2–17.9)	REF
Yes	1111	211	21.4 (18.4–24.8)	1.33 (1.01–1.75)
Hypercholesterolemia				
No	16,867	1797	12.5 (11.8–13.3)	REF
Yes	2277	1062	42.6 (39.3–45.9)	2.85 (2.36–3.45)
Diabetes mellitus				
No	17,784	2163	13.9 (13.1–14.8)	REF
Yes	1336	683	52.2 (47.9–56.4)	2.95 (2.39–3.65)

Reported statistics (other than frequencies) represent weighted values according to PATH Study specifications. Due to missing data points, subgroup frequencies do not all add up to the full analytic sample (n = 19,147). Details provided in supplement file. aOR = adjusted odds ratio; CI = confidence interval.

Multivariable results from modeling smoking and vaping as a composite variable are shown in Figure 2. Former smokers, current exclusive smokers, and current dual users had 28%, 36%, and 77% higher odds of hypertension than never smokers, respectively. No significant differences were observed in the odds of hypertension with former smokers or current exclusive smokers as the referent group. Point estimates in Figure 2 analyses were generally higher for current vapers who formerly smoked than for those who never smoked, but no statistically significant findings were observed.

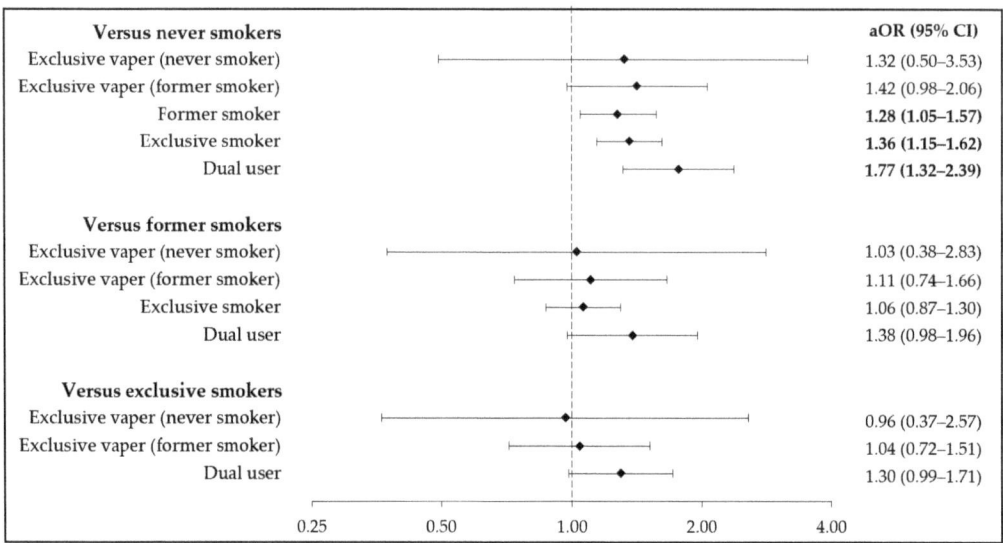

Figure 2. Multivariable odds for hypertension among the analytic sample, modeling smoking and vaping as a composite variable. All results come from weighted logistic regression models controlling for age, race-ethnicity, sex, annual household income, education, leisure-time physical activity, BMI, heavy alcohol use, insurance status, marital status, hypercholesterolemia, and diabetes mellitus. aOR = adjusted odds ratio; CI = confidence interval.

4. Discussion

In this nationally representative cross-sectional study of US adults aged 18–54 years, both current vaping and current smoking were significantly associated with self-reported diagnosed hypertension when modeled as separate parameters and controlling for potential confounding variables. The strength of association was similarly modest for both factors: current vapers had 31% higher odds of hypertension than those who did not currently vape, while current smokers had 27% higher odds of hypertension than those who did not currently smoke. Additionally, when modeling a combined smoking and vaping variable that accounted for former smoking, current dual users had 77% higher odds of hypertension, while current exclusive smokers had 36% higher odds. Although the small number of vapers in the analytic sample limited statistical power upon additional stratification, the association between current exclusive vaping and hypertension appeared slightly stronger among those who formerly smoked.

This was the first epidemiologic study to comprehensively evaluate the association between vaping and hypertension in an adult sample. Vaping is most common among three distinct groups of individuals: (a) youth and young adults, many of whom have never been habitual cigarette smokers, (b) adult current smokers who are interested in quitting, and (c) adult former smokers who have successfully quit smoking but continue vaping in place of cigarettes [24,25]. Whereas adult current and former smokers are often interested in using e-cigarettes to reduce harmful effects of smoking [26], this is clearly not the case for tobacco-naïve vapers. Therefore, it is important to evaluate potential harms of vaping on both an absolute level as well as relative to smoking cigarettes. Under the assumption that these cross-sectional results can be extrapolated to approximate risk estimates, our findings would suggest both vaping and smoking have a similar detrimental influence on blood pressure regulation, while utility of e-cigarettes for harm reduction in smokers may be limited with respect to hypertension. However, this interpretation should be met with scrutiny; even the most adept cross-sectional studies are ill-suited for causal inference. Specific to this study, data from earlier waves of the PATH Study have indicated that e-cigarette use is frequently a transient phase [27], whereas cigarette smoking is more persistent. Combined with the recency of e-cigarettes in the marketplace, differential levels in cumulative exposure to the two products is important to note when interpreting prevalence odds ratios [28]. Furthermore, even when attempting to control for former smoking in our models, some level of residual confounding is likely among current exclusive vapers due to varying levels of lifetime exposure to cigarette smoking (e.g., some current exclusive vapers had smoked 'a pack a day' for 20 years and just recently quit, others had quit smoking 5 years ago). The possibility of reverse causality playing a role in our results also cannot be dismissed, as smokers with prevalent hypertension might be more interested in switching to vaping than someone who has not been diagnosed with hypertension.

Even with these limitations in mind, our findings are concerning from a public health perspective. Hypertension is a relatively common condition [29] and plays a causative role in the pathogenesis of atherosclerosis [30]. As such, it remains a leading cause of disease burden worldwide [3,31], and even minor differences in disease risk would have significant ramifications at the population level [32]. That current dual users had the highest odds of hypertension is unsurprising, given previous research indicating higher rather than lower exposure to toxicants among current dual users compared with current exclusive smokers [33]. Our results comparing current vaping with current smoking are especially interesting, as previous cross-sectional studies have also observed similar point estimates for current smoking and current vaping when evaluating associations with major adverse cardiovascular endpoints (e.g., stroke, myocardial infarction) [11,13,14]. This contrasts with cross-sectional studies of respiratory outcomes (e.g., asthma, COPD, chronic wheezing), which have reported relatively smaller point estimates for current vaping than for current smoking [34–36]. Two recent studies have also examined inflammatory biomarkers relevant to cardiovascular health, observing similar levels among exclusive vapers and non-tobacco users while exclusive smokers and dual users had higher levels [37,38]. Additionally, while our analysis evaluated hypertension solely as an outcome variable, the potential for vaping to act synergistically with blood pressure in influencing overall cardiovascular risk is plausible and important to consider in future studies. This has been the prevailing hypothesis for the relationship between smoking and blood pressure for some time [39–41].

4.1. Previous Research on Vaping and Blood Pressure

4.1.1. Absolute Harms

Given the recency of e-cigarettes, the long-term health effects of vaping remain unclear. Thus far, evidence supporting a hypothetical role for vaping in hypertension development primarily stems from animal models. A handful of mechanisms have been established in studies of mice regularly exposed to high levels of e-cigarette emissions. These include overactivation of the renin–angiotensin–aldosterone system via vaping-induced increases in circulating levels of inflammatory cytokines [42] and heightened aortic pulse wave velocity via vaping-induced increases in aortic stiffness [16]. Additionally, human experimental studies have evaluated the acute blood pressure response to vaping in small samples of adult current vapers. A recent meta-analysis of these studies reported mean increases of 2.0 mmHg for both systolic blood pressure and diastolic blood pressure following vaping sessions of 5–30 minutes in duration [15]. Only one of the studies included in the meta-analysis reported on longevity of vaping-induced blood pressure elevations: following a five minute vaping session, systolic blood pressure returned to baseline levels after an average of 25 minutes at resting (diastolic blood pressure was not measured) [43]. With regard to the chronic blood pressure adaptations which characterize hypertension, the applicability of these studies is uncertain; similar acute blood pressure responses are observed for other exposures including physical activity, which is known to be protective against hypertension development [44,45].

4.1.2. Relative Harms

While knowledge of the absolute harms of e-cigarettes remains limited, there have been some randomized controlled trials (RCTs) that provide valuable insight towards the relative harms of vaping compared to smoking, including two that explored blood pressure as a secondary outcome. The ECLAT study was a 1-year smoking cessation trial where adult smokers were given one of three e-cigarettes of varying nicotine concentrations with the aim of quitting smoking. Among respondents who fully abstained from smoking from week 12 to the end of follow up (n = 18), no significant changes in systolic blood pressure were observed for baseline normotensive participants (systolic blood pressure < 130 mmHg and diastolic blood pressure < 85 mmHg), while those with baseline elevated blood pressure saw an average 16.3 (standard deviation: ±11.3) mmHg reduction in systolic blood pressure [46]. In the more recent VESUVIUS trial, adult smokers were randomized to a control group (continued smoking; n = 47) or one of two e-cigarette intervention arms, one group transitioning to nicotine-containing e-cigarettes (n = 37) and the other to nicotine-free e-cigarettes (n = 37). After a 4-week follow up, the mean change in systolic blood pressure differed significantly across the 3 arms: continued smokers saw a reduction of 1.9 mmHg, while the nicotine-containing intervention arm saw a reduction of 4.2 mmHg and the nicotine-free intervention arm saw a reduction of 9.7 mmHg [47]. Notably, both trials enrolled participants who smoked an average of 18–20 cigarettes daily, and the nicotine-containing e-cigarette intervention arms utilized early generation products with nicotine concentrations of 5.4–16.0 mg/ml. Given the rising popularity of e-cigarettes with substantially higher nicotine concentrations (e.g., 56 mg/ml) [48], future RCTs evaluating these newer products as well as studies that enroll less frequent smokers will expand understanding of potential cardiovascular harm reduction.

In addition to the aforementioned RCTs which have considered blood pressure as a secondary outcome, Polosa et al. explored blood pressure changes in a 2016 prospective analysis of 89 baseline hypertensive smokers (43 e-cigarette adopters, 46 continued exclusive smokers) [49]. 20 of the e-cigarette adopters abstained from cigarettes completely during follow-up, while the other 23 decreased their daily cigarette consumption from 20 to 5 cigarettes on average. After a 12-month follow-up, the 43 participants that adopted regular e-cigarette use saw respective decreases of 10 mmHg for systolic blood pressure and 6 mmHg for diastolic blood pressure. Stratified analyses indicated meaningful blood pressure reductions were possible for those e-cigarette adopters who reduced rather than quit smoking cigarettes, albeit to a lesser degree than those who fully abstained from cigarette smoking.

4.2. Strengths and Limitations

In addition to being the first epidemiologic study of vaping and hypertension, our study has a handful of strengths. The PATH Study is an exceptionally comprehensive data source with respect to tobacco use, even including biomarker data for a large subset of participants. This affords a unique opportunity to validate self-reported tobacco use measures that other epidemiologic datasets may not have. Indeed, prior assessments of specificity and sensitivity for self-reported smoking and vaping status instill confidence that exposure misclassification is not a major concern in our analysis [50]. PATH's detailed tobacco information also makes it ideal for studying novel products and accounting for use of multiple products. In order to examine the "pure" associations of vaping and smoking with hypertension, we used two strategies to mitigate the potential confounding influence of other tobacco products: (a) primary models excluded users of tobacco products other than cigarettes or e-cigarettes; (b) in sensitivity analyses, we re-introduced the 'other' tobacco product users and adjusted for other tobacco products as potential confounders (Figure S2; results were consistent with those from the Figure 2 analyses). We also excluded people aged 55+ years to avoid survivorship bias, as the current research paradigm indicates that smoking and hypertension have combined effects on risk of cardiovascular disease mortality [39–41]. This would disproportionately influence survival among middle and older age smokers, introducing a bias among the 55+ age group. This phenomenon was likely observed in supplemental analyses of Wave 3 PATH respondents that were 55+ years old, for whom the observed association with hypertension was null for current smoking and inverse for current vaping (Table S4).

Along with previously mentioned limitations, a constraint of PATH is the lack of dietary information, which is particularly relevant for hypertension (e.g., sodium and potassium intake) [51]. As health behaviors tend to cluster [52], smokers may have been more likely to maintain nutrition habits associated with higher risk of developing hypertension, as previously reported in other studies [53]. While we are unaware of publications assessing the relationship directly, this could also be true for vapers, the majority of which are current or former smokers. Regarding the outcome of interest, self-reported diagnosed hypertension has not yet been validated within the PATH Study. However, similar hypertension case-finding questions have demonstrated reproducibility and substantial agreement with clinical blood pressure measurements in other representative samples of the US adult population [54,55]. Furthermore, the prevalence of self-reported hypertension at Wave 3 of the PATH Study was consistent with those reported by the Centers for Disease Control and Prevention in 2015–2016 [29]. It is also important to consider a potential detection bias due to the outcome variable's reliance on physician diagnosis of hypertension. Blood pressure measurement is a common screening procedure across a broad set of health professional visits (e.g., annual physicals, emergency room visits, etc.). This means those who see a physician more frequently could have more opportunities to be diagnosed with hypertension, even if their visits are for reasons seemingly unrelated to high blood pressure. As it pertains to our study, it is possible that tobacco users and non-users differ in their frequency of health professional visits. We conducted a sensitivity analysis looking at the proportion of each tobacco user group who selected "Yes" to the question "In the past 12 months, have you seen a medical doctor?" at Wave 3 of PATH, as well as at the two previous waves for our study's analytic sample (Table S5). There were statistically significant differences across the 6 tobacco use categories overall for doctor visitations at each wave (χ^2 p <0.001), however the absolute differences in proportions between groups were for not especially large. Finally, the e-cigarette marketplace has evolved since the time of this survey to include devices of varying power as well as substantial ranges in nicotine concentration [56,57]. It will be important to re-evaluate associations with health outcomes as e-cigarette technology continues to evolve.

5. Conclusions

In summary, this cross-sectional analysis of young and middle-age adults in Wave 3 of the PATH Study found a positive albeit weak association between vaping and self-reported hypertension, of similar magnitude to that of cigarette smoking and hypertension. Our findings underscore the importance of more rigorous longitudinal research into the health effects of e-cigarettes, reinforcing the uncertainty surrounding long-term ramifications of vaping. Moreover, the results suggest important distinctions should be made between respiratory and cardiovascular outcomes when considering the harm reduction potential of e-cigarettes.

Supplementary Materials: The following are available online at https://www.mdpi.com/2305-6304/9//52/s1, Figure S1: Flow diagram describing the analytic sample and detailing the study's case definition for hypertension, Figure S2: Multivariable odds for hypertension among PATH Wave 3 respondents aged 18–54 years including users of 'other' tobacco products, modeling smoking and vaping as a composite variable, Table S1: Descriptive statistics of the analytic sample, according to a composite variable accounting for current vaping status, current smoking status, and former smoking status, Table S2: Missing data in the analytic sample, Table S3: Respondents excluded from regression analyses due to missing data points during primary analyses of the analytic sample, Table S4: Prevalence of hypertension and multivariable odds for hypertension among Wave 3 PATH respondents, stratified by age.

Author Contributions: Conceptualization, C.R.M., H.S., D.L., and M.L.G.; methodology, C.R.M., H.S., D.L., and M.L.G.; formal analysis, C.R.M. and H.S.; writing—original draft preparation, C.R.M. and H.S.; writing—review and editing, D.L. and M.L.G.; visualization, C.R.M.; supervision, D.L. and M.L.G. All authors have read and agreed to the published version of the manuscript.

Funding: This research was supported by the National Cancer Institute of the National Institutes of Health (NIH) and the Center for Tobacco Products of the Food and Drug Administration (FDA) under Award Number U54CA228110. This work was also supported by the University of Rochester CTSA award number UL1 TR002001 from the National Center for Advancing Translational Sciences of the National Institutes of Health (DL). In addition, this work was supported by the University of Rochester Infection and Immunity: From Molecules to Populations (IIMP) award number BWF-1014095 from the Burroughs Wellcome Fund of Institutional Program Unifying Population and Laboratory Based Sciences (HS). The content is solely the responsibility of the authors and does not necessarily represent the official views of the NIH or the Food and Drug Administration (FDA).

Institutional Review Board Statement: Ethical review and approval were waived for this study because it involved only secondary data analysis of de-identified PATH survey data. PATH was conducted according to the guidelines of the Declaration of Helsinki, and approved by the Westat Institutional Review Board.

Informed Consent Statement: Informed consent was obtained from all subjects involved in the study.

Data Availability Statement: Publicly available datasets were analyzed in this study. This data can be found here: [https://www.icpsr.umich.edu/icpsrweb/NAHDAP/search/studies?q=PATH] (accessed on 8 March 2021).

Conflicts of Interest: M.L.G. has received a research grant from Pfizer, Inc. and served as a member of the scientific advisory board to Johnson & Johnson. The other authors declare no conflicts of interest. The funders had no role in the design of the study; in the collection, analyses, or interpretation of data; in the writing of the manuscript, or in the decision to publish the results.

References

1. GBD 2015 Tobacco Collaborators. Smoking Prevalence and Attributable Disease Burden in 195 Countries and Territories, 1990–2015: A Systematic Analysis from the Global Burden of Disease Study 2015. *Lancet* **2017**, *389*, 1885–1906. [CrossRef]
2. World Health Organization. *WHO Report on the Global Tobacco Epidemic, 2019*; World Health Organization: Geneva, Switzerland, 2019.
3. GBD 2017 Risk Factor Collaborators. Global, Regional, and National Comparative Risk Assessment of 84 Behavioural, Environmental and Occupational, and Metabolic Risks or Clusters of Risks for 195 Countries and Territories, 1990–2017: A Systematic Analysis for the Global Burden of Disease Study 2017. *Lancet* **2018**, *392*, 1923–1994. [CrossRef]
4. US Department of Health and Human Services. *The Health Consequences of Smoking—50 Years of Progress: A Report of the Surgeon General*; Centers for Disease Control and Prevention, National Center on Chronic Disease Prevention and Health Promotion, Office on Smoking and Health: Atlanta, GA, USA, 2014.
5. US Department of Health and Human Services. *How Tobacco Smoke Causes Disease: The Biology and Behavioral Basis for Smoking-Attributable Disease: A Report of the Surgeon General*; Centers for Disease Control and Prevention, National Center on Chronic Disease Prevention and Health Promotion, Office on Smoking and Health: Atlanta, GA, USA, 2010.
6. Ezzati, M.; Henley, S.J.; Thun, M.J.; Lopez, A.D. Role of Smoking in Global and Regional Cardiovascular Mortality. *Circulation* **2005**, *112*, 489–497. [CrossRef]
7. Wagner, K.A.; Flora, J.W.; Melvin, M.S.; Avery, K.C.; Ballentine, R.M.; Brown, A.P.; McKinney, W.J. An Evaluation of Electronic Cigarette Formulations and Aerosols for Harmful and Potentially Harmful Constituents (HPHCs) Typically Derived from Combustion. *Regul. Toxicol. Pharmacol.* **2018**, *95*, 153–160. [CrossRef]
8. Helen, G.S.; Liakoni, E.; Nardone, N.; Addo, N.; Jacob, P., III; Benowitz, N.L. Comparison of Systemic Exposure to Toxic and/or Carcinogenic Volatile Organic Compounds (VOCs) during Vaping, Smoking, and Abstention. *Cancer Prev. Res.* **2019**, *13*, 153–162. [CrossRef] [PubMed]
9. Farsalinos, K.E.; Gillman, G. Carbonyl Emissions in E-Cigarette Aerosol: A Systematic Review and Methodological Considerations. *Front. Physiol.* **2018**, *8*, 1119. [CrossRef] [PubMed]
10. Romijnders, K.A.; Van Osch, L.; De Vries, H.; Talhout, R. Perceptions and Reasons Regarding E-Cigarette Use among Users and Non-Users: A Narrative Literature Review. *Int. J. Environ. Res. Public Health* **2018**, *15*, 1190. [CrossRef] [PubMed]
11. Alzahrani, T.; Pena, I.; Temesgen, N.; Glantz, S.A. Association between Electronic Cigarette Use and Myocardial Infarction. *Am. J. Prev. Med.* **2018**, *55*, 455–461. [CrossRef] [PubMed]
12. Osei, A.D.; Mirbolouk, M.; Orimoloye, O.A.; Dzaye, O.; Uddin, S.I.; Benjamin, E.J.; Hall, M.E.; DeFilippis, A.P.; Stokes, A.; Bhatnagar, A. Association between E-Cigarette Use and Cardiovascular Disease among Never and Current Combustible-Cigarette Smokers. *Am. J. Med.* **2019**, *132*, 949–954. [CrossRef]

13. Farsalinos, K.E.; Polosa, R.; Cibella, F.; Niaura, R. Is E-Cigarette Use Associated with Coronary Heart Disease and Myocardial Infarction? Insights from the 2016 and 2017 National Health Interview Surveys. *Ther. Adv. Chronic Dis.* **2019**, *10*, 1–10. [CrossRef] [PubMed]
14. Parekh, T.; Pemmasani, S.; Desai, R. Risk of Stroke with E-Cigarette and Combustible Cigarette Use in Young Adults. *Am. J. Prev. Med.* **2020**, *58*, 446–452. [CrossRef]
15. Skotsimara, G.; Antonopoulos, A.S.; Oikonomou, E.; Siasos, G.; Ioakeimidis, N.; Tsalamandris, S.; Charalambous, G.; Galiatsatos, N.; Vlachopoulos, C.; Tousoulis, D. Cardiovascular Effects of Electronic Cigarettes: A Systematic Review and Meta-Analysis. *Eur. J. Prev. Cardiol.* **2019**, *26*, 1219–1228. [CrossRef]
16. Olfert, I.M.; DeVallance, E.; Hoskinson, H.; Branyan, K.W.; Clayton, S.; Pitzer, C.R.; Sullivan, D.P.; Breit, M.J.; Wu, Z.; Klinkhachorn, P. Chronic Exposure to Electronic Cigarettes Results in Impaired Cardiovascular Function in Mice. *J. Appl. Physiol.* **2017**, *124*, 573–582. [CrossRef]
17. Gerloff, J.; Sundar, I.K.; Freter, R.; Sekera, E.R.; Friedman, A.E.; Robinson, R.; Pagano, T.; Rahman, I. Inflammatory Response and Barrier Dysfunction by Different E-Cigarette Flavoring Chemicals Identified by Gas Chromatography–Mass Spectrometry in e-Liquids and e-Vapors on Human Lung Epithelial Cells and Fibroblasts. *Appl. Vitro Toxicol.* **2017**, *3*, 28–40. [CrossRef] [PubMed]
18. Oparil, S.; Zaman, M.A.; Calhoun, D.A. Pathogenesis of Hypertension. *Ann. Intern. Med.* **2003**, *139*, 761–776. [CrossRef] [PubMed]
19. Groppelli, A.; Giorgi, D.M.; Omboni, S.; Parati, G.; Mancia, G. Persistent Blood Pressure Increase Induced by Heavy Smoking. *J. Hypertens.* **1992**, *10*, 495–499. [CrossRef] [PubMed]
20. Virdis, A.; Giannarelli, C.; Fritsch Neves, M.; Taddei, S.; Ghiadoni, L. Cigarette Smoking and Hypertension. *Curr. Pharm. Des.* **2010**, *16*, 2518–2525. [CrossRef]
21. Conklin, D.J.; Schick, S.; Blaha, M.J.; Carll, A.; DeFilippis, A.; Ganz, P.; Hall, M.E.; Hamburg, N.; O'Toole, T.; Reynolds, L. Cardiovascular Injury Induced by Tobacco Products: Assessment of Risk Factors and Biomarkers of Harm. A Tobacco Centers of Regulatory Science Compilation. *Am. J. Physiol. Heart Circ. Physiol.* **2019**, *316*, H801–H827. [CrossRef]
22. US Department of Health and Human Services; National Institutes of Health; National Institute on Drug Abuse; United States Department of Health and Human Services; Food and Drug Administration Center for Tobacco Products. *Population Assessment of Tobacco and Health (PATH) Study*; [United States] Public-Use Files, User Guide 2017; FDA: Washington, DC, USA, 2017.
23. Hyland, A.; Ambrose, B.K.; Conway, K.P.; Borek, N.; Lambert, E.; Carusi, C.; Taylor, K.; Crosse, S.; Fong, G.T.; Cummings, K.M. Design and Methods of the Population Assessment of Tobacco and Health (PATH) Study. *Tob. Control* **2017**, *26*, 371–378. [CrossRef]
24. Dai, H.; Leventhal, A.M. Prevalence of E-Cigarette Use among Adults in the United States, 2014–2018. *JAMA* **2019**, *322*, 1824–1827. [CrossRef] [PubMed]
25. Hammond, D.; Reid, J.L.; Rynard, V.L.; Fong, G.T.; Cummings, K.M.; McNeill, A.; Hitchman, S.; Thrasher, J.F.; Goniewicz, M.L.; Bansal-Travers, M. Prevalence of Vaping and Smoking among Adolescents in Canada, England, and the United States: Repeat National Cross Sectional Surveys. *BMJ* **2019**, *365*, l2219. [CrossRef] [PubMed]
26. Coleman, B.N.; Rostron, B.; Johnson, S.E.; Ambrose, B.K. Electronic Cigarette Use among US Adults in the Population Assessment of Tobacco and Health (PATH) Study, 2013–2014. *Tob. Control* **2017**, *26*, e117–e126. [CrossRef] [PubMed]
27. Coleman, B.; Rostron, B.; Johnson, S.E.; Persoskie, A.; Pearson, J.; Stanton, C.; Choi, K.; Anic, G.; Goniewicz, M.L.; Cummings, K.M. Transitions in Electronic Cigarette Use among Adults in the Population Assessment of Tobacco and Health (PATH) Study, Waves 1 and 2 (2013–2015). *Tob. Control* **2019**, *28*, 50–59. [CrossRef] [PubMed]
28. Reichenheim, M.E.; Coutinho, E.S. Measures and Models for Causal Inference in Cross-Sectional Studies: Arguments for the Appropriateness of the Prevalence Odds Ratio and Related Logistic Regression. *BMC Med. Res. Methodol.* **2010**, *10*, 66. [CrossRef] [PubMed]
29. Fryar, C.D.; Ostchega, Y.; Hales, C.M.; Zhang, G.; Kruszon-Moran, D. *Hypertension Prevalence and Control among Adults: United States, 2015–2016*; NCHS Data Brief; National Center for Health Statistics: Hyattsville, MD, USA, 2017; Volume 289.
30. Fuchs, F.D.; Whelton, P.K. High Blood Pressure and Cardiovascular Disease. *Hypertension* **2020**, *75*, 285–292. [CrossRef]
31. Forouzanfar, M.H.; Liu, P.; Roth, G.A.; Ng, M.; Biryukov, S.; Marczak, L.; Alexander, L.; Estep, K.; Abate, K.H.; Akinyemiju, T.F. Global Burden of Hypertension and Systolic Blood Pressure of at Least 110 to 115 Mm Hg, 1990–2015. *JAMA* **2017**, *317*, 165–182. [CrossRef]
32. Rose, G. Sick Individuals and Sick Populations. *Int. J. Epidemiol.* **2001**, *30*, 427–432. [CrossRef]
33. Goniewicz, M.L.; Smith, D.M.; Edwards, K.C.; Blount, B.C.; Caldwell, K.L.; Feng, J.; Wang, L.; Christensen, C.; Ambrose, B.; Borek, N. Comparison of Nicotine and Toxicant Exposure in Users of Electronic Cigarettes and Combustible Cigarettes. *JAMA Netw. Open* **2018**, *1*, e185937. [CrossRef]
34. Bhatta, D.N.; Glantz, S.A. Association of E-Cigarette Use with Respiratory Disease among Adults: A Longitudinal Analysis. *Am. J. Prev. Med.* **2020**, *58*, 182–190. [CrossRef]
35. Hedman, L.; Backman, H.; Stridsman, C.; Bosson, J.A.; Lundbäck, M.; Lindberg, A.; Rönmark, E.; Ekerljung, L. Association of Electronic Cigarette Use with Smoking Habits, Demographic Factors, and Respiratory Symptoms. *JAMA Netw. Open* **2018**, *1*, e180789. [CrossRef] [PubMed]
36. Li, D.; Sundar, I.K.; McIntosh, S.; Ossip, D.J.; Goniewicz, M.L.; O'Connor, R.J.; Rahman, I. Association of Smoking and Electronic Cigarette Use with Wheezing and Related Respiratory Symptoms in Adults: Cross-Sectional Results from the Population Assessment of Tobacco and Health (PATH) Study, Wave 2. *Tob. Control* **2020**, *29*, 140–147. [CrossRef]

37. Stokes, A.C.; Xie, W.; Wilson, A.E.; Yang, H.; Orimoloye, O.A.; Harlow, A.F.; Fetterman, J.L.; DeFilippis, A.P.; Benjamin, E.J.; Robertson, R.M. Association of Cigarette and Electronic Cigarette Use Patterns With Levels of Inflammatory and Oxidative Stress Biomarkers among US Adults: Population Assessment of Tobacco and Health Study. *Circulation* **2021**, *143*, 869–871. [CrossRef] [PubMed]
38. Mainous, A.G., III; Yadav, S.; Hong, Y.-R.; Huo, J. E-Cigarette and Conventional Tobacco Cigarette Use, Dual Use, and C-Reactive Protein. *J. Am. Coll. Cardiol.* **2020**, *75*, 2271–2273. [CrossRef] [PubMed]
39. Khalili, P.; Nilsson, P.M.; Nilsson, J.-A.; Berglund, G. Smoking as a Modifier of the Systolic Blood Pressure-Induced Risk of Cardiovascular Events and Mortality: A Population-Based Prospective Study of Middle-Aged Men. *J. Hypertens.* **2002**, *20*, 1759–1764. [CrossRef] [PubMed]
40. Nakamura, K.; Barzi, F.; Lam, T.-H.; Huxley, R.; Feigin, V.L.; Ueshima, H.; Woo, J.; Gu, D.; Ohkubo, T.; Lawes, C.M. Cigarette Smoking, Systolic Blood Pressure, and Cardiovascular Diseases in the Asia-Pacific Region. *Stroke* **2008**, *39*, 1694–1702. [CrossRef]
41. Hara, M.; Yakushiji, Y.; Suzuyama, K.; Nishihara, M.; Eriguchi, M.; Noguchi, T.; Nishiyama, M.; Nanri, Y.; Tanaka, J.; Hara, H. Synergistic Effect of Hypertension and Smoking on the Total Small Vessel Disease Score in Healthy Individuals: The Kashima Scan Study. *Hypertens. Res.* **2019**, *42*, 1738–1744. [CrossRef] [PubMed]
42. Crotty Alexander, L.E.; Drummond, C.A.; Hepokoski, M.; Mathew, D.; Moshensky, A.; Willeford, A.; Das, S.; Singh, P.; Yong, Z.; Lee, J.H. Chronic Inhalation of E-Cigarette Vapor Containing Nicotine Disrupts Airway Barrier Function and Induces Systemic Inflammation and Multiorgan Fibrosis in Mice. *Am. J. Physiol. Regul. Integr. Comp. Physiol.* **2018**, *314*, R834–R847. [CrossRef]
43. Vlachopoulos, C.; Ioakeimidis, N.; Abdelrasoul, M.; Terentes-Printzios, D.; Georgakopoulos, C.; Pietri, P.; Stefanadis, C.; Tousoulis, D. Electronic Cigarette Smoking Increases Aortic Stiffness and Blood Pressure in Young Smokers. *J. Am. Coll. Cardiol.* **2016**, *67*, 2802–2803. [CrossRef] [PubMed]
44. Pescatello, L.S.; Buchner, D.M.; Jakicic, J.M.; Powell, K.E.; Kraus, W.E.; Bloodgood, B.; Campbell, W.W.; Dietz, S.; DiPietro, L.; George, S.M. Physical Activity to Prevent and Treat Hypertension: A Systematic Review. *Med. Sci. Sports Exerc.* **2019**, *51*, 1314–1323. [CrossRef] [PubMed]
45. Miller, C.R.; Wactawski-Wende, J.; Manson, J.E.; Haring, B.; Hovey, K.M.; Laddu, D.; Shadyab, A.H.; Wild, R.A.; Bea, J.W.; Tinker, L.F.; et al. Walking Volume and Speed Are Inversely Associated with Incidence of Treated Hypertension in Postmenopausal Women. *Hypertension* **2020**, *76*, 1435–1443. [CrossRef]
46. Farsalinos, K.; Cibella, F.; Caponnetto, P.; Campagna, D.; Morjaria, J.B.; Battaglia, E.; Caruso, M.; Russo, C.; Polosa, R. Effect of Continuous Smoking Reduction and Abstinence on Blood Pressure and Heart Rate in Smokers Switching to Electronic Cigarettes. *Intern. Emerg. Med.* **2016**, *11*, 85–94. [CrossRef] [PubMed]
47. George, J.; Hussain, M.; Vadiveloo, T.; Ireland, S.; Hopkinson, P.; Struthers, A.D.; Donnan, P.T.; Khan, F.; Lang, C.C. Cardiovascular Effects of Switching from Tobacco Cigarettes to Electronic Cigarettes. *J. Am. Coll. Cardiol.* **2019**, *74*, 3112–3120. [CrossRef] [PubMed]
48. Huang, J.; Duan, Z.; Kwok, J.; Binns, S.; Vera, L.E.; Kim, Y.; Szczypka, G.; Emery, S.L. Vaping versus JUULing: How the Extraordinary Growth and Marketing of JUUL Transformed the US Retail e-Cigarette Market. *Tob. Control* **2019**, *28*, 146–151. [CrossRef]
49. Polosa, R.; Morjaria, J.; Caponnetto, P.; Battaglia, E.; Russo, C.; Ciampi, C.; Adams, G.; Bruno, C. Blood Pressure Control in Smokers with Arterial Hypertension Who Switched to Electronic Cigarettes. *Int. J. Environ. Res. Public Health* **2016**, *13*, 1123. [CrossRef]
50. Tourangeau, R.; Yan, T.; Sun, H.; Hyland, A.; Stanton, C.A. Population Assessment of Tobacco and Health (PATH) Reliability and Validity Study: Selected Reliability and Validity Estimates. *Tob. Control* **2018**, *28*, 663–668. [CrossRef]
51. Sacks, F.M.; Svetkey, L.P.; Vollmer, W.M.; Appel, L.J.; Bray, G.A.; Harsha, D.; Obarzanek, E.; Conlin, P.R.; Miller, E.R.; Simons-Morton, D.G. Effects on Blood Pressure of Reduced Dietary Sodium and the Dietary Approaches to Stop Hypertension (DASH) Diet. *N. Engl. J. Med.* **2001**, *344*, 3–10. [CrossRef]
52. Chiolero, A.; Wietlisbach, V.; Ruffieux, C.; Paccaud, F.; Cornuz, J. Clustering of Risk Behaviors with Cigarette Consumption: A Population-Based Survey. *Prev. Med.* **2006**, *42*, 348–353. [CrossRef]
53. Alkerwi, A.; Baydarlioglu, B.; Sauvageot, N.; Stranges, S.; Lemmens, P.; Shivappa, N.; Hébert, J.R. Smoking Status Is Inversely Associated with Overall Diet Quality: Findings from the ORISCAV-LUX Study. *Clin. Nutr.* **2017**, *36*, 1275–1282. [CrossRef]
54. Mentz, G.; Schulz, A.J.; Mukherjee, B.; Ragunathan, T.E.; Perkins, D.W.; Israel, B.A. Hypertension: Development of a Prediction Model to Adjust Self-Reported Hypertension Prevalence at the Community Level. *BMC Health Serv. Res.* **2012**, *12*, 312. [CrossRef]
55. Vargas, C.M.; Burt, V.L.; Gillum, R.F.; Pamuk, E.R. Validity of Self-Reported Hypertension in the National Health and Nutrition Examination Survey III, 1988–1991. *Prev. Med.* **1997**, *26*, 678–685. [CrossRef] [PubMed]
56. O'Connor, R.J.; Fix, B.V.; McNeill, A.; Goniewicz, M.L.; Bansal-Travers, M.; Heckman, B.W.; Cummings, K.M.; Hitchman, S.; Borland, R.; Hammond, D. Characteristics of Nicotine Vaping Products Used by Participants in the 2016 ITC Four Country Smoking and Vaping Survey. *Addiction* **2019**, *114*, 15–23. [CrossRef] [PubMed]
57. Havermans, A.; Krüsemann, E.J.; Pennings, J.; De Graaf, K.; Boesveldt, S.; Talhout, R. Nearly 20 000 E-Liquids and 250 Unique Flavour Descriptions: An Overview of the Dutch Market Based on Information from Manufacturers. *Tob. Control* **2021**, *30*, 57–62. [CrossRef] [PubMed]

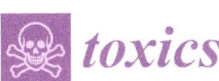

Review

Critical Review of the Recent Literature on Organic Byproducts in E-Cigarette Aerosol Emissions

Sebastien Soulet [1,†] and Roberto A. Sussman [2,*,†]

1. Ingesciences, 2 Chemin des Arestieux, 33610 Cestas, France
2. Institute of Nuclear Sciences, National Autonomous University of Mexico, Mexico City 04510, Mexico
* Correspondence: sussman@nucleares.unam.mx
† These authors contributed equally to this work.

Abstract: We review the literature on laboratory studies quantifying the production of potentially toxic organic byproducts (carbonyls, carbon monoxide, free radicals and some nontargeted compounds) in e-cigarette (EC) aerosol emissions, focusing on the consistency between their experimental design and a realistic usage of the devices, as determined by the power ranges of an optimal regime fulfilling a thermodynamically efficient process of aerosol generation that avoids overheating and "dry puffs". The majority of the reviewed studies failed in various degrees to comply with this consistency criterion or supplied insufficient information to verify it. Consequently, most of the experimental outcomes and risk assessments are either partially or totally unreliable and/or of various degrees of questionable relevance to end users. Studies testing the devices under reasonable approximation to realistic conditions detected levels of all organic byproducts that are either negligible or orders of magnitude lower than in tobacco smoke. Our review reinforces the pressing need to update and improve current laboratory standards by an appropriate selection of testing parameters and the logistical incorporation of end users in the experimental design.

Keywords: e-cigarettes; vaping; aerosol emissions; puffing protocols; organic byproducts

Citation: Soulet, S.; Sussman, R.A. Critical Review of the Recent Literature on Organic Byproducts in E-Cigarette Aerosol Emissions. *Toxics* **2022**, *10*, 714. https://doi.org/10.3390/toxics10120714

Academic Editors: Andrzej Sobczak and Leon Kośmider

Received: 3 October 2022
Accepted: 14 November 2022
Published: 22 November 2022

Publisher's Note: MDPI stays neutral with regard to jurisdictional claims in published maps and institutional affiliations.

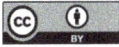

Copyright: © 2022 by the authors. Licensee MDPI, Basel, Switzerland. This article is an open access article distributed under the terms and conditions of the Creative Commons Attribution (CC BY) license (https://creativecommons.org/licenses/by/4.0/).

1. Introduction

Electronic cigarettes (ECs) have become popular substitute products of conventional cigarettes in the framework of tobacco harm reduction, as there is a broad consensus that the aerosol they generate contains far fewer toxic and carcinogenic compounds than tobacco smoke [1–3] (see [4] for a diverging opinion). However, users of the devices ("vapers") are still exposed to the inhalation of harmful or potentially harmful compounds (HPHCs), particularly carbonyls, nitrosamines, metallic compounds and possibly carbon monoxide (CO) and free radicals or Reactive Oxygen Species (ROS). For vaping to fulfill a beneficial harm reduction goal, it is necessary to assess and evaluate laboratory studies that have examined the presence of these HPHC byproducts in vaping emissions.

In a previous paper [5], we reviewed 12 studies targeting metal content in EC emissions. We found that all studies reporting high metal levels (e.g., nickel, lead, chromium and manganese) surpassing toxicological markers suffered from serious methodological shortcomings, especially (but not only) testing high-powered sub-ohm devices at high wattages with the puffing parameters of the CORESTA Method 81 [6,7]) or slight variations of it (i.e., "CORESTA-like"). Almost all laboratory testing is currently conducted by means of these puffing protocols, which were conceived and developed for testing low-powered devices using an airflow rate around 1 L/min and puff volumes below 70 mL. However, these puffing parameters are inadequate for testing sub-ohm devices that require much larger airflow and puff volume to evacuate and condensate efficiently the large amount of vaporized e-liquid produced by the large supplied power. Pending on the wattage range, the combination of high power with low airflow rate and puff volume is either prone or certain to lead to a device testing under overheating conditions. It is also unrepresentative of consumer usage, as sub-ohm devices are mostly used and widely recommended (by manufacturers, vaping magazines and forums) for the 'direct to lung' (DTL) vaping style that involves much larger airflows and puff volumes [8,9] (see also [5]).

It is not expected that laboratory testing will reproduce the wide individual diversity (devices, e-liquids, puffing habits) of real-life vaping behavior, but it is necessary and desirable that its experimental setup must be conceived to provide the best possible approximation to the representative characteristics of consumer usage. These facts are recognized by all stakeholders: the official documents of the CORESTA protocol, regulators, academics and consumers (see summary, discussion and references in [10]). A necessary task to evaluate the limitations of the current CORESTA based standard (and suggest upgrades and improvements) is a thorough technical criticism of current laboratory testing largely based on this standard.

To assess current laboratory testing of EC emissions, we apply in the present review a critical analysis of experimental methodology analogous to the one undertaken in [5] but now focusing on laboratory studies detecting nonmetallic byproducts. We provide an extensive review of a literature consisting of 38 articles published since 2018, listed and classified by subject in Table 1 below:

Table 1. Classification by subject of studies under review

Reviewed studies	Section	References
2 previous review articles	Section 5	[11,12]
22 studies on carbonyls and byproducts	Section 6	[13–34]
3 studies on CO	Section 7	[35–37]
4 studies on ROS	Section 8	[38–41]
5 studies on byproduct formation	Section 9	[42–46]
2 studies on carbonyls vs. nicotine	Section 10	[47,48]

Together with the revision of each individual study cited in Table 1, we also provide an extensive discussion of the physical principles underlying the optimal regime of operation of ECs, the conditions that define representative vaping habits and a summary and evaluation of this literature.

For any given device and e-liquid composition, the appropriate power range for laboratory testing can be determined in the laboratory by an optimal regime characterized by a linear relation between the mass of e-liquid vaporized (MEV) and supplied power W [8]. Underheating occurs below this range with no vaporized e-liquid, while overheating occurs above this range as the relation becomes nonlinear. In the optimal regime, an equilibrium of heat exchange is maintained when a sufficient airflow provides the necessary forced convection (inhalation) to form the aerosol by condensation of the vaporized e-liquid [8,9,49]. Overheating occurs when nucleate boiling gives way to film boiling [22] in which a layer of gas surrounds the coil, propitiating radiative heating exchange, which rapidly increases the rate of vaporization of the e-liquid, breaking the equilibrium sustained by forced convection in the linear regime. While the wick capillarity and e-liquid viscosity decrease as the rate of e-liquid consumption increases with increasingly higher temperatures, the liquid supply to the coil also decreases in parallel with the development of film boiling. The process continues until the coil is dry and thermal energy is radiated (potentially reaching up to 1000 °C) and the wick material (typically cotton) is pyrolyzed at about 450 °C. These conditions produce in end users a burning sensation in the aerosol identified as a "dry puff" or "dry hit".

The specific power ranges of the optimal regime are device-dependent and can exhibit wide variation in terms of the coil alloys, e-liquid composition and flavors. However, manufacturers provide recommendations of power ranges and usage of the devices and the optimal regime (as described before) provides a laboratory testable procedure to assess these power ranges. When puffing parameters are inappropriate (specially insufficient airflow), these power ranges become narrower, thus facilitating the overheating process even at power settings below the upper limits of manufacturer recommendations. This process can be abrupt in low-powered devices (ciga-likes, pods, second-generation models) whose optimal regime is delimited by narrow wattage ranges. Thus, a small extra supplied power can trigger a rapid onset and development of overheating, especially in devices lacking an inbuilt mechanism preventing this problem. For high-powered devices, the optimal regime occupies a wider range of power settings, so overheating is likely to occur in a more gradual way, making it harder for users to detect it.

Most laboratory testing of emissions has been conducted without carefully monitoring that their experimental setup avoids overheating and unrealistic testing, often (but not always) by testing high-powered devices with insufficient airflow and high power settings above a narrowed power range of the optimal regime. While the emergence of overheating conditions is potentially detectable by sensorial perceptions of users, either by a flavor deterioration or by inhaling an aerosol that becomes too hot, it is well known that users always identify the burning repellent sensation of a "dry puff" that occurs at the end state of an overheating when e-liquid depletes and the wick is pyrolyzed. As shown in a recent study [34], incorporation of end users provides useful guidelines to select the appropriate parameters for realistic and user relevant testing, especially with low-powered devices for which an extra watt can initiate overheating. Unfortunately, few emission studies incorporate input from users in their experimental design. These methodological problems were already identified in the important review by Farsalinos and Gillman [11] of 32 studies on carbonyl byproducts published up to 2017. We find it concerning that five years afterward, these issues still need to be addressed.

The literature on organic byproducts in EC emissions contains detailed and impeccable chemical experiments in reaction pathways associated with the production in the laboratory of these compounds but fail to verify if these chemical processes are plausible or if they are compatible with the physical constraints of the optimal regime. Evidently, an impeccable chemical analysis of EC aerosols might be valuable in itself, but without anchoring its experimental design on the optimal regime, the authors might find results that have little relevance to most end users. The possibility to replicate and reproduce experimental outcomes is a crucially important criterion to evaluate experimental research. Unfortunately, some studies that we revised do not comply with this criterion by failing to disclose sufficient information on important details of their experimental design (puffing parameters, tested devices and e-liquids). Some studies test old devices without providing information on their storage conditions or current state. All this information is relevant to interpret experimental results and possibly replicate them.

Besides comparison between products, evaluation of quality control and fulfillment of regulatory requirements, one of the main tasks of laboratory testing is to assess potential health risks to end users from the presence in EC emissions of potentially toxic byproducts. All studies that we reviewed highlight the toxicity potential of these byproducts, with most studies testing sub-ohm devices concluding serious harm potential to end users from their experimental outcomes. However, our findings in this review suggests that the severity of these risk assessments requires a careful and skeptical evaluation. In some cases, the conclusions of severe risks are questionable, as they emerge from studies that have tested the devices under completely unrealistic and user irrelevant conditions, though in other studies, the risk severity would not apply to the majority of users but only (possibly) to a minority of users with unrepresentative or unsustainable vaping habits.

The section-by-section development of the review is as follows. In Section 2, we explain the physical considerations that define the optimal regime. In Section 3, we discuss various ways to describe and approximate realistic vaping behavior, while in Section 4, we present a methodological description of our review, discussing the conditions of experimental consistency and toxicological realiability as references to evaluate laboratory studies . We summarize in Section 5 two previously published reviews, including a landmark review that examined carbonyl studies published before 2018, providing various key elements of the methodological criticism that we are following in the present review. In Section 6, we review 22 studies focusing on the detection and quantification of carbonyls and other byproducts; in Sections 7 and 8, studies respectively focusing on CO and ROS; in Section 9, we revise 5 studies whose main focus is the understanding of chemical pathways of byproduct formation from solvent degradation and in Section 10, two studies looking at the relation between carbonyl production and the compensatory behavior associated with low nicotine concentrations. In Sections 11–13, we discuss various relevant theoretical issues addressing misunderstandings found in the revised literature, an assessment of risk communication and our conclusions.

2. Foreword: The Optimal Regime of Vaping

ECs have been subject to intense scrutiny from their harm reduction role as a substitute product that facilitates smoking cessation. Concerning issues have been raised on their usage among adolescents, impact on health and the pharmacokinetics of nicotine, among many other topics. Unfortunately, there has been little interest in understanding the physical processes that govern the proper functional operation of EC devices.

Since chemical reactions are enhanced by the temperature, many articles have performed temperature measurements of the coil as an attempt to observe the device functionality. However, temperature is an intensive state variable that results from specific conditions that are difficult to control. In the case of a vaping device, the power supplied by the battery heats the wire, transfering heat to the e-liquid and allowing its vaporization into the air induced by the user inhalation. Essentially, the fundamental physical process is heat transfer, and it should then be understood from studying the various involved heat fluxes, especially from the power supplied into the wire surface.

However, few studies have remarked that vaping devices have effective functioning limits: a minimal and a maximal power setting that depends on the wire and device design, the e-liquid composition and also on the airflow rate. These limits are quantifiable by a rigorous relation between the mass of e-liquid vaporized (MEV) vs. supplied power (W). In 2020, Talih et al. [22] published the first article that provides a physical explanation of these limits. Boiling occurs in different form when there is heat flux. Under nucleate boiling (thermal equilibrium between minimal and maximal powers), bubbles are formed on the wire, whereas in film boiling, a local layer of gas surrounds the wire, initiating an efficient process of radiative heat transfer.

Talih et al. [22] also found that the maximal power marking the beginning of the film-boiling regime also marks the starting point of an exponential increase in aldehyde production. Their observations were the same for all tested devices, the two high-powered devices (SMOK TF-N2 0.12 Ohm and V12-Q4 0.15 Ohm) and also for the low-power device (VF platinium 2.2 Ohm). This exponential behavior in reaction rates, also found in articles on CO, is fundamentally linked to Arrhenius relations and reveals a significant temperature increase above the temperatures of optimal conditions. In an optimal regime, e-liquid vaporization occurs under thermal equilibrium or close to it [50]. Therefore, above these equilibrium conditions, e-liquids are overheated in the gas phase by radiative heat transfers. Putting together this knowledge leads us to consider several assumptions based on experimental observations:

- Overheating conditions in which e-liquids undergo temperatures above the boiling temperature of glycerol (VG) leads to significant increase in e-liquid degradation reactions, wick pyrolysis and wire oxidation, leading to a hotter aerosol than that in optimal conditions.
- Overheating conditions are not restricted to high-powered devices, they can also affect low-powered devices. This is illustrated in Figure 1, showing the optimal regime for low- and high-powered devices: a linear relation between mass of e-liquid vaporized (MEV) and supplied power W. The difference is that the optimal regime extends for

a wider range of power settings in high-powered devices, while it is restricted to narrow power ranges in low-powered devices. Therefore, it is relatively easy in these devices to enter an overheating condition with little extra supplied power, while for a high-powered device, the deviation from the optimal regime can be more gradual. Several studies have shown that overheating and dry puffs occur in low-powered devices [51].

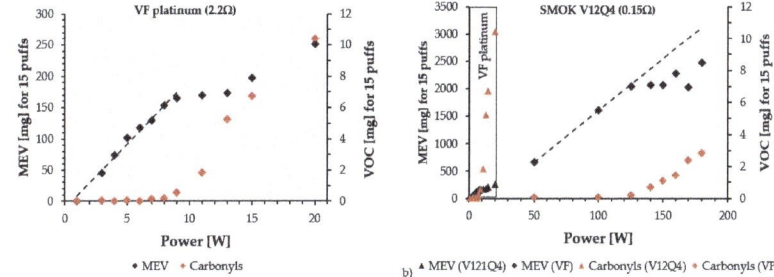

Figure 1. Both panels display vaporized e-liquid mass (MEV) in mg vs. supplied power in W (black squares), with data taken from the experimental results listed in the supplementary file of Talih et al. [22]. Both panels show how in a laboratory setting it is possible to detect the power ranges where the MEV vs. W relation is linear and the appearance of overheating conditions when it becomes nonlinear, coinciding with the onset of an exponential increase of aldehyde production (red squares). The left panel (**a**) shows how for a low-powered device, the optimal regime occupies a narrow power range, while for a high-powered device (right panel (**b**)), the power range is wide. Notice that the power range of the optimal regime of the low-powered device is compressed in the extreme left-hand side of the graph of panel (**b**).

- The use of a CORESTA regime on devices intended for DTL vaping leads to the narrowing of the power range of the optimal regime range by decreasing its maximal power. This has been confirmed by experimental results reported by Soulet et al. [8] (see Figure 2a below) and Floyd et al. [52]. Therefore, experiments of this type can lead to overheating conditions, even under the power range required by the manufacturer.
- The manufacturer-recommended power range is evaluated before releasing a device into the market, with users identifying a dry puff by perceptions if used above these ranges. Since the boiling point of pure VG (288 °C) and autoignition temperature of an organic material like cotton (350–400 °C) are close, the onset of overheating will initiate cotton degradation, leading to a "dry puff". In a recent study, which we review in Section 6, Visser et al. [34] matched the chemical characterizations of carbonyls in emissions and the human perceptions of dry puffs in the generated aerosol. Their findings support the claim that dry puff conditions are perceived as a repellent sensation that degrades the pleasant taste of vaping aerosol that prevails under normal conditions [34,53].

A common misconception in several studies (see [20,21,30,38–41]) comes from testing a device by fixing power W at a single value and varying airflow rate (or puff volume with a fixed puff duration or opening the airflow vents system with fixed puff volume and puff duration). Proceeding in this way necessarily leads to an incomplete account of the involved variables and thus an incorrect characterization of the effects of the airflow. The inhalation induced airflow produces a forced convection on the wire and its influence should be characterized with regards to the supplied heat flux. This fact renders the airflow rate (and more fundamentally air velocity) as a key dynamical parameter that can modify the entire functioning curve of a vaping device (i.e., the minimal and maximal powers and the slope in the MEV vs. W graph of the optimal regime).

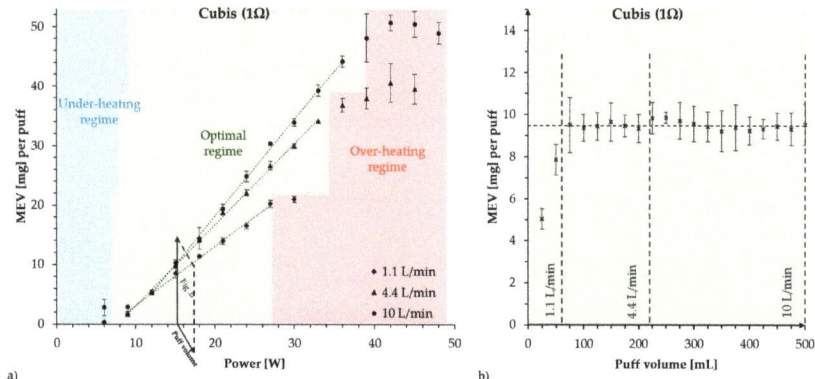

Figure 2. Comparison of two functionality curves for the Cubis 1Ω device: MEV vs. W for fixed airflow (left panel (**a**)) and MEV vs. puff volume in mL for fixed power at 15 W (right panel (**b**)). Panel (**a**) displays the effects of increasing the fixed airflow from 1.1 L/min (CORESTA conditions), 4.4 L/min to 10 L/min (extracted from [8]). A higher airflow rate increases the slope of the linear relation between MEV and W, allowing for a wider power range under the optimal regime, with appearance of overheating conditions at higher power settings. For low airflow (smaller slope), the optimal regime is limited by a narrow power range. The right panel (**b**) shows MEV to be insensitive to increasing puff volume, apparently suggesting that airflow has no effect on MEV. However, varying airflow under a single fixed power is an artificial testing combination that does not define the optimal regime (see explanation in the text).

As an example of how the effect of airflow can be misunderstood, Figure 2b displays the dependence of the vaporized e-liquid mass MEV on puff volume (i.e., related to the airflow rate for a puff duration fixed at 3 s). Below 100 mL airflow increases MEV, reaching an approximately constant value all the way to 500 mL. This funcional dependence could prompt the conclusion that large airflows (from larger puff volumes at fixed puff duration) bear no influences on the amount of MEV, which any user of the 'Direct to Lung' (DTL) style inhaling large puff volumes knows is untrue. In reality, Figure 2a shows that airflow bears a strong influence on the functioning curve, but this must be tested supplying a range of fixed values of W, a single value is not sufficient to characterize the optimal regime. Additionally, we remark that MEV would also have reached a constant value on the same range of tested puff volumes if the experiments depicted in Figure 2 would have been done at other power values, for example, 12 W.

Mathematically, setting the experimental variables as only 'MEV vs. airflow' or 'MEV vs. puff volume' with a single fixed W results in curves (as in Figure 2b) in a 2-dimensional cross section defined by the plane W constant in the 3-dimensional plot of MEV as a function of W and airflow. Focusing only on a constant W plane obscures the understanding of the role of airflow in balancing the heat transferred by W to condense MEV to form the aerosol under thermodynamically efficient conditions [8]. Experiments fixing W and varying puff volume or airflow might also under (or over) estimate the physical limits of the values that these variables can reach, as these limits are determined by the efficiency of the balance between W, MEV and airflow.

From the arguments presented above, it is clear that experiments with inappropriate air flow will necessary overestimate the risk from exposure to aldehydes over normal conditions. As explained before, the decrease of maximal optimal regime powers due to testing a high-powered device with a low airflow regime (for example 1 L/min) leads to an early onset of the exponential increase of aldehydes that are released and potentially inhaled by the user, but this would not happen in the same power with the proper high intensity air flow (around 10 L/min) used in DTL vaping. Then, a low puff volume instead of a volume consistent for DTL vaping leads to concentration of these quantities in a smaller volume of evacuated e-liquid vapor. This inconsistency between puffing parameters and device power is likely to lead to biased results in a toxicological evaluation, but it does not reflect the representative usage of sub-ohm devices for DTL vaping (see further discussion in Sections 3.1, 3.2, 11 and 13).

This section provides the necessary background to understand the main criticism of the studies that we revise in this review. The inconsistency between laboratory testing with a CORESTA or CORESTA-like protocol and majority representative usage of high-powered sub-ohm devices was already mentioned in the review by Farsalinos and Gillman of 2018 [11] of studies on carbonyl byproducts published before 2017. Unfortunately, many recent studies continue testing the devices under these inappropriate conditions, which puts forward the urgency to provide upgraded methodological standards and also to correctly evaluate the consistency of the experiments during the peer review process.

3. Realistic Testing vs. Realistic Vaping

Puffing parameters in laboratory testing of EC emissions must mimic as best as possible realistic usage. However, it is necessary to provide robust criteria for what can be understood as "realistic", since there is a wide diversity of vaping habits. We address this issue in this section.

3.1. Vaping Styles: MTL and DTL vs. Device Characteristics

There are two main forms of puffing ECs: the 'mouth to lung' (MTL) style (inhalation into the oropharyngeal cavity, momentaneous retention followed by lung inhalation) and 'direct to lung' (DTL) style (direct lung inhalation without oral cavity retention). The existence of these two main styles among the diversity in vaping behavior is not an issue of fashion, it has been observed (for example) in studies analyzing videos and films of many vapers in social media (see references in [10]), particularly a large study [54] was able to clearly distinguish the two styles after analyzing 300 videos containing 1200 puffing events from 252 vapers in 14 countries.

Although there is no published demographic evidence directly linking device type with preference of MTL or DTL styles, there are plausible arguments supporting the high compatibility of MTL style with low-powered devices with high resistances and DTL style with high-powered sub-ohm devices. This vaping style vs. device type connection has been long known by retailers, manufacturers and many consumers, with the following arguments put forward and commented in highly trusted vaping forums and magazines [55,56]:

- Low powered devices (ciga-likes, second generation clearomizers, cartridge and refillable pods, tank stating kits) typically operate at powers well below 20–25 W, have narrow mouthpieces and thus involve lower puffing volumes under high air resistance, similar to smoking. Beginner vapers (many of whom are still current smokers) tend to adopt the MTL style that is close to the puffing habits and puff volumes of cigarette smoking [57,58]. Typically, vapers using low powered devices for MTL style use PG dominated e-liquid solutions with higher nicotine concentrations.

- High powered sub-ohm devices operating at W > 40–50 W, use external batteries, often allow users to set up power/temperature, are more bulky and expensive than low powered devices, thus requiring higher level of maintenance and expertise. Their mouthpieces are wide and thus their low air resistance facilitates drawing large puffing volumes that need not be retained in the reduced volume of the oropharyngeal cavity. Therefore, they are not likely preferred by beginners or vapers simply trying to quit and remain smoke-free, but by veteran vapers who have quit smoking long ago and thus tend to enjoy the recreational hobby-like aspect of vaping, often puffing large clouds, using low nicotine concentrations and e-liquids with predominantly VG content.

Evidently, the rapid development of vaping technology and the growth and diversity of the vaping market have introduced a continuum of device types, including those of intermediate power (20–40 W) compatible with both MTL and DTL style and sub-ohm and supra-ohm resistances. with many vapers gradually becoming able to practice both styles: DTL with a sub-ohm device in situations in which emission of large aerosol clouds is not disturbing to bystanders (at home) and MTL when they need to vape discretely. Vapers gradually learn to follow their sensorial faculties to adapt to the diversity of devices according to their personal needs, though naive beginners or smokers trying to vape may experience unpleasant extreme situations when puffing a given device with the wrong 'technique' (see candid descriptions in [55]). Unfortunately, there is still insufficient published demographic data to assess vaping behavior.

In spite of the increasing diversity of vaping behavior, consumer magazines and forums comment that the two main vaping styles and their connection with device types still remain roughly well defined and distinguishable. These anecdotal accounts agree, in general, with available observations in studies cited by [10]. It is also consistent with the footage material examined in [54]: 80% of users of sub-ohm devices practice DTL and 98% of DTL vapers use sub-ohm devices, while 95% of users of low-powered supra-ohm devices practice MTL. However, the rapidly evolving dynamics of the vaping market might lead to substantial changes in the prevalence of these styles, such as a gradual increase of consumer preference for new low powered pod devices in the US [59], the UK [60] and Germany [61], as well as increasing popularity of low powered disposable devices, specially among young adults and teenagers [60,62,63].

The connection between vaping style and device type is relevant to assess emission studies, most of which have been carried on with CORESTA or CORESTA-like protocols, which should be appropriate for testing low powered devices used with low airflows and puff volumes comparable to cigarette smoking. However, as we argued in Section 2, testing high powered sub-ohm devices with the low airflows and puff volumes used by these protocols can be very problematic, as it increases the likelihood of overheating by narrowing the power range of optimal regime (approaching overheating conditions might be detected as a flavor deterioration, see Section 3.3). CORESTA or CORESTA-like protocols might be inconsistent with the majority consumer usage of sub-ohm devices for DTL vaping that involves large airflows (see Section 3.2). As we show in Sections 6-10 and summarize in Section 11, at least half of all revised laboratory emission studies have tested sub-ohm devices with CORESTA or CORESTA-like protocols. We discuss the shortcomings of this testing in Section 12 and the implications for health risk assessment in Section 13.

3.2. Inhalation Behavior

Inhaling through an EC device involves overcoming a specific pressure drop that must be added to the pressure of rest breathing a tidal volume around 500 mL, roughly 10% of vital capacity, with deeper inhalation involving more exerted pressure and inhaled volume. Every device has a specific air resistance coefficient linking the pressure drop generated to the airflow rate passing through. The physiological limits of full vital capacity (10 kPa) and this device-specific air resistance determine the physiological range of airflow rate in real life vaping. The volume capacity of the oropharyngeal cavity (100–170 cm^3 [64]) places physical limits to the amount of air diluted aerosol that can be puffed and flushed with a given puff duration for the mouth retention in MTL vaping, while no such limit occurs in DTL vaping.

Devices used for MTL vaping are mainly designed with small air inlet holes (diameters around 1–2 mm), which leads to a high air resistance that significantly reduces range the range of possible airflows. As an example [49], the Eroll device from Joyetech allows an airflow range of 0–2.8 L/min, with the user inhales very small volume even at the top value 2.8 L/min. Assuming a middle value of this range at 1.4 L/min and a puff with the rest tidal inhalation volume of 500 would imply a puff duration above 20 s, a long duration that is not only unrepresentative, but uncomfortable (normal breath lasts less than 5 s). Therefore, a user necessarily has to inhale a lesser aerosol volume that dilutes in air.

As a contrast, devices meant for DTL vaping have larger air inlet holes or a groove, all of which significantly reduces their air resistances, even leading to negligible values.

Therefore, the user will be able to generate significantly higher airflow rate. As an example, in the tests conducted in [49] most of the DTL devices only reached 20% of the maximal pressure of the lung at at airflow of 10 L/min, thus suggesting that the airflow rate can be, at least theoretically, significantly higher. Average adults under rest conditions breath 12–16 inhalations per minute, with breaths lasting on average 3.75–5 s and airflow rates of 7.5–10 L/min, with both frequency and volume increasing with effort.

However, vaping is mostly a recreational activity that tends to occur at an intensity close to resting conditions, so we can assume that, given the low to negligible air resistance of sub-ohm devices, DTL vaping involves inhalation through puffs whose volume will be close to that of the average resting tidal volume (500 mL), as the body does not require an extra consumption of oxygen. A "cloud chasing" competition or a presentation of a device might trigger an extra "performing" effort involving higher puff volume, but these are infrequent extreme situations. Additionally, given the extra effort needed to overcome the pressure drop of the device, we can also assume that puff duration will tend to be shorter than in a resting inhalation. While we do recognize the wide variation in puffing habits (even within DTL and MTL styles), we believe that a puff volume of 500 mL and puff duration of 3 s, with a resulting airflow rate of 10 L/min, seems to be appropriate to characterize on average DTL as a plausible hypothesis that needs to be tested experimentally.

3.3. Organoleptic Perceptions

Flavouring compounds emulating fruity, mint, tobacco and sweet desert tastes [65] are essential for e-liquids solutions to generate a pleasant aroma/taste sensation during vaping. The deterioration of these sensorial experiences can also signal users that their device might not be functioning normally. Under optimal conditions e-liquids are heated at temperatures below the boiling temperature of pure glycerol VG (288 °C), with heating elements still wet, at least close to the e-liquid, with the porous structure in the wick also wetted. Passing towards overheating conditions leads to local drying that increases with increasing power. The porous structures are built up with a sheet of cotton, mainly composed (>90%) of cellulose, which is a biopolymer made of a linear chain of D-glucose. Since the 1980s, the wood industry has undertaken well documented studies of cellulose pyrolysis through a heating process from 20 °C to 800 °C. This pyrolysis is not uniform and can be separated in four main stages [66,67]:

- Below 100 °C, cellulose loses water that is contained in its fibers.
- Between 150 °C and 290 °C, dehydration reactions occur resulting in a small weight lost.
- Between 290 °C and 380 °C, fast depolymerisation of cellulose happens releasing close to 80% of volatile condensable compounds (boil-oil) as levoglucosan reaching 60%, furans as 5-hydroxymethylfurfural (5-HMF), 5-methylfurfural (5-MF), furfural, furfuryl alcohol and gaseous compounds as CO, CO_2 and small chain compounds (glycolaldehyde, acetaldehyde, acetol).
- Between 380 °C and 800 °C, boil-oil also contains phenols and ketones compounds formed by the charring process of the remaining solid structure, with an important release of methane and CO resulting in a carbon mass at 800 °C.

An extensive discussion of the different processes during cellulose pyrolysis can be found in the review of Collard and Blin [68]. Bearing in mind the pyrolysis process outlined above, is is not outlandish to assume that the onset of overheating conditions in vaping can easily initiate the fastest stages of cellulose pyrolysis, resulting in additional mass loss that can be measured during the generation of emissions. Under such conditions, extra condensable and non-condensable compounds might be added to the gas phase of the aerosol generated by the vaporization of the e-liquid. Some of these new molecules are furans, like furfural and 2-furanmethanol, producing bread/burnt type of odors and a bitter taste. These organoleptic properties of condensable compounds are also well documented by the food industry, which uses wood burning to provide some specific flavours to various food items: smoked fish, meat, cheeses and other food items [69,70]. Additionally, some polycyclic aromatic hydrocarbons (PAHs), classified as respiratory HPHCs, are also produced mainly at temperatures above 400 °C [71].

Although the physicochemical processes linking the dry puff phenomenon to the cotton pyrolysis process have not been well researched, there is solid evidence documented in the literature of cellulose pyrolysis and wood burning, processes that release new chemicals that affect sensorial perception. While there is no experimental evidence that these effects are noticeable in vaping, it is not far fetched to assume that earlier stages of an overheating regime (temperatures around 280–300 °C) could trigger the early stages of this process through a deterioration of flavorings due to the extra release of chemicals. However, MTL devices have small heating coil surfaces and the passage from the optimal regime to overheating might occur more abruptly in more compressed power ranges (see Figure 1), but this passage can be gradual enough in DTL devices designed with significantly larger coil surfaces and normally used with large airflows (which favors lowering temperatures). Therefore, dry-puff conditions can be perceived as a local abrupt event in low power devices, but in DTL it should be sufficiently gradual to be perceived as a kind of taste deterioration by users.

3.4. Puffing Frequency and Duration

Given the advance in EC technology, it is not surprising to find a wide variation in puffing habits among the millions of vapers worldwide. Evidently, the standardized and regimented laboratory testing parameters will never provide a precise fit to real life vaping, but to evaluate how good an approximation it can be, it is unavoidable to consider averages and representative puffing parameters obtained in observational studies of vapers under natural conditions, with an understanding of their scope and limitations.

Early original observational studies of vaping habits (see review by Prasad [72]) showed similar mean numbers of daily puffs (mean ± SD): 225 ± 59 in [73], 163 ± 138, median = 132 in [74] and 78 ± 162 in [75], though reporting an enormous variability in the full range of daily puffs, for example: 24–1091 in [73] and 1–1286 in [74]. Vapers in these studies used first and second generation devices whose nicotine delivery rate was inefficient. Subjects in more recent studies [47,76,77] used second and third generation devices that allowed modifying power setups and with better nicotine deliver, thus reporting a compensatoty effect with more daily puffs for lower nicotine levels (see Section 10). These studies also report higher numbers of daily puffs, for example, we have from [47] (mean ± SD): 338 ± 161 (low nicotine level fixed power), 308 ± 135 (low nicotine level variable power), 279 ± 127 (high nicotine level fixed power), 272 ± 128 (high nicotine level variable power), where low and high nicotine level respecively given by 6 mg/mL and 18 mg/mL.

Besides counting daily puffs, it is important to remark that real life vaping follows circadian patterns that are not regimented. As shown in [74,78] puffs numbers cluster at daily hours of wakefulness (8 h to 23 h), identifying certain usage patterns: relatively regular puffing with large interpuff separation, short periods of very frequent short duration puffs (likely reminiscent of "cigarette breaks") and longer periods with long duration infrequent puffs (these patterns are also supported by videos of vapers [54]).

Considering the puffing data that emerges from these observational studies, we believe that the upper range of daily puff numbers (over 1000) found in [73,74] are unrepresentative outliers that can be ruled out. Assuming a wakefulness time of 16 h, 1000 puffs imply puffing every minute 1000 times, an excessive regime, more so considering the fact that vaping is not allowed in most work places, which significantly reduces the circadian period when vaping is possible.

Given the daily puffs outcomes from more recent studies and considering circadian variation comprising periods of frequent and infrequent puffing, we believe that a useful mean value that is most representative of vaping usage is 250–300 daily puffs, obviously understood as an estimator that roughly incorporates daily variation. This value is useful as a criterion to evaluate qualitatively how much interpuff lapses and puff duration in laboratory testing can be a reasonable approximation to observed patterns in a daily time frame. It is also useful to evaluate daily exposure doses given experimental outcomes expressed as a "per puff" basis. Thus, it is misleading to extrapolate to realistic vaping a study involving 50, 100 or 300 regimented puffs with a 10 s interpuff interval, as this frequent puffing has been observed to occur in a short timeframe involving 10–20 puffs, but it is not representative of daily behavior. Likewise, we can regard as unrealistic very long puff duration times, even if reported in observational studies (5.6 s is reported as 95% percentyl in [54]). Rather, we will consider as representative values 2–4 s puff duration.

4. Methodology: Towards a Consistency Standard of Laboratory Testing

This extensive review focuses on published articles on emissions form vaping products, with experiments aimed at characterizing byproducts generated by EC aerosol. We used the PubMed database applying the algorithm illustrated in Figure 3 with the following terms:

- electronic cigarette(s) OR e-cigarette(s) OR vaping product(s)
- AND aerosol(s) OR emission(s)
- AND (aldehyde(s) OR carbonyl(s) OR formaldehyde OR acetaldehyde OR acrolein OR acetone OR crotonaldehyde) OR (carbon monoxide) OR (free radical(s))

Since the review by Farsalinos and Gillman [11] has already revised studies published up to 2017, we excluded studies published before January 2018. From this searching process we found the 38 articles cited and listed in Table 1, mostly dealing with aldehydes, but also CO and and free radicals. We will evaluate these articles under the following criteria which we believe can provide a useful guideline for improving the quality of laboratory testing of EC emissions:

1. **Experimental consistency.** The consistency between the experimental procedure (puffing parameters, devices, analytic methods) and the best approximation available to user behavior. Experimental inconsistencies occur mainly between the type of device tested and (i) the puffing protocol, (ii) a supplied of power higher than the limits recommended by the manufacturer as inferred from the optimal regime.
2. **Reproducibility of the experiments.** The articles under revision must provide sufficient information that allows, in principle, a possible replication of the experiments. Vaping aerosol requires for its generation the usage of: a device (mod and atomizer), an e-liquid and a vaping regime (puffing). The authors must also provide the commercial name of the devices, as well as the technical information on the coil used (if it is a removable part), the commercial name of the e-liquid with as full information as possible, including the e-liquid composition if it is an in-lab production, all this together with the vaping regime: puff duration, the airflow rate, puff frequency, number of puffs/series. Experiments conducted with rebuilt devices ("Do It Yourself" devices) cannot be considered relevant to approximate real usage, as they are handmade coils.
3. **Toxicological confidence.** The authors must provide detailed account of the experimental outcomes to correctly compute daily exposure (with the right time frame and air dilution volume) and compare it with toxicological threshold limits published by official organizations. The utility and relevance of this comparison is closely tied to how well the study complies with the criteria of Experimental Consistency and Reproducibility, otherwise the risk assessment is either an over (or under) estimation, speculative, irrelevant to end users or only applicable/relevant to special minority niches.
4. **Old and/or used devices.** Authors testing such devices must communicate their storage conditions and current state, as well as justify the reason why such devices are tested. This is important, as there is evidence that devices older than 2–3 years (used or new) may degrade and undergo leaking corrosion (see full discussion of this issue in [79]).

We provide in Section 11 a color/symbol code system (tick marks and traffic lights) to evaluate how well the studies we review in the following sections comply with these quality criteria.

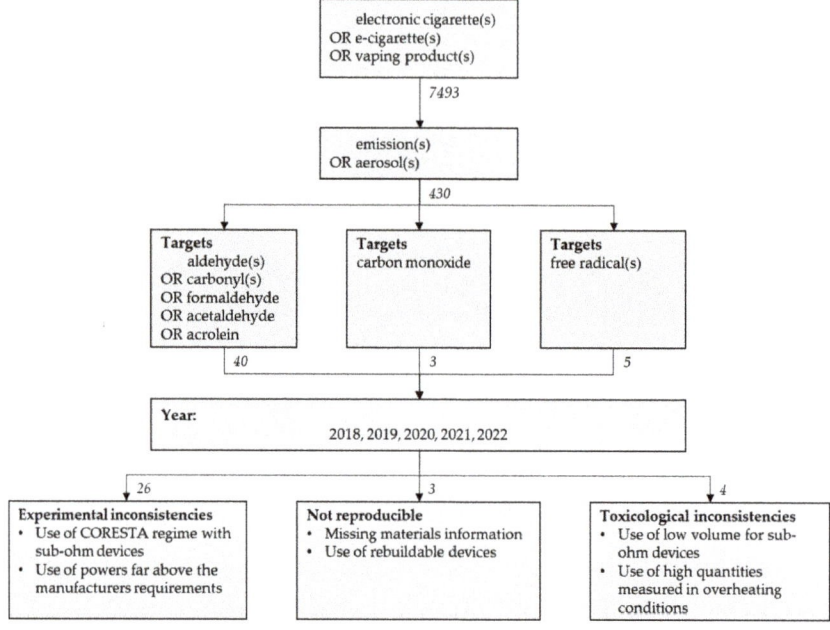

Figure 3. Methodological algorithm used to selecte the papers of this review.

5. Previously Published Review Articles

5.1. A Groundbreaking Review

Farsalinos and Gillman published [11] in 2018 an important review of 32 studies obtained by a PubMed search of studies published between 2013 and 2017 focusing on carbonyl byproducts. The authors comment on the wide (ad hoc) diversity experimental procedures, producing an enormous range of outcomes in concentrations, all of which is symptomatic of a lack of a consensual testing standard in this extensive literature, thus hampering the possibility of an objective comparison and interpretation of obtained results. While the overwhelming majority of the 32 reviewed studies tested the low-powered devices that were of common usage before 2017 (first and second generation ciga-likes and clearomizers), all of which are today either obsolete or of marginal use, the methodological critique by Farsalinos and Gillman is still relevant in assessing present day lack of proper standards in laboratory testing. As we argue in Sections 2–4 (and in our recent review of metal studies [5]), unrealistic testing, overheating and possible dry hits can also occur in emission studies testing devices available today (specially, but not only, third generation sub-ohm models).

In discussing the methodological considerations, the authors remark that excessively large concentrations of carbonyl byproducts (specially, but not only, formaldehyde) detected in some studies might be a consequence of machine testing the devices under inappropriate and/or unrealistic conditions, such as: puffing parameters that bear no connection with real life habits of consumers: too short inter-puff lapses and/or excessively long duration puffs, low puff volumes for third generation tank devices that were available commercially at the time of the review (2017). The authors place special emphasis on the specific "dry puff" phenomenon, a terminal overheating condition that arises as the e-liquid in the atomizer depletes and the supplied power pyrolyzes the wick (see Sections 2 and 3.3), all this taking place while vaping machines continue operating. The authors emphasize that only 4 of the 32 reviewed articles explicitly verified absence of a dry puff during testing. They argue that the simple ad hoc assumptions made by most authors on puffing parameters or ranges of supplied power would be insufficient to prevent or identify a dry puff during the experiments, but actual vapers participating in the testing can easily identify it by its "organoleptic" or sensory effects (a burning repellent taste). However, as we show in Section 2, the authors' claim that dry puffs dramatically increase carbonyl production is not speculative, but a fact verified experimentally, which complements sensorial testing by actual vapers as in [34].

Farsalinos and colleagues conducted in 2015 an observational laboratory experiment, aided by voluntary vapers, showing that excessively high aldehyde production only occurs under dry puff conditions [80]. However, they published replication studies (summarized in [11]) to reproduce the outcomes of two laboratory studies, Jensen et al. [81] and Sleiman et al. [82], which generated controversy and alarmist media headlines by detecting extremely large aldehyde concentrations much higher than in cigarette smoke:

- The experiment by Jensen et al. [81], published as a letter to the editor, examined the emissions of a top coil C4 device (now obsolete), detecting extremely high levels of formaldehyde hemiacetals, not formaldehyde, yet using the outcomes of their tests they estimated a lifetime cancer risk for formaldehyde inhalation in vaping that was 15 times higher than that from estimates from cigarette smoking. The replication in [83] showed using the same device and e-liquid that such levels only occur for abnormal usage under overheating and human identifiable dry puffs. Given the implications and the widespread diffusion of [81], there were calls for its retraction [84]. The team of Jensen et al. responded to this criticism in this communication [85], but as stated in [86], they could not deny that these worrying levels of byproducts did happen under abnormal usage conditions.

- Sleiman et al. [82] tested two devices: a top-coil and a bottom-coil, both with a silica wick atomizer filled with a commercial tobacco-flavored liquid. High levels of carbonyls were found (in ng/mg): formaldehyde 1300–48,200, acetaldehyde 260–19,080, acrolein 120–10,060, acetone 70–1410 and crotonaldehyde 10–720, with levels in the upper end of the ranges far exceeding the respective emissions from tobacco cigarettes, leading to warnings about serious risks from vaping. For the replication in [87] Farsalinos and colleagues used the same devices and aided by volunteering vapers showed that such high emissions happened under clear dry puff conditions, with usage in the normal ranges producing outcomes closer to the low end of the ng/mg ranges well below respective levels in cigarette smoke. They also tested a more recent device mentioned in [82] finding even lower aldehyde levels.

Another study by Khlystev and Sambureva [88], also reviewed in [11], claimed that flavorings by themselves generically dominate carbonyl production and lead to excessively large aldehyde production in comparison with testing the same device with nonflavored e-liquids. This study was also replicated in a comment by Farsalinos and Voudris [89], using the same device and (what seemed to be) the same e-liquids, showing that flavorings did not produce this large enhancement of aldehydes. This lead to an interesting exchange with Khlystev and Samburova replying to the comment [90] and Farsalinos and Voudris countering that reply [91]. In a more recent study in 2020 Gillman et al. [92] found that flavorings do contribute to aldehyde abundance, but at much lower levels of enhancement than those reported in [88].

5.2. A Recent Descriptive Review

Ward et al. (2020) [12] present a descriptive review summarizing the extensive literature on potentially harmful chemicals in ECs emissions, commenting very briefly only on the main outcomes. Toxicants are classified in 6 major categories: carbonyls, volatile organic chemicals, trace elements (metals), reactive oxygen species and free radicals, polycyclic aromatic hydrocarbons and tobacco-specific nitrosamines. The review contains 92 articles selected through the PRISMA search protocol. All studies we are revising in the present review (and in our review on metals in [5]) are also cited by Ward et al.

The review is a valuable source for references, but the reviewed articles are barely described without any critique. Given the large amount of cited studies, a merely descriptive approach is understandable and justified, though readers should be aware that substantial information is missing when presenting outcomes of studies without evaluation. To illustrate this point, we use an example taken from the section Trace elements of Ward et al, who cite a study by Ting et al. [93] (their reference 54) mentioning that it "identified that 5% of ECs and e-liquid combinations tested emitted Cr at levels that exceeded permissible daily exposure limits". However, the study of Ting et al. shows several serious flaws, making their outcomes completely unreliable: they did not identify the tested ECs and characteristics (brands, coil resistance, power/voltage ranges), did not specify the power levels in which the devices were tested and assumed an unrealistic amount of 1200 daily puffs to compute exposures. Evidently, this study has no utility or relevance to end users, yet readers will assume that it has the same quality as other cited studies.

6. Studies Focused on Quantifying Carbonyls and Other Byproducts

We present in this section an extensive revision of 22 studies mostly focused on laboratory experiments to quantify the presence of carbonyl byproducts in EC emissions, though some of the studies also discuss in detail pathways of thermal degradation for specific compounds. We exclude studies published before 2018, most of which were reviewed by Farsalinos and Gillman [11].

6.1. Studies Published in 2018

Vreeke, Peyton and Strogin. The authors [13] used NMR spectroscopy to examine the role of the chemical Triacetin (TA, used in "do it yourself" and in commercial e-liquids) in the enhancement of the production PG and VG degradation aldehydes (formaldehyde hemiacetals, acrolein and acetaldehyde), to explore the possibility that this enhancement might be derived directly from the flavoring molecules. They tested a sub-ohm device SMOK Alien 220 W with a SMOK Baby 0.4 Ω single vertical coil (at 55 and 65 W) and with a Kanger Protank 2 Clearomizer with a 2.2 Ω single horizontal coil (at 9 and 11 W), using a CORESTA protocol: 3 s puff, 30 s interpuff period and a 55 mL puffing volumes. Compared with an e-liquid with a 50:50 P/G mix and no TA, both devices with e-liquid containing 10% TA produced a significant increase in aldehyde levels, of up to 185% (about twice as much). Noticeably, save for the device with 2.2 Ω at 11 W, acrolein and acetaldehyde were only detected when TA was present in the e-liquid and the enhancement was larger for that device.

Information about aldehyde enhancement from specific flavoring chemicals is certainly useful for e-liquid manufacturers, regulators and consumers. The enhancement of aldehyde production was found in this study for the sub-ohm device at 55 and 65 W was. While these power levels might be within manufacturers recommendations when the device is used with airflows of DTL vaping, they should be in the overheating region when puffed with a reduced CORESTA airflow that narrows the power ranges of the optimal regime. Hence, these experimental outcomes were very likely obtained under overheating conditions that are either unrealistic or only relevant for a minority niche of users (see Sections 2, 3.1 and 12.1). The other combination of a powerful mod battery with an outdated clearomizer is very odd, as users would normally attach this clearomizers to low-powered mods.

Korzun et al. The authors [14] examined the effect of flow rates and levels of specific aerosol toxicants produced in EC emissions, arguing that their wide variation among users can be a confounding element in aerosol chemistry. Large airflows can lower coil temperatures and thus decrease toxicant production, a relevant fact for users of sub-ohm devices doing the DTL vaping style that involves large airflows and puff volumes (to generate "large clouds"). The authors argue that large airflows do not favor intermediate aldehyde formation compounds along the chemical paths of PG and VG degradation.

However, the authors' choice of the largest airflow in their experiments, 36 mL/s (roughly 2 L/min), is far below the typical airflows used in DTL vaping (about 170 mL/s or about 10 L/min [8]).

The tested device was a Tesla Invader III with a KangerTech SubTank Mini atomizer with operational power of 15–30 W, single bottom coils with a 1.26 Ω and 50:50 PG/VG e-liquids, tested at 11, 13, 17 and 24 W. Sessions of 20 puffs with two protocols: CORESTA (3 s puff duration, 30 s puff interval, 55 mL puff volume) and two Custom Square Mode (3 s puff duration, 30 s puff interval, 21 and 198 mL puff volume), flow rates of 18.3, 7.0 and 36 mL/s, respectively. Analytic determination by quantitative NMR (qNMR).

While testing at 11–17 W showed toxicants with concentrations below LOQ and LOD, the authors argue that the main hazard to end users is the excessive exposure to the solvents, particularly PG. The tested device at 24 W and 18.3 ml/s emits 18.5 mg/puff of PG/VG, assuming a 50:50 PG/VG partition as in the e-liquid and 25 puffs/h leads to 115.6 mg/h of inhaled PG. The authors compare this value with 75 mg/h inhaled PG, the dose from the 1 h inhalation threshold of the Spacecraft Maximum Acceptable Concentration of the NASA, concluding that PG inhalation poses a serious harm to users. This risk assessment is highly questionable, as the cited SMAC document warns that its threshold values are only applicable to a spacecraft environment (an extremely enclosed and isolated environment that bears no relation with real life vaping scenarios). Using a more reliable source looking at respiratory effects of PG aerosol inhalation in healthy human subjects [94], mild exposure related symptoms only occur at 871 mg/m^3 which (for 20 m^3 daily air breathing by adults) implies an inhalation of 725 mg/h of PG, 7 times above the inhaled PG from the tested device.

El Hellani et al. This study [15] assesses nicotine and carbonyl yields in popular low-powered devices in the U.S. market as of 2017: they tested 27 devices, disposables, pr-filled cartridges and tank models of 10 brands. E-liquids were in three flavors: tobacco and menthol a third different one, with 7.11–20.90 mg/mL nicotine concentration and a wide variation of VG/PG ratios and power ranges around a 5 W average. Sessions of 15 puffs were conducted, with puffing parameters selected to "represent an experienced user": 4 s puff duration and 10 s inter-puff duration with a puff velocity of 1.5 L/min. However, this excessively high puffing frequency is unrepresentative of EC users (though it may be representative of smoking breaks of cigarette smokers). It also increases the possibility of high carbonyl yields and even dry puffs [11,16].

In total 12 carbonyls in the gas phase were targeted for HPLC analysis, including formaldehyde, acetaldehyde, acetone, acrolein. However, the way the authors report and compare carbonyl yields and concentrations is misleading. They report a range 3.72–48.85 µg/15 puffs of carbonyl yields (also in the abstract), without mentioning that (from their Table 2 and Figure 2), the high end value of this range corresponds to only two unrepresentative outlier values (in 27 measurements) with 24 quantifications below 11 µg/15 puffs. As the authors recognize, such outliers are necessarily produced by dry puffs, and thus denote abnormal usage. They report formaldehyde concentrations of 0.58–5.05 mg/m^3, again without mention that the high end of this range corresponds to the same 2 unrepresentative outliers. These concentrations are lower than those in tobacco smoke (4.6–148.9 mg/m^3), but above measured human breath (<0.5 mg/m^3) and the short term 15 min exposure limit (REL of NIOSH) 0.123 mg/m^3. However, comparison with formaldehyde in human breath is irrelevant to assess exposures from ECs and the right occupational marker to compare EC emissions is not the 15 min SREL-NIOSH, but the PEL-NIOSH 0.92 mg/m^3 (or 0.75 ppm) for time averaged 8 h lifetime exposure, which is above the representative quantified formaldehyde concentrations around 0.6 mg/m^3.

6.2. Studies Published in 2019

Beauval et al. The authors [16] show that, together with multiple other factors (power, temperature, device architecture, e-liquid composition, flavorings), the choice of puffing parameters (specially puff duration and interpuff frequency) significantly influences aerosol yields and outcomes of aldehydes, a fact that complicates an objective comparison between studies and interpretation of their results. They also provide a summary of reported concentrations (in ng/puff) of formaldehyde, acetaldehyde, acetone, acrolein, propionaldehyde and methyl-glyoxal, reported in 20 studies published between 2013 and 2017 (all of which were reviewed by Farsalinos and Gillman).

Aerosol was generated from a single e-liquid (PG:VG 65/35, mint flavour; 16 mg/mL nicotine) by operating two devices from the French manufacturer NHOSS: a second generation "Lounge" model, 2.8 Ω nichrome top-coil, 4.6 W and a third generation "Mod box TC" model with Air Tank claromiser, 0.5 Ω kanthal bottom-coil and power supply 7–50 W, tested at ranges recommended by the manufacturer 18–30 W. They used DNPH cartridges for carbonyl collection and HPLC-UV for analysis. Aerosol temperature at the mouthpiece was measured by a NTC 3950 thermistor in separate tests under same conditions. Overheating and dry puff were controlled by monitoring also e-liquid consumption and replacing atomizers after each 20 puff session. Environmental contamination controlled by blank collections before each experiment.

Seven puffing regimes were defined for the tests, the standard CORESTA regime (puff volume: 55 mL, puff duration 3 s, puff frequency: a puff every 30 s) by the following modified parameters: puff volumes 35 and 100 mL (PV− and PV+, airflow 0.21 and 0.6 L/min), puff duration: 2 and 6 s (PD− and PD+) and puff frequency: 1 puff every 60 and 14 s (PF+ and PF−). The alteration of EC components after 480 puffs was also considered (the initial and final CORESTA, IC AND FC).

For the Lounge and TC 18 W consumed e-liquid was 5–10 mg/puff, with largest values produced by longer puff PD+, while the TC 30 W consumed 15–25 mg/puff with largest values produced by larger puff volume PV+. Regarding carbonyl outcomes, if we remove unrealistic PD+ and TC 30 W (a sub-ohm device tested with a low airflow) then concentrations are negligible (well below 1 µg/puff). Concentrations ranges (ng/puff): 20–255 (formaldehyde), 29–364 (acetaldehyde), 4.4–28 (Acetone), ND-40 (acroleine), 1.0–32 (propionaldehyde) and 4.5–141 (methyl-glyoxal).

The measured temperatures at the mouthpiece show smooth logarithmic-like curves that increase during the fist 5 puffs and reach a sort of plateau. These temperature measurements were not validated and are not reliable, since aerosol temperature time variation must be sensitive to the puffing sequence, producing saw teeth profiles. Nevertheless, it is interesting to qualitatively compare the temperature curves between the different graphs, as all were obtained with the same instrument and method. This comparison shows higher plateau temperatures for longer and more frequent puffs (PD+ and PF+) for both tested devices and all power settings. Also, the largest plateau temperatures occurs for the TC 30 W, which provides qualitative support to the inadequacy of testing a sub-ohm tank model at its higher power level with a low flow rate of at most 0.6 L/min.

Ooi et al. The authors [17] first sample emissions with a device made of an Innokin Iclear 30 S (Shenzhen, China) atomizer with a Kanthal coil and an Istick 30 W battery with a variable voltage of 2.0–8.0 V (no information is provided on power levels and coil resistance). E-liquids with various VG/PG ratios were used for GC-MS analysis, with the E-cig was operated at 4.80 V and vaped at 3 s per puff for a total of 12 puffs, with 30 s interpuff lapse and airflow 2.0 L/min (they refer their puffing parameters to their reference [14] published in 2014, which did not not use this airflow). The authors only report increasing presence (through GC-MS spectra) of carbonyls in aerosol emissions from e-liquids with a higher VG/PG ratio, but do not quantify the analytes, reporting only carbonyl outcomes from old studies published between 2010 and 2014.

After describing the limitations of the GC-MS analytic technique (analyte condensation inside sampling bags absorption into the aerosol phase prior to sample analysis), the authors sample and analyze the vapor phase by Fourier Transform Infrared Spectrometry (FTIR) in the emissions of a sub-ohm device Joyetech eVic-VT E-cig device with variable temperature control (ranges 200–600 F), at two temperatures: 500 F (260 °C) and 600 F (316 °C). No information is supplied on the puffing protocol. Emissions were generated for immediate analysis by FTIR, and thus (according to the authors) the obtained concentrations were much higher than the nondisclosed ones obtained with GC-MS and the other device: 1236 ± 361 mg/m^3 at 260 °C and 3250 ± 449 mg/m^3 at 315 °C, as well as 8.91 ± 0.07 mg/m^3 for CO at 315. However, these concentrations are meaningless without knowing the puffing parameters used for the Joyetech eVic-VT, a sub-ohm device that can run to high power up to 230 W and that they tested at its maximal temperature. The authors remark that their CO emissions were lower than those reported by El Hellani et al. [36] which surpass National Ambient Air Quality Standard, but (as we show in our comments on that study in Section 7) these outcomes correspond to unrealistic puffing parameters and thus are irrelevant for end users.

Balushkin et al. This comprehensive study [18] was funded by Philip Morris International. Thirty-four samples were tested of commercial devices purchased in 2015, 2017, and 2018: closed disposable "cigalike", cartridge systems and open tanks models (brands listed in supplementary file) and analyzed with 57 e-liquids brands and flavors, together with an internally prepared reference e-liquid (39.1% PG, 39.1% G, 1.8% nicotine, and 20% water) used in testing open tank systems.

The authors focus on carbonyls, specially: acetaldehyde, acrolein, and formaldehyde, though other HPHCs (nitrosamines, metals) were also targeted and generally found not quantifiable. The devices were tested from maximal e-liquid levels until full depletion, in horizontal position and at the highest temperature or power setting (for devices with variable temperature or power). Carbonyl compounds were analyzed using HPLC-UV. The study follows the CORESTA method 81 standardized aerosol generation and collection protocol, though slight variations of this protocol were used only for 9 closed systems, but these small puffing protocol deviations had little effect in their carbonyl emissions.

The authors define the "end of life" criterion for e-liquid depletion (12.5 mg mass loss per blocks of 50 puffs) to allow for a direct comparison of products and avoidance of dry puffs. Outcomes are reported on a per-puff basis computed from the lifetime average yields. The study shows that generally low-powered closed systems produce the lowest levels of lifetime average yields of carbonyl emissions (18.9–10,700, formaldehyde (see their Table 3), while these emissions are in general higher in open tank systems (538–53,400 ng/puff, formaldehyde (see their Table 4). However, these outcomes might be overestimations with respect to real life usage, as users might feel a foul flavor well before high lifetime percentages arise. Also, some of the tested devices were acquired as far back as 2015, which does not rule out corrosion and leaching effects, given the lack of information on their storage conditions.

Some of the results of the study provide very useful information to consumers. As shown in the examples displayed in Figures 4 and 5 of Baluskin et al., outcomes of formaldehyde in a closed system increase by an order of magnitud as the device reaches 50% of its lifetime, thus suggesting the need to avoid toxicants as best as possible by using the devices with high e-liquid levels in cartridges and tanks. Also, as shown in the supplementary file, usage of the device at 45 degrees inclination in general produces less carbonyl yields. The authors also stress the use of air blanks to avoid misrepresentation of the data in laboratory testing.

The study confirms facts that follow from the considerations we have presented in Section 2 on an optimal regime for aerosol generation and the realistic usage of devices, namely: negligible to low carbonyl yields occur in low-powered devices tested with an appropriate verification of absence of dry puffs, under CORESTA or CORESTA-like puffing protocols that are appropriate for the design of these devices. The authors do recognize that such puffing protocols are inadequate for testing sub-ohm open tank systems, which as we have stated, drastically reduce the power ranges of the optimal regime and do not provide (specially at high power settings) sufficient airflows and puff volumes that these devices require for an efficient aerosol generation to be used for DTL vaping.

Reilly et al. The authors [19] examine carbonyls and nicotine yields, as well as free radicals in aerosol emissions from four different flavors of Juul devices. The four flavors available at the time of the study (currently only tobacco and menthol are available) exhibited no difference in nicotine yields (164 ± 41 µg/puff), formaldehyde (0.20 ± 0.10 µg/puff), acetone (0.20 ± 0.05 µg/puff) and PG/VG ratio (PG/VG 30:70). To quantify free radicals the e-liquid in the cartridges were refilled with nicotine-free PG/VG ratios 30:70 or 60:40 with or without citral, leading to a concentration of 5.85 ± 1.20 pmol/puff ~10^{11} nmol/puff (5–6 orders of magnitude below cigarette smoke). Juul devices produce free radicals and carbonyls at substantially lower levels lower than those observed in other e-cig products.

6.3. Studies Published in 2020

Son et al. This study [21] evaluated the effects of device settings, vaping topographies and e-liquid compositions on the levels of carbonyl compounds. For the tested power settings devices with bottom coils generated 10–10,000 less formaldehyde than cigarette smoke. As the authors argue, aerosol emissions are affected by the patterns of of EC usage: puffing parameters (puff duration, frequency, volume), power settings, coils and e-liquids. As a guideline to determine their experimental settings from a wider variety of these patterns, the authors resort to the same parameters they have used in previous studies [40,95], based on observational data obtained from the same sample of 23 recruited vapers (we review [40] in Section 8).

All experiments were conducted with values from this observational data. For power and puff volume, the median (average, 95% percentile) were 6.4 (14.7, 31.3) W and 90 (35, 170) mL, puff duration 2.0 and 3.8 s (24 s interpuff interval). The EC was also the same is in [40,95]: refillable tank with replaceable Nichrome heating dual-bottom coils with 0.8 Ω, with two batteries Apollo Valiant battery (Apolo E-cigarette, Concord, CA, USA) and Sigelei-100W battery (Sigelei US, Pomona, CA, USA), range of power outputs 3–80 W, with wattage obtained by varying voltage for the 0.8 Ω coil. Collection and analysis: DNPH cartridges and an HPLC/UV system. To assure better control, e-liquids were prepared in situ in three compositions 100% VG, PG/VG 50:50 mixture and 100% PG, with 8 flavors freshly prepared by adding 10% of the corresponding flavoring agents.

As expected, aldehyde yields increased with power (6.4 W to 31.3 W), with larger rates for PG and PG:VG than for VG e-liquids, since PG boiling temperature is lower and byproduct formation initiates at lower temperatures as power increases. Formaldehyde yields increased for all e-liquids at increasing power (6.4–31.3 W), but (as expected) with a larger rate for PG and PG/VG 50:50 e-liquids than VG e-liquids. Acetaldehyde did not increase in 6.4–31.3 W in the VG e-liquid, but increased 2.7 and 8.5 times in PG/VG 50:50 and PG e-liquids. Acrolein yields increased 2 times between 6.4 W and 31.3 W. Fruit flavored e-liquids produced higher formaldehyde yields than mint/menthol and creamy/sweet flavored ones.

In terms of vaping topography, formaldehyde yields increased with increasing puff volume (35 mL to 90 mL) for fixed puff duration, but not significantly in 90–170 mL, increasing also with puff duration for fixed volume. However, as shown in their Table 3 for a pure VG e-liquid at 6.4 W, these combinations of puff volume and duration do not involve significant increase of aldehyde yields: for puff duration increasing 2 s to 3 s at average 90 mL puff volume formaldehyde goes from 790.0 ± 32.3 to 903.0 ± 56.2 ng/puff, with much smaller yields in all parameters for the remaining aldehydes.

This study is valuable because the authors have made an effort to incorporate in their experimental design a much wider set of vaping parameters (puffing, power settings, e-liquids, flavors) than most emission studies, which simply choose a fixed set for the whole testing. However, the authors' choice of parameters is still too limited, even if referred to the data of the small sample of 23 vapers they are considering. For example, instead of considering e-liquids with pure PG and VG (which are not realistic) a better choice would have been PG/VG 30:70 and PG/VG 70:30 mixtures.

Also, Table S2 of their Supplementary File shows that up to a 75 percentile of the 23 vapers use power settings below 13 W, while the upper value 31.3 W corresponds to a 95 percentile (one of the 23 vapers). Also, the authors mention in [95] that "These selected power output levels (6.4, 14.7, 31.3 W) have been characterized as *safe*, *hot*, and *extremely hot* on a popular consumer Web site that provides users with vaping tutorials". This is information from users based on their sensorial perception, it should not be dismissed (at least it should be considered). This information suggests that the lowest experimental value, 6.4 W, is representative (i.e., "safe"), not only of this sample but of consumers of this type of devices, while the upper experimental value 31.3 W is not only an outlier in this sample, but it is very likely a power setting that consumers would avoid ("extremely hot").

Evidently, the possibility that 31.3 W could be an unrepresentative outlier (likely used in the reference sample by one or two vapers) should have been verified by inquiring with end users. Consultation with end users and considering the output from their sensorial experiences can be extremely useful to set up realistic and relevant experimental parameters (see [34,53]). This is important, since at 31.3 W the levels of all carbonyls (specially formaldehyde) that were found in this study are much higher (specially for the unrealistic pure PG e-liquid). Considering 31.3 W as still representative, but without verifying it, might lead to artificially high estimations of ranges of carbonyl yields and exposure levels.

Considering as the most realistic parameters the V:G 50:50 mixture at 6.4 W, the values of carbonyl yields reported in Table 4 of their supplementary file of experimental outcomes for the combinations of power and e-liquid composition, shows a maximal formaldehyde yield of about 1 µg/puf, which for 250 average daily puffs leads to a daily formaldehyde exposure of 250 µg/day which is close to the strict AFNOR and OEHAA thresholds (assuming 20 m^3 of daily breathed air), but well below the occupational PEL-NIOSH of 18.45 mg/day.

Zelinkova and Wenzl The authors [23] tested the Voopoo Drag with its 0.25 Ω and 0.5 Ω and Vaporesso SWAG device with 0.15 Ω and 0.5 Ω coils. The devices were filled with PG/VG 50:50 e-liquids and the puffing protocol was a CORESTA regime. Formaldehyde, acetaldehyde, acrolein, propionaldehyde, acetone, butyraldehyde, crotonaldehyde and 2-Butanone were quantified for each power tested and matched with the mass of e-liquid vaporized. Power levels were varied from the lower one recommended by the manufacturers to levels above their recommendation. Each experiment was conducted in triplicate. Although the usage of a CORESTA protocol for testing two sub-ohm devices is either unrealistic or only relevant for a minority niche of users (see Sections 3 and 4), the study results are valuable, as they allow for the estimation of a maximal supplied power marking the outset of the exponential increase of aldehydes production. This study together with [22] illustrate the link between the optimal regime and a minimal aldehyde production (see Section 2).

Talih et al. The authors [22] examine and discuss the link between boiling processes and carbonyls formation. They tested 3 devices: a TF-N2 (0.12 Ω), a TFV12-Q4 (0.15 Ω) and a VF platinum (2.2 Ω), all filled with pure glycerol e-liquid, applying a 1 L/min airflow over 15 puffs of 4 s duration and 10 s interpuff interval (an excessively intense regime). This is an important study, which (as we discussed in Section 2) provides a significant contribution to the understanding of the physical processes of an overheating regime linked to film boiling. Although its experimental setup is unrealistic: two sub-ohm devices tested under a CORESTA-like regime with intense puffing, with all 3 devices tested at maximal power above the manufacturers recommendations, the authors' results illustrate that maximal supplied powers leads to an exponential increase in carbonyl production, specially formaldehyde, whereas these byproducts remain at minimal levels under specific power ranges that define optimal operational conditions.

Uchiyama et al. The authors [24] examine the effects of power and temperature on the generation of byproducts resulting from the thermal degradation pathways of PG and VG from 3 comercial devices. The 3 tested devices were not fully identified (no information whatosoever is supplied on models and brands), but from the described characteristics of the mods and atomizers it is evident they are powerful sub-ohm devices. For their denomination as Brands A, B, C respectively, battery voltage (V): 3.7, 3.7, 37, power range (W): 1–75, 7–75, 7–85, coil type and resistance (Ω): stainless steel 0.1–3.5, stainless steel 0.1, stainless steel and zinc alloy 0.3–3, recommended power range (W): 40–50, 15–60, 30–60. New atomizers were used in all e-cigarettes. Only one commercially available e-liquid consisting of PG (approx. 30%), and VG (approx. 70%) containing nicotine (approx. 0.3%), menthol, and apple flavor was used for all e-cigarettes.

Aerosol generation and collection was conducted according to the CORESTA protocol: 55 mL puff volume, 3-s puff duration, and 60-s puff interval. The latter interval was modified from 30 s to 60 s, since puffing had to be interrupted after approximately 10 puffs because of overheating and so the EC switch was turned on 2 s before puffing and turned off 10 s later. Analysis was conducted with QP 2010 Plus GC/MS and LC-20(HPLC) systems (Shimadzu, Kyoto, Japan).

Generation of carbonyl byproducts was very low with total particulate matter (TPM) 13 mg/15 puffs at supplied power of 10 W, but above 40 W byproduct generation exponentially increased. Testing the devices at 50 W shows (their Table 4) that device B emits much higher mass levels (in µg) in the gas phase than those of tobacco smoke (CM6 cigarette) of formaldehyde (2300 ± 220 vs. 15 ± 0.5), acetaldehyde (1800 ± 580 vs. 1200 ± 150) and acrolein (830 ± 87 vs. 120 ± 3.2).

The authors recognize that such high outcomes are associated with high temperatures (determined by temperature programs of the mods but not validated by the authors) exceeding 500 °C at 60–75 W reached by the atomizer of the device B, while the maximum temperature of the atomizer Brands A and C was approximately 250 °C with small variations above 40 W (this differences in temperatures are displayed in their Figure 7), While formaldehyde, acetaldehyde and acrolein reached for Brands A and C much lower levels than those with Brand B, these levels are still comparable to those of tobacco smoke (in their Table 4).

Evidently, several flaws can be identified in this study. Failure to properly identify the devices makes it more difficult to interpret outcomes and prevents any replication of the experiments. An odd result is finding formaldehyde split in the gas and particle phases, when its high volatility suggests it should be predominantly in the gas phase (an explanation of this odd result in terms of the aerosol collection methods was suggested in [30]).

However, the main shortcoming of this study is the usage of a CORESTA puffing protocol for testing sub-ohm devices at high power settings, as this leads to user irrelevant experimental conditions that are prone to overheating, as the authors recognize when setting up the puffing procedure sequence by turning off the device puffing 10 s after each puff. While carbonyl outcomes from devices Brands A and B were much lower, they were also extremely likely artificial overestimations due to testing under inadequate parameters. The authors' risk assessments are not relevant for real life vaping, as end users of these devices vape the DTL style with airflows and puffing volumes far larger than those of CORESTA protocol used to test them. A final remark, the authors refer to usage of EC's as "smoking" and vaping aerosols as "smoke". This a profoundly mistaken and misleading terminology.

Cunningham et al. This extensive study [25] by industry funded authors (British American Tobacco BAT) analyzes toxicant content in EC emissions from five EC manufactured by BAT, looking at the effects on the emissions from the variation of wicks, atomizer coils and benzoic acid content. After quantifying 97 aerosol constituents and 84 smoke compounds, 16 of the 19 HPHCs identified by FDA were absent in the emissions of all tested ECs. A comparison with two tobacco cigarettes showed that levels of the nine World Health Organization (WHO) TobReg priority cigarette smoke toxicants were more than 99% lower in the emissions of the ECs. No evidence was found of toxic byproducts formed from the thermal decomposition of benzoic acid in the e-cigarettes tested or from enhanced thermal decomposition of propylene glycol or glycerol by the nickel–iron coil.

The tested devices were BAT products: Vype ePen2 and Vype ePen3 (both Nicoventures Trading Ltd., Blackburn, UK). The study tested the Vype ePen2 at high power setting 4.4 W, but a low one 2.8 W is available. The device is button activated and is formed by a reusable section with a 650-mAh rechargeable battery and a disposable flavor cartridge, a silica rope wick and an NiCr coil. The Vype ePen3 operates at 5.9 W with a NiFe coil resistance 1.95–2.36 Ω, it is a closed system with a rechargeable 650-mAh battery and a flavored e-liquid pod of 2 mL capacity. The devices contains protect circuit board (PCB) to prevent over current and over charging. A fully charged battery provides 200 puffs.

The devices use e-liquids with different ratios of nicotine vs. benzoic acid and slightly different PG/VG ratio. For the comparison of the aerosol chemistry the ePen2 and ePen3 are filled with Blended Tobacco (18 mg/mL nicotine) and only the ePen3 with Master Blend (18 mg/mL nicotine with medium benzoic acid). The two cigarette products were: Kentucky reference 1R6F and Benson & Hedges Skyblue (Japan Tobacco International).

EC devices were tested with the puffing protocols of the CORESTA method 81 EC. For the tobacco cigarettes Canadian Modified conditions (55-mL puff volume, 2-s puff duration, 30-s interval, vents blocked). Aerosol collection: glass fiber filter disc (pad) followed by an impinger. Analysis by GC-MS. The authors provide measurements of background air/method samples and emphasize their importance to avoid confounding the quantification of toxicants at low concentrations with contamination from laboratory air and analytical methodology equipment and reagents.

Quantified outcomes are displayed as mass per puff for the ECs and tobacco cigarettes (Tables 3 and 4). For the ECs, besides aerosol collected matter, water, nicotine and the solvents PG and VG, most carbonyls appear BLD or NQ, with formaldehyde, acetaldehyde, acetone, methylglyoxal, isobutyraldehyde appearing at ng/puff levels. The remaining compounds (triacetin, menthol, PAHs, VOCs, TSNA, phenols, flavorants, acids and CO) are also BLD or NQ. The authors display the outcomes of same compounds for EC emissions as mass normalized by nicotine in their Tables 4 and 5. Depending on the nicotine concentration in the e-liquids, the ePen2 had 3–7 times lower nicotine yields per-puff than the ePen3 and 81% lower than those from both cigarettes, while the ePen3 with high levels of benzoic acid produced larger nicotine yields than the cigarettes.

The authors discuss various forms of comparing EC emissions with tobacco smoke, all of which showing a 2–3 orders of magnitude reduction in toxicant content. The lack of detection of benzene, phenols and PAHs rules out degradation products from benzoic acid, while absence of byproducts of wick materials (cotton and silica) in both EC devices disproves the hypothesis that silica is thermally more stable than cotton and provides evidence that wicks of both devices are stable under standard EC operating conditions.

Noël et al. The authors [26] examine the production of three aldehydes (formaldehyde, acetaldehyde and acrolein) from an unspecified EC device, undertaking a comprehensive cytotoxicity analysis on gene expression in human bronchial epithelial cells exposed at the air–liquid interface to the device emissions.

The authors do not disclose the device model and brand, they only mention that it operates with atomizers set up with 9 distinct resistance/voltage combinations: 0.15, 0.5 and 1.5 Ω and 2.8, 3.8 and 4.8 V, which leads from Ohm's law to these power ranges for each voltage: 52, 96, 153 W for 0.15 Ω, 16, 28, 46 W for 0.5 Ω and 5, 10, 15 W for 1.5 Ω. E-liquids with 36 mg/mL of nicotine were used (to mimic exposure of heavy smokers), PG/VG 50:50 ratio, and with either butter or cinnamon flavors. The puffing protocol was CORESTA 81: 3-s puff duration, and a 55-mL puff volume every 30-s. Samples were collected in 10-puff sessions. Quantification by gas chromatography with a flame ionization detector (GC- FID). Analysis HPLC.

Nicotine, acetaldehyde, formaldehyde, and acrolein levels (µg/puff) were flavor dependent. Large increase occurs when comparing 0.15 vs. 1.5 Ω at 4.8 V (15, 46, 153 W). Lesser increase was found for cinnamon flavor (acrolein was below LOD). Carbonyl yields were low for 1.5 Ω at all voltages (5, 10, 15 W). From the bars in their Figure 1, the three aldehydes have negligible levels (approx. 0.5 µg/puff) for all tests with 1.5 Ω and all voltages, with formaldehyde, acetaldehyde and acrolein, respectively, reaching 18, 10, 10 µg/puff for the combination 0.15 Ω at 4.8 V (153 W), with values for 0.5 Ω closer to those with 1.5 Ω.

The authors claim that sub-ohm vaping induces flavor dependent detrimental effects to human lung epithelial cells. They conclude that taking together their experimental results could help policymakers to "take the necessary steps to prevent the use or manufacturing of sub-ohm (i.e., 0.15 Ω) atomizers", as their emissions induce flavor-specific detrimental effects on lung cells due to cytotoxicity, enhanced oxidative stress, low levels of nitric oxide, diminished transepithelial electrical resistance (TEER), and altered expression of key genes associated with biotransformation, oxidative stress, and inflammation, all this besides cellular toxicity via oxidative stress mechanisms. Further, they claim that their data also suggests that ECs may not be a "safe" alternative to conventional cigarettes.

Evidently, the authors are issuing completely unwarranted and disproportionate statements. The claim that the type of laboratory cytotoxic experiments they have performed can somehow predict actual clinically verified harm in sub-ohm vapers, which would merit such a harsh regulation, is extremely speculative. The resulting increase of aldehyde levels, as well as their connection with deleterious cytotoxic effects from the sub-ohm device, simply follow from the authors' inappropriate and unrealistic experimental design: using a CORESTA puffing protocol to test this type of device at high power settings (153 W), which as we explained in Section 2 are the testing conditions that lead to overheating and possibly dry puff, producing an aerosol that end users most likely would find repellent.

Mallock et al. This German study [27] compared the US and European versions of Juul. While the early European version did not compensate for a much lower e-liquid nicotine concentration in this version, the modified version shows an increased vaporization that provides a better approximation to the nicotine delivery of the US version. Notably, carbonyl levels remain comparable to those of the US product. In general, carbonyl and other emissions byproducts are detected in Juul devices in lower levels than in other pod devices.

6.4. Studies Published in 2021

Chen et al. This comprehensive study [28] of Juul emissions by from Juul Labs, tested 4 Juul devices in terms of 4 product combinations available in the US market in 2021: nicotine concentrations 35/59 mg/mL in two favors: Virginia Tobacco (VT) and Menthol (Me). Carbonyls are in the Group I of analytes based on FDA guidance for in its Pre Market Tobacco Authorization (PMTA) process for vaping products. Aerosol was collected for Group I only in the "nonintense" (NI) regime with 3 s puff duration and 30 s interpuff interval. Ten replicate measurements were performed from each of each product combination. More than 40 of the 53 targeted analytes were below detection or below quantification. Mass per puff was analyzed over three 50-puff collection blocks: beginning, middle and one at the end. The outcomes were displayed in Table 3, showing the largest mass yields for formaldehyde and acetaldehyde at $\sim 10^{-2}$ µg for all product combinations.

Crosswhite at al. This study [29] was also funded by Juul Labs. It applied a nontargeted analysis to obtain a more complete list of aerosol constituents in the aerosol generated by the 4 varieties of Juul devices: Virginia Tobacco pods with 3.0% and 5.0% nicotine concentrations (VT3 and VT5). Aerosol was generated in sequential 50 puff blocks for a nonintense (3 s puff duration, 30 s interpuff lapse, 55 mL puff volume) and intense (6 s puff duration, 30 s interpuff lapse, 110 mL puff volume) regimes.

The analysis employs two complimentary nontargeted analytic methods: GC–MS methods optimized and adequate for analysis of for volatile/polar, including flavor and aroma compounds, together with LC–MS-based methods amenable to characterize semi/non/volatile, semi/non/polar and higher-molecular-weight compounds that might be contained in the liquid droplets making the particulate phase of EC aerosol. hieve a quantity estimation across multiple compounds. While these complementary analysis methods cover a broad chemical space, they cannot detect all chemicals in the aerosol (metals and nonionizable compounds). Aerosol trapping methods were adapted for each analytic technique. Blank samples were also analyzed.

Nicotine, PG, VG and benzoic acid were not detected. All detected compounds were above 0.7 µg/g for GC–MS analysis and above 0.5 µg/g for LC–HRMS analysis and differing from blank measurements were identified and semiquantified. Tentatively identified analytes were grouped in five groups: flavorants, HPHCs (from the FDA tobacco product supplied list), extractable and leachables, byproducts of chemical reactions and unidentifiable compounds. For VT3 the five groups formed 0.23% (intense) and 0.2% (non intense) of the aerosol mass, itemized as flavorants: 70% (intense) and 75% (nonintense), reaction byproducts: 16% (intense and nonintense). HPHCs were not detected in the nonintense regime. Similar outcomes were obtained for the VT5 in both intensity regimes. The numbers of detected compounds were 88 (VT2) and 91 (VT5), of which 67 are common in both intensity regimes, while compounds common with the 5162 compounds of tobacco smoke were 29 (VT3) and 32 (VT5).

Li et al. The authors [30] tested mainstream aerosols from a third generation device, Evolv DNA 75 color modular vaping device (Evolv LLC., Hudson, Ohio) with replacement single mesh vaping coils (SS316L, FreeMax Technology Inc., Shenzhen, China) that have a coil resistance of 0.12 Ω.

Emissions were tested for puffing parameters close to the CORESTA protocol: fixed flow rate 1.186 ± 0.002 and puff volume 59.3 ± 0.1 mL, but with variable puffing rate (2, 3, 4 puffs/min) and puff duration (2, 3, 4 s) at a fixed flow rate, both at 191 °C, 3 s puff and e-liquid with PG/VG = 30/70 and 3 mg/mL nicotine. Temperature was set for the tests at 157, 191, 216, 246 and 266 °C with the temperature control software supplied by the manufacturers. The authors recognize that this modified CORESTA protocol cannot be extrapolated to real vaping scenarios, but claim that increasing puff duration and controlling temperature can somehow compensate this limitation. However, it is unrealistic to keep fixed a CORESTA airflow and the temperature (assuming the device temperature control is accurate) while increasing puff duration. As we elaborate in Sections 2 and 12, this is the main drawback of this study.

The chemical characterization of carbonyl byproducts is undertaken by targeted and nontargeted analyses using LCHR-MS (liquid chromatography high-resolution mass spectrometry), GC gas chromatography, besides in situ chemical ionization mass spectrometry, and gravimetry. The authors provide a comprehensive discussion of the thermal degradation reaction pathways involved in carbonyl production in the normal temperature range of realistic vaping (below 266 °C), arguing that the heat-induced dehydration mechanism is dominant over the path of H-abstraction by radicals such as OH, the latter playing a minor but not negligible role.

The results of the study reinforce known outcomes: most aerosol components are volatile or semivolatile, with over 99.5% of emissions made of PG and VG in both aerosol phases. The study finds that PG mostly tends to be found in the gas phase, with the particle phase containing substantial part of VG and all nicotine (the nicotine phase partition depends on the e-liquid PH). Volatile carbonyls (including formaldehyde) tend to be in the gas phase. Other outcomes are:

- The temperature dependence of carbonyl production is very sensitive to the coil metal alloy (the authors' Figure 2), an expected result given the different heat conducting coefficients of these metals.
- The mass yields (in µg/puff) displayed in their Figure 3 show formaldehyde, hydroxyacetone, acetaldehyde, acrolein, and propionaldehyde, characterized by an exponential dependence on temperature that is seen to become steep at the upper temperature range (266 °C), while the dependence is linear for acetone, dihydroxyacetone, and glyceraldehyde.
- The PG/VG and nicotine ratios and nicotine proportion in the particle phase closely mirrors the PG/VG e-liquid ratio, with the 30/70 mixture (at 191 °C) leading to roughly 3/4 VG and 1/4 PG with 0.3% nicotine.
- As expected the mass concentration of 7 carbonyls increase with an increasing puff duration at same temperature (191 °C) and with fixed airflow (which makes these values unrealistic).

These results are consistent with the reaction modeling suggesting a higher efficiency of the heat-induced path at the tested temperature range, while the linear dependence (which may become exponential at temperatures higher than those tested) is consistent with the radical pathway dominating at temperatures above 360 °C. Although computerized modeling supports the heat-induced pathway from VG to be more efficient than the radical pathway at normal EC usage temperatures, formaldehyde, hydroxyacetone and acrolein can be formed from either pathway and from both PG and VG.

In discussing health impacts, the authors recognize that the doses for both solvents PG and VG are below toxicological makers and that the carbonyl concentrations they found are way below those of tobacco cigarettes (even in their higher range of tested temperatures). However, they develop questionable speculations on inhaling excessive doses of acrolein from the fact that this aldehyde is mainly a byproduct of VG, which becomes the dominant compound in the emissions as vaping proceeds.

Assuming an 8:1 ratio of VG to PG mass aerosolization for a PG/VG 30:70 mixture, they estimate (based on the outcomes they found in the study) that only 30–40% of the e-liquid will be consumed (well before liquid depletion) when it becomes entirely VG with likely a high acrolein content. This is very questionable, first because this hypothetical acroleine exposure is not applicable to actual vapers, since (as the authors admit) the puffing setup that they used cannot be extrapolated to real vaping scenarios (we discuss this issue in Section 12). Second, since sub-ohm tank devices are normally vaped with PG/VG 30:70 ratios and low nicotine concentrations for direct to lung style, serious deleterious effects from such an acrolein excess would have likely been noticed by end users who (following the authors' hypothesis) would end up vaping almost pure VG at high power ranges. However, so far the main reported concerning carbonyls are formaldehyde and acetaldehyde, with acrolein playing a minor role and (as far as we are aware) there is no evidence that sub-ohm vaping of VG dominated e-liquids intrinsically produces more adverse respiratory effects than other vaping styles and e-liquids.

Yan et al. The authors [31] apply orbitrap MS for a nontargeted analysis of EC emissions. They identify more than 30 "features" characterized by pairs of the mass to-charge ratio of the compound and the retention time. Compounds are identified containing nicotine and PG (NIC-PG) with increasing abundance relative to nicotine increasing supplied power.

Devices: OD1: an iStick 25 (Eleaf, Shenzhen, China) with power range 1–85 W and equipped with a HW2 coil (recommended range 20–70 W), and OD2: a SMOK Alien 220 Mod device (Shenzhen IVPS Technology Co, Shenzhen, China) with P = 6–220 W and equipped with a TFV8 Baby Tank and a SMOK V8 Baby-Q2 coil (recommended power range: 20–50 W). E-liquid was VG/PG 80:20 mixture. Aerosol was collected by a system of tubes and pipettes to a peristaltic pump. The devices were tested at high powers, OD1: 20, 40 and 80 W, OD2: 40, 120 and 200 W. The puffing protocol was: 4 s puffs, interpuff time 26 s at a flow rate of 1 L/min.

Except for the use of a different analytic technique (orbitrap MS) and a nontargeted approach, the authors used exactly the same experimental setup (devices, power settings, puffing parameters) as a study that we reviewed in [5] by Zhao et al. [96], which tested by means of the same low airflow CORESTA-like protocol the same high-powered sub-ohm devices at high power settings, even well above the settings recommended by the manufacturers. As we argue in Section 2, this experimental setting is a blue print for detecting large byproduct yields produced by laboratory testing under unrealistic and clearly overheating conditions that are prone to produce large levels of toxic byproducts. As with the sub-ohm devices tested in the study reviewed in [5], the experimental results of this study have no relevance for end users.

Tehrani et al. The authors [32] apply LC-HRMS, a sensitive analysis technique, to a nontargeted study of e-liquids and EC aerosols from 4 devices. The number of detected compounds and the proportion of combustion associated hydrocarbons in e-liquids increased when in aerosol form. Lipids and hazardous additives and contaminants, such as tributylphosphine oxide and the stimulant caffeine were also detected in e-liquids and aerosols.

The authors tested the following 4 devices: a third-generation modifiable-power (Smok ProColor 225W with TFV8 Big Baby Beast Tank, Shenzhen Ivps Co., Ltd., Shenzhen, China), two fourth-generation cartridge ("pods"): Juul, Juul Labs, San Francisco, CA and Vuse Alto, British American Tobacco, London, UK), and a disposable pod device (Blu Disposable, Imperial Brands, Bristol, UK). E-liquids covered a wide range of nicotine levels (whether base or salts) but only with tobacco flavor.

Aerosol was generated at 1.1 L/min airflow with puff topography based on the International Organization for Standardization 20768:2018 method 1541: 3 s puff duration and a shortened interpuff interval of 10 s. The shorter interpuff interval was found to be necessary to produce sufficient condensed aerosol sample volumes for Blu, Juul, and the PG/VG base e-liquid. Three blocks of consecutive 100 puffs each were machine puffed for each device, recharging after each block, with aerosols generated from a single pool of e-liquid for each product for the 3 blocks. Slightly higher aerosol mass was generated in the final 100-puff interval for the Juul, whose maximal set by manufacturers is 200 puffs.

It is not surprising that such a vast array of compounds were detected, given the high resolution of LC-HRMS and the enormous amount of generated aerosol from such an extremely intense puffing regime: 3 blocks of 100 puffs taken each 10 s. Since demographic studies of vapers in natural conditions [72–75] show on average 200–300 daily puffs, such a regime would involve compacting all daily puffing during 12–16 h of wakefulness into 30–50 min. This is evidently an unrealistic experimental setup geared to detect as much compounds as possible, even if this is achieved under conditions completely unrelated and detached from real life.

Besides being unrealistic, this regime is an artificial way to magnify detection of byproducts in emissions, even from the trapping material or the environment. As shown in the study by Belushkin et al. [18], production of byproducts in the aerosol significantly increases as a device is consuming e-liquid that is progressively "aging", even without depletion. This aging can be critical for low-powered pod devices being puffed with the same e-liquid 300 times every 10 s.

Regarding the Smok ProColor 225W with a TFV8 Big Baby Beast Tank, a powerful sub-ohm device, the authors fail to disclose the power settings and coil resistance with which it was tested, an essential information to interpret and possibly replicate their results. Also, the use of an airflow of 1.1 L/min is completely inappropriate for such a device designed and used for DTL vaping. Testing this device with this puffing regime most likely leads to overheating conditions even if puffed within the recommended power settings (see Section 2). Furfural and various fatty acids are byproducts of cellulose (wick) pyrolysis (see Section 3), but are also among the compounds detected in this study, which would confirm testing under dry puff conditions.

The authors present a very detailed examination and classification of the detected compounds, validation tests and calibrations. However, this comprehensive study is completely unrealistic and irrelevant for end users.

Cancelada et al. The authors [20] quantified HPHCs in aerosols emissions generated using a SMOK V8 kit designed with a TFV8 Big Baby tank and five coils M2 (0.15 Ω and 0.25 Ω), X4 (0.15 Ω), T8 (0.15 Ω) and Q2 (0.6 Ω) filled with a commercial e-liquid Euro Gold from Naked 100. The experiments were conducted using a fixed nominal voltage of 3.8V (i.e., 98 W for 0.15 Ω coils, 58 W for 0.25 Ω coil and 24 W for 0.6 Ω coil) varying puff volume (50 mL, 100 mL, 250 mL, 350 mL and 500 mL) and a fraction of airflow vent system opening (0%, 25%, 75% and 100%). The first series of experiments reported the masses of e-liquid vaporized (MEV) according to the puff volumes for the different opening fractions tested using the M2 0.15 Ω. Because the results are close to each other (except at very low puffs volume), the authors reported that the puff volume and opening fraction did not affect the mass of e-liquid vaporized. As we argue in detail in Section 2, this interpretation of the results is erroneous, as the experiments were conducted with a single power. This is even more confusing, as the M2-0.15 Ω coil is normally recommended by the manufacturer to operate between 25 W and 80 W and the one tested here was running at 96 W (based on manufacturer information).

The authors further graphed an open airflow system vs. puff volume in a grid, with formaldehyde levels quantified and reported in terms of the mass of e-liquid vaporised in the emissions. The resulting graph shows some higher formaldehyde levels with small puff volume and reduced airflow than with high puff volume and fully open vent system. Even more interesting, iso-lines can be estimated with a picture at 0% and 50 mL and tends to a very low limit approaching 500 mL and/or 100%. The authors argue that increasing airflow rate can reduce the degree of decomposition of e-liquid components. In reality, changing the puff volume or the airflow opening fraction modifies the same parameter: the speed of air, as they change the pressure drop in the device. With the characterizations of the air resistance for each opening fraction these results would have highlighted that the iso-values are due to experiments carried out with the same speed of air and the same heat exchange by forced convection. The remaining graph would be a classic one with the speed of air in the x-axis and the formalehyde ratio in the y-axis. As for MEV, the interpretation of the results is confusing because it was obtained with a single fixed power.

Finally, the authors tested the five coils using two opening fractions 50% and 25% with a 50 mL puff volume and reported the MEV and the quantities of some HCHPs with 50% fraction. Based on the previous experiments, the authors would provide results obtained with a CORESTA-like vaping regime unless they made experiments using a puff volume (i.e., airflow rate) consistent with DTL. The MEV of the 0.6 Ω coil (24 W) is lower than 0.25 Ω (58 W), itself lower than 0.15 Ω dual and quadruple coils (96 W), still lower than the octuple coils. As these classification is now surprising, it should be noted that they are initially recommended for power range of respectively 40 W–80 W (Q2), 30–50 W (M2), 25–80 W (M2), 30–70 W (X4) and 50–110 W (M2) highlighting that Q2 was tested below the requirements, T8 under the range required and M2, X4 above the requirements. Based on this observation, it is also not surprising that so high levels of carbonyls were found for M2 0.25 Ω and that 0.15 Ω dual coil has high deviations compared to the results of the others coils suggesting that dry puff occurs for one device.

6.5. Studies Published in 2022

Xu et al. The authors [33] quantified HPHCs in aerosols emissions of four market-leading flavoured e-cigarettes available in the Chinese market. Levels of eight carbonyls, five volatile organic compounds (VOCs), four tobacco-specific nitrosamines (TSNAs), 16 polycyclic aromatic hydrocarbons (PAHs), and seven heavy metals where quantified and compared with their presence in mainstream tobacco smoke. Small variations of mass yields of carbonyls were found among the different ECs, but the vast majority of targeted HPHCs were either undetected or found in significantly lower yields than in cigarette smoke (commercial or reference 3R4F).

Two devices were tested, each with nonrefillable cartridges in two flavors: RELX Classic (mung bean and tobacco) and RELX Infinity (coke and watermelon), both operating at 6.5 W. Aerosols were generated and collected by 100 puffs with the CORESTA Recommended Method No. 81: a square-wave puff profile, 55 mL puff volume, 3 s puff duration, and 30 s interpuff interval. Aerosol condensate was passed either through a collection vessel containing suitable solvent for the analysis of carbonyls, VOCs or heavy metals (lead, stibium, arsenic, nickel, chromium, cadmium, and mercury). TSNAs and PAHs were collected through a Cambridge filter pad. For comparison with tobacco smoke a cigarette was counted as 10 EC puffs.

Quantification of formaldehyde, acetaldehyde, acrolein, acetone, propionaldehyde, butanol, butyraldehyde, and butanone was based on CORESTA Recommended Method No. 7414 and the AFNOR XP D90-300-3 standard. Samples were analyzed by ultraperformance liquid chromatography (UPLC). The study also targeted and quantified VOCs, TSNAs, PAHs and heavy metals. The mass yields as µg/100 puffs and µg/10 cigarettes were displayed in Table 2.

For carbonyls, the largest mass yield (ng/puff) in the ECs was for formaldehyde: 0.017–0.15, acetaldehyde: 0.017–0.092, acetone: 0.005–0.048, acrolein: 0.015–0.042, with the remaining carbonyls below detection. VOCs, TSNAs, PAHs were all below detection limits, while negligible yields were quantified for heavy metals (the largest for nickel at 1.78 ng/puff). Carbonyls yields were three orders of magnitude smaller than their corresponding yields in tobacco smoke.

In the neutral red uptake and Ames assays, aqueous extracts of the e-cigarette aerosols did not induce obvious cytotoxicity or mutagenicity, whereas CS aqueous extract showed dose-related cytotoxicity and mutagenicity.

Visser et al. The authors [34] present a 'human volunteer-validated' approach that can provide user relevant conditions in laboratory testing of EC emissions. The study matches the dry puff assessment from 13 volunteering experienced vapers with carbonyl detection laboratory testing. This approach can reduce the possibility of reporting excessively high toxicant levels that emerge in tests conducted under unrealistic conditions, producing EC aerosols that end users would find unpleasant and even repellent (specially the dry puff 'burned out' sensation).

Vapers used the same EC devices (JustFog Q16C with 1.2 and 1.6 Ω coils and eLeaf Pico batteries). Power ranges recommended by the manufacturer were 6.4–12.1 W (1.6 Ω coil) and 8.5–16.1 W (1.2 Ω coil). The e-liquids were: menthol, vanilla and fruit, with PG/VG ratio 50/50, 30/70, 30/70 and nicotine levels 0, 0, 3 mg/mL, respectively. The vapers were instructed to vape in 'mouth to lung' style (to avoid as much as possible excessive deviation in airflows and puff volumes), sampling six combinations of coils, e-liquids and power levels (10 W–25 W in 3 W steps), reporting the absence/presence of a dry puff sensation through a 100-unit visual analog scale. Every combination was classified as either "dry puff flavor" (10% of the puffs reporting this sensation) or "no dry puff flavor" (otherwise).

As expected, dry puff sensation was not reported in any coil/liquid combination at lower power ranges 10–13 W, but above 13 W a complicated pattern emerged that depends on the e-liquids and coils. In parallel with this assessment, laboratory testing was conducted for the same combinations of coils, e-liquids and power settings assessed by the vapers, targeting carbonyl compounds through a HPLC-DAD (high-performance liquid chromatography—diode array detection) analysis. The puffing parameters were blocks of three 3-second puffs with 1-minute intervals and puff volume of 55 mL. The analysis detected only at higher power ranges 11 carbonyl species: formaldehyde, two acetaldehyde isomers, acrolein and lactaldehyde (the remaining were not identified). These compounds were denoted "dry puff markers" and a cutoff for each one was defined as its maximal quantified value (in µg/puff) in the power range (in each combination of coils/liquids) where the vapers assessed "no dry puff flavor". For every coil/liquid combination, outcomes of these 11 markers above the cutoff were regarded as dry puffs (a very conservative approach, since the vapers did not report a dry puffs in 90% of the puffs).

The criterion to test the matching between vapers' sensorial assessment and the chemical analysis was given by 11 carbonyl markers being above their cutoff values, which identified the corresponding coil/liquid/power combinations as dry puffs. This matching was consistent for 83% of puffs with 17% false negatives, with the largest divergence occurring in the fruit flavored e-liquid with the 1.6 Ω coil (60% dry puffs from the carbonyl test vs. 20% for the sensorial evaluation at about 20 W).

This study represents a fist step in the incorporation of end user input in the improvement of laboratory testing of EC emissions. The authors recognize the obvious limitations of the study (small sample of users, e-liquids, coils and a single EC device, subjectivity of sensorial validation). However, the study has other limitations not mentioned by the authors. The dry puff is not a sudden isolated event, it can emerge gradually, with overheating before a dry puff producing variation of sensorial experiences in users (the authors did not verify e-liquids depletion, so it can not be ruled out that users reported these variations). Evidently, as the authors suggest, studies with larger samples of vapers and devices should follow since human assistance can increase the accuracy and quality of emission testing.

7. Carbon Monoxide (CO)

The present section provides a review of three studies that detected CO in EC aerosol emissions. Since CO is a hazardous byproduct of incomplete combustion, it is important to understand under which experimental conditions it has been detected when testing ECs.

Casebolt et al. (2019). The authors [35] used a Cleito device with a 0.2 Ω coil filled with two commercial e-liquids of 50:50 PG/VG ratio. Despite the fact that this device is designed for DTL inhalation, the experimental airflow rate was 0.85 L/min, which is inconsistent with real use of the device (it is even below that of the CORESTA protocol for the low intensity vaping regime ISO20768: 1.1 LT/min). The recommended power specifications for this device can be found in the internet: between 55 and 70 Watts. Ignoring this information they conducted the experiments applying powers from 40 to 180 Watts by steps of 20 Watts. Their results reveal an exponential increase in the maximal concentration of CO from 60 Watts onwards, though it is close to zero for power below 60 Watts. Casebolt et al. [35] concluded by an alarmist warning on CO production in commercial devices, despite the fact that their results show that CO was not quantifiable under the normal operational power of the devices, only under unrealistic tested conditions.

El-Hellani et al. (2019). The authors [36] used a rebuildable atomizer to test the presence of CO in emission from sub-ohm electronic cigarettes. For this purpose they designed a coil from different alloys (nichrome, nickel, stainless steel and Kanthal) by wrapping a 24 or 26 Ga wire (diameters of 0.511 mm and 0.405 mm) around an inner diameter of 3 mm leading to 10 or 13 wraps. Japanese cotton was wetted with a 30/70 PG/VG e-liquid ratio and an air flow rate of 1 L/min was applied. All their coils had the same surface, though their geometric shape was different. In their Figure 3 they reported the detection of CO in the aerosol when applying powers from 25 to 175 Watts by steps of 25 Watts. No CO was detected below 100 Watts and levels started to be detected from 125 Watts with an increasing peak according to the supplied power. Then, in their Figure 1, they compared the use of different coil geometries (keeping their surface constant) at 125 Watts. For the same geometry (denoted by A in their paper), CO was quantified with its reported values displaying a high dispersion, thus suggesting that this is not a reproducible experiment. This might be due to the fact that 125 Watts is the minimal starting point of production. Finally, they designed an additional geometry to compare CO daily exposure at 75, 125 and 200 Watts to the CO exposure from a conventional cigarette. The geometry they used represents half of the initial geometry (5 wraps instead of 10), leading to a surface divide by 2. As boiling is a thermal phenomenon and the coil surface is a key parameter, the functioning limits using 5 wraps can be estimated by dividing them at 10 wraps by the same order of magnitude. Therefore, from the detection of CO using 10 wraps beginning at 100–125 Watts, we can assume that these limits would be between 50 and 63 Watts using 5 wraps.

The authors assumed glycerol pyrolysis as the source of CO production. Their results from an experimented study [97] on the degradation of glycerol in the gas phase shows production of CO and also CO_2 from 675 C onwards, which are temperatures well above those of a vaping device in which glycerol is heated and vaporized from its liquid phase. As it reaches gas phase conditions, it mixes with fresh air and cools almost instantaneously. Rather, CO production can be explained by another source of pyrolysis. As film boiling is initiated, it creates a layer of gas around a small part of the wire creating an associated volume of dried fibers under conditions that are adequate for cellulose pyrolysis for which CO and CO_2 formation is well documented and reported at temperatures above 400 C [98,99]. Therefore, there is a high probability that the authors detected CO under dry puff conditions that are repellent to end users.

Son et al. (2019). The authors [37] investigated CO productions using a pod (JUUL), a ciga-like (V2 VMR products), a top-coil (Ego CE4) and a mod (Cleito 0.4 Ω). Ciga-likes are now obsolete and the Ego CE4 is no longer available due to capillary issues, but the Juul and Cleito devices are still marketed. The Cleito is recommended for DTL vaping and for power between 40 and 60 Watts. The airflow rate during the experiments (1.5 L/min) is inconsistent with the real use of the device. Together, the JUUL and Cleito produced a quantity of CO below 10 µg per puff, leading to a daily inhalation of CO below 2.5 mg (assuming 250 puffs per day). The WHO recommends a maximal allowed concentration of 103 mg/m^3 during 15 consecutive minutes (in a volume inhaled of 0.2 m^3 in 15 min). Even if a user vapes 250 daily puffs in 15 min (an impossible feat), the exposure concentration is 12 mg/m^3, representing 12% of the WHO recommendation. It is evident that spacing the puffs through a day leads to the dilution of local peaks of concentrations in CO and to an exposure concentration representing 2% of the daily requirement (7 mg/m^3). Using the most worrying result obtained in the paper, CO does not exceed this toxicological limit. In comparison with a conventional cigarette (10 cigarettes per day, 13 puffs per cigarette, 0.75–1.73 mg of CO per puff), a daily use of a vaping device leads to the inhalation of at most 1/161 of the CO inhaled from a conventional cigarette.

8. Reactive Oxygen Species (ROS)

Reactive Oxygen Species (ROS), specially Hydroxyls and OH compounds, in EC aerosol have been the subject of several studies [38–41,100,101] (we exclude [101], as its experimental procedure is too obscure and EC devices were not identified). Free radicals are an important group of potentially toxic byproducts, as they are a major constituent of reactive oxygen species (ROS) and reactive nitrogen species (RNS) responsible for oxidative stress affecting many physiological functions. We review five studies focused on free radical detection in EC aerosol emissions.

Bitzer et al. (2018a). The authors [38] tested a powerful sub-ohm device: Wismec Reuleaux RX200S Mod, powered by three 18650 batteries and endowed with "constant control temperature" and "constant control power" modes, which allow the user to operate the device by fixing a target constant temperature or power in the ranges 100–315 °C and 1–200 W. The tests were conducted in both modes. As in previous studies [39,100], the authors conducted experiments with CORESTA-like puffing parameters: 40 puffs, 5 s puff duration, 30 s interpuff lapse and airflow rate of 500 mL/min = 8.33 mL/s.

The study spin trapped and analyzed free radicals through a nontargeted species approach by electron paramagnetic resonance (EPR). The detected free radical abundance was $\sim 10^{13}$–10^{14} molecules/puff. A previous 2016 study by the same group of authors [100] using a low-powered device detected an abundance of $\sim 10^{13}$. These free radical levels are between 1/100 and 1/1000 of the free radical abundance of $\sim 10^{16}$–10^{17} molecules/puff detected in tobacco smoke with the same EPR technique (see [38,39,100]). Free radical production increased as follows:

- close to 2-fold between 100 and 300 °C under constant-temperature regime.
- at even steeper rate from 10 to 50 W under constant wattage, with coil temperatures higher than those of the constant-temperature regime.
- close to 3-fold in e-liquid mixtures with higher PG content in comparison with ratios of PG/VG 0:100 and PG/VG 100:0. This was associated with an increases in aerosol-induced oxidation of biologically relevant lipids.

These results show that reactive free radical production in e-cigarette aerosols is highly solvent. While radical production depended on aerosol generated at higher temperatures, disproportionately high levels were observed at close to 100 °C despite limited aerosol production.

However, there are various problems with the experimental setup. Coil temperature controls from instruments in sub-ohm devices are not very reliable: they are based on applying Fourier law to flat homogenous medium whose conductive properties are given by simplified empiric relations between power and resistance for different alloys (the formula in equation 1 of the study). To address this problem the authors should have provided an experimental validation of temperature measurements. There is also a conceptual problem with fixing the temperature (See Section 12), which is a thermodynamical intensive state variable whose evolution is determined (see Section 2) by the heat flux exchange balance between e-liquid vaporization close to thermal equilibrium and its condensation (and aerosol formation) by forced convection. Fixing the temperature at an arbitrary value (assuming it is experimentally validated and accurate) would force an isothermal process that is most likely, either incompatible with the heat exchange balance, or conducing to contrived conditions on coil resistance or power.

The constant power regime is more consistent, as power is an extensive state variable that can be set up externally. However, the authors used a CORESTA-like puffing protocols with an extremely small airflow rate (0.5 L/min). As we argue in Sections 3 and 4, such diminished airflow is problematic for testing a powerful sub-ohm device, as it should lead to a severely narrowed power range of the optimal regime (see Figure 2), with a high likelihood that its upper power end (which determines the outset of overheating) lies within the 10–50 W ranges in which the authors conducted the tests. Not surprisingly, the authors detected a steep increase of free radical production as the device was tested along 10–50 W. The authors mention that this increase was due to high temperatures, but we would add that this is a further sign of testing in clear overheating conditions.

While the experimental settings of this study might allow for certain combinations of power, temperature and resistance that correspond to real life usage or at least conditions relevant to a majority of users, the authors do recognize (and we argue in Sections 3 and 4) that it might also lead to combinations that are completely unrealistic or only applicable to a minority of vapers who might use sub-ohm devices for MTL style. This is a valuable study, but its experimental outcomes are likely applicable only to a minority niche of vapers (see Sections 2, 3.1 and 12.1).

Bitzer et al. (2018b). This is a study [39] by the same group of authors as [38], focusing on the effect of flavorings compounds on the production of free radicals. The authors use the same device as [38], a device endowed with a constant temperature mode that permits setting up its operation at a fixed temperature. The puffing protocols was also the same as in [38]: 5 s puff duration, 30 s interpuff lapse and 500 mL/min = 8.33 mL/s. Hence, our critique on [38] is directly applicable to this study (see our comments further ahead).

The authors analyzed (with GC-MS) 49 commercially available nicotine-free food grade flavor concentrates (β-damascone, δ-tetradecalactone, γ-decalactone, citral, dipentene, ethyl maltol, ethyl vanillin, linalool, and piperonal), as well as food grade ethyl vanillin propylene glycol acetal (found in more than 45% of flavors). Nearly 300 unique chemicals were identified in the concentrates. To examined thermal degradation of flavored aerosols, the concentrates were diluted to 20% into a mixture PG/VG 60:40 in similar concentrations found in commercial e-liquids.

Close to 43% of the flavors resulted in significant increases in radical production as compared to the base PG:GLY (60:40) mixture: from 46% (lemon) to 122% (vanilla custard), but significant reductions in radical production below baseline were observed as a result of adding Vanilla flavoring. The radical inhibition effects of ethyl vanillin suggest its possible use an additive in e-liquids reduce free radical production during aerosol formation.

Relative abundance of the different flavorants in each e-liquid concentrate was correlated with radical production. Strong correlations between found for β-damascone, δ-tetradecalactone, γ-decalactone, citral, dipentene, ethyl maltol, ethyl vanillin, ethyl vanillin PG acetal, linalool, and piperonal. Dipentene, ethyl maltol, citral, linalool, and piperonal promoted radical formation in a concentration-dependent manner. However, interestingly, ethyl vanillin inhibited the radical formation also in a concentration dependent manner. The capacity to oxidize biologically-relevant lipids was closely linked with free radical production.

To assess the results of this study we remark that all experiments were conducted with the tested EC device setup at 225 °C and 50 W, but aerosols were generated by a very low airflow, a rate 50% lower than that of the CORESTA 1 L/min airflow. This is important, since as we argued in the revision of [38] (and as shown in Figure 2 and discussed in Section 2) such a small airflow rate should produce a significant reduction of the power range of the optimal regime, rising the probability that the fixed 50 W used in the testing could be in the overheating region. Hence, it is not possible to rule out that the device was tested under overheating conditions and even a dry puff.

Son et al. (2019). The authors [40] utilize the same experimental set up as in their 2020 study on carbonyls [21] and in a 2018 study [95] (see section), except that in the present study they only considered two power settings: 6.4 and 31.3 W. The main difference with other ROS studies is that they did not follow a nontargeted approach through EPR, but one targeting OH free radicals by the reaction of captured aerosol with disodium terephthalate (TPT) to form 2-hydroxyterephthalic acid (2OHTA), the known reaction product of OH and TPT. Their outcomes, given as nmol/puff of 2OHTA, are about $\sim 10^{14}$–10^{15} molecules/puff, an order of magnitude higher than those reported in [38,39,100]. However, this result is questionable, as it follows from the outcomes produced with a tested device puffed with a pure VG e-liquid, which is completely unrealistic in end users. Also, this large value occurs at maximal power of 31.3 W (see the high vertical box in the authors' Figure 1). As we argue when reviewing the authors' carbonyl study [21], it is very likely (on the grounds of their sample of vapers) that this maximal power level is an unrepresentative outlier (95 percentile). If the boxes for the pure VG e-liquid and this maximal power level are removed from their Figure 1, then 2OHTA levels become of magnitude $\sim 10^{14}$ like those found by EPR methods. However, the technique used by the authors is based on the 35% yield of the 2OHTA reaction that reflects the amount of OH radicals formed available for fluorescence detection. Letting all radical species from the degradation products remain in the reaction environment could give rise to further radical chains and lead to the formation of excess OH (through, for example, the Haber–Weiss reaction that produces hydroxyl radicals-OH from hydrogen peroxide-H_2O_2 and superoxide-O_2^-). This technique of quantifying OH free radicals might introduce uncertainties in OH quantification if not undertaken carefully (see details in [102]).

To estimate the exposure to OH radicals from ECs (from their outcomes) the authors assume the number of daily puffs for vapers to be in the range 10–1000. Taking 1000 puffs per day then they claim that OH exposure from ECs can be as high as (or higher than) that from tobacco cigarettes. Evidently, 1000 daily puffs is an extreme outlier that does not justify this alarming conclusion, besides the fact that their upper end outcome 10^{15} molecules/puff is an overestimation by an order of magnitud. Taking their representative values at 6.4 W, OH exposure from vaping is at most 1/100 of the exposure from smoking.

Haddad et al. (2019). The authors [41] applied an optimized acellular 2′,7′-dichlorofluorescin (DCFH) probe technique to measure ROS in EC aerosols in sub-ohm and supra-ohm devices, varying power, e-liquid composition and nicotine concentrations. ROS emissions were quantified in the total particulate matter (TPM) of ECIG aerosols and tobacco smoke. For all device types ROS emissions were uncorrelated with power but were highly correlated with power per unit area. An increase in the e-liquid VG content produced higher ROS flux, but nicotine did not affect ROS emissions.

The devices used were: supra-ohm VaporFi platinum tank (5 and 11 W) and a sub-ohm Smok TFV8 device with a V8-T8 coil head (eight coils). Vaping sessions: 5 puffs (VaporFi platinum tank) and 2 puffs (Smok TFV8). Puffing protocol: 4-s puff duration, 10-s interpuff interval, 1 L/min flow rate for both EC devices and for cigarettes 10 puffs with ISO puffing protocol.

To assess the effects of power, the Smok TFV8 was vaped at 50, 75, 100, 150 and 200 W with a PG/VG 50:50 solution and 12 mg/mL nicotine concentration. The Smok TFV8 at fixed 50 W was used to assess the effect of different coil heads: V8-Q4 (4 coils), V8-T8 (8 coils), V8-T10 (10 coils) and TF-Q4 (4 coils). To examine the effects of e-liquid composition and nicotine concentration, the authors the following set up: PG/VG (100/0, 50/50 and 0/100 PG/VG) and (0, 6 and 12mg/mL) in a 50/50 PG/VG solution, all tested at 5 and 11 W (VaporFi platinum tank) and 50 and 150 W (Smok TFV8). Results are reported as the mean of three measurements after blank subtraction.

It is evident that the authors conducted the tests in this study under extreme and unrealistic conditions. A powerful sub-ohm device (Smok TFV8) is recommended for DTL vaping, but it is puffed with a CORESTA-like protocol with 1 L/min airflow and a short interpuff lapse (10 s) and at high powers 50, 75, 100, 150 and 200 W. Even if 50 W might be within the recommended power range of the manufacturers for DTL vaping, puffing this device at 1 L/min airflow narrows the power range of the optimal regime (see Section 2 and Figure 2) making it almost certain that the device was puffed under overheating conditions even at this lowest power used by the authors.

Regarding the VaporFi platinum tank, the authors mentioned it was activated by the aerosol lab vaping instrument (ALVIN) of The American University of Beirut, citing their reference (43) of a study the same author group published in 2015 [103], which describes such a device operating in the power range 3.0–7.5 W. However, the authors tested this instrument with the VaporFi tank at 5 and 11 W, which is above the operation power range, making it almost a certainty that at least some of the tests were conducted under dry puff conditions. Therefore, the experimental outcomes of these study for the sub-ohm Smok TFV8 device and the VaporFi platinum tank are completely irrelevant for end users.

9. Chemical Pathways of Solvents Degradation

We review in this section 5 studies whose main focus is not quantifying carbonyl byproducts in EC emissions, but improving the understanding of their production process from the chemical pathways of the thermal degradation of e-liquid solvents (PG and VG).

Jensen, Strogin and Peyton (2017). This study [42] was not reviewed in [11], its main novelty and significance is its usage of spectral analysis from nuclear magnetic resonance (NMR) (instead of the usual analysis with LC MS or GC MS) to conduct an extensive probing of the chemical pathways of byproducts derived from thermal degradation of vaporized PG and VG. Compounds not previously detected were found in the pathway reactions with HCHO compounds, though only acetaldehyde and hydroxyacetone were quantified. The authors used a second generation Innokin iTaste VV4 with a KangerTech Protank-II claromizer, bottom coil 1.8–2.5 Ω and e-liquid PG/VG 50:50. Puff volume was kept fixed 55 mL, collecting 6–22 mg of aerosol by single puffs of varying duration: 3, 5 and 10 s. The wick was wetted and intervals between puff were 5 min or more as an attempt to avoid dry puffs and overheating.

However, varying puff duration with fixed puff volume leads for 5 and 10 s puffs to a very diminished airflow (11 and 5.5 mL/s). Even for such a low-powered device and without liquid depletion (verified by the authors), this puffing regime necessarily leads, as power increases 6–14 W, to overheating from insufficient evacuation of vaporized e-liquid and is also an artificial way to enhance carbonyl production (see large aldehyde outcomes for extended puff duration DP+ trials in [16]), besides the fact that 10 s puffs are extreme and unrealistic. The presence of overheating can be appreciated by the nonlinear relation obtained by plotting PG/VG generation (about >99.9% or aerosol mass) vs. power from the data in Table S1 of the Supplementary File. Evidently, the quantified acetaldehyde yields per puff for 10 s puffs are overexposures under abnormal conditions.

Wang et al. (2017). The authors [43] examine the production of toxic volatile carbonyl compounds from PG and VG at varying a controlled temperature ranging up to 318 °C, by means of a "device-independent test method" utilizing a stainless steel, tubular reactor in flowing air that simulates a generic EC device.

The authors used e-liquids with pure PG and VG, a 50:50 PG/VG mix and two commercial ones. Acrolein was only detected in e-liquids containing VG and above 270 C. Formaldehyde and acetaldehyde were detected at reactor temperatures of 215 °C for both PG and VG, but at same temperature (318 °C) pure VG produced significantly higher yields: (in µg per mg of liquid): 21.1 $\pm$ 3.80 vs. 2.03 $\pm$ 0.80 (formaldehyde), 2.40 $\pm$ 0.99 vs. 2.35 $\pm$ 0.87 (acetaldehyde) and 0.80 $\pm$ 0.50 vs. traces (acrolein). The authors claim that at 215 °C the estimated daily exposure to formaldehyde from e-cigarettes surpasses the USEPA and OEHHA toxicological thresholds.

The experimental set up is as follows: 5–10 mg of test e-liquid was loaded at the center of a 0.3 g piece of glass wool, which was then carefully transferred to the middle of a stainless steel, tubular reactor (25 cm long and 1 cm in inner diameter) housed in a horizontal, split-sided furnace. Contact between liquid and inner surface of the reactor was avoided. One end of the tube reactor was connected to compressed air with a regulated constant flow rate of 200 mL/min, to produce a 2.9 s transition time of e-liquid with air in the reactor to mimic a 3 s puff duration. Aerosols were collected onto DNPH cartridges and analyzed by HPLC.

The authors define as "reactor temperature" the temperature in the glass wool inside the reactor, fixed by a temperature controller and measured by a thermocouple. Although the test outcomes are shown in graphs at various fixed temperatures (215, 270, 315 °C), most likely these temperatures are reached by heating the reactor for a short time (the "transition time" mentioned before).

The displayed graphs for these fixed temperatures for 5 e-liquids show negligible yields of the 3 aldehydes below 215 °C, with yields rising at >215 °C (with larger increase for formaldehyde). Yields from VG are an order of magnitude larger than those of PG, which is in contradiction to results in other studies, a contradiction that the authors suggest can be explained by potential interaction of VG with reactor materials (stainless steel). The graphs for the PG/VG 50:50 mixture and a commercial e-liquid show the same qualitative behavior, but in the PG/VG mixture the rise of yields occurs below 215 °C and for the commercial liquid up to 250 °C.

This study is valuable for showing the temperature dependence of aldehyde production, even if it is evident that the tubular reactor used in this study is a poor simulator of an EC device (a fact the authors recognize). A steady flow of compressed air carrying e-liquid vapor at very low fixed airflow (3.33 mL/s) is an extremely crude inhalation model. As a consequence, the detected aldehyde yields cannot be extrapolated to those emerging from testing EC devices and the authors' risk assessments are not relevant for end users.

Finally, the authors' temperature measurements were not validated and thus do not seem to be reliable. However, even if temperature measurements were accurate, the temperature dependence of a process like aldehyde production is a thermodynamic process that cannot be modeled by temperature measurements from a sequence of fixed temperatures and a fixed airflow. We discuss this common conceptual error in Section 12.

Li et al. (2020). The authors [44] present in detail a theoretical quantification model that can significantly contribute to a better understanding of the chemical pathways of carbonyl production in EC emissions.

Conventionally, carbonyl quantification is done by derivatizing with 2,4-dinitrophenyl hydrazine (2,4-DNPH) to produce hydrazone adducts, followed by LC or GC chromatography analysis with calibration of chromatographic peak areas guided by carbonyl-DNPH standards. Additional purification steps are required to isolate the mono and multi hydrazones in the DNPH synthesis. However, some carbonyls are not commercially available and further require a separate synthesis. The authors propose two goals: (1) to use high mass resolving power coupled to chromatography to better identify DNPH hydrazones of functionalized and simple carbonyls and acids, and (2) to develop a quantification for cases when analytical standards are unavailable.

To validate this technique the authors use a disposable device blu (Imperial Brands Inc., Bristol, United Kingdom), with non-refillable "Classic Tobacco" e-liquid cartridges. The device comprises a rechargeable 140 mA h battery and an atomizer with coil resistance of 3.5 Ω. Puffing protocol: two devices were puffed in tandem (4 puffs for each e-cigarette), puff duration 2 s with 8 puffs/min (7.5 s inter-puff lapse), average flow rate 2.3 L/min and puff volume 77 mL.

All analytes were separated in the chromatographic spectrum using accurate single ion cromatography, which once integrated into the full ion chromatography avoids coelusion and misidentification of spectral peaks that might lead to overestimation of abundance. A total of 19 DNPH hydrazones were identified: six hydroxycarbonyls, four dicarbonyls, three acids, and one phenolic carbonyl, with the most abundant being hydroxyacetone, formaldehyde, acetaldehyde, lactaldehyde, acrolein, and dihydroxyacetone. As the authors remark, an important finding from this quantification method is that hydroxycarbonyls are just as important as simple carbonyls in the byproducts content of emissions.

The obtained carbonyl yields are displayed in their Table 2 (µg/puff): 0.15 formaldehyde, 0.11 acetaldehyde, 0.071 lactaldehyde, 0.061 acrolein, 0.037 dihydroxyacetone. By assuming 250 daily puffs they compute a daily formaldehyde exposure of 37.5 µg/day which is below the OEHHA daily exposure threshold of 180 µg/day. However, while the levels of mass abundances for the blu device were low, they are likely overestimations, as the authors' puffing parameters are unrealistic: 2.3 L/min airflow and 77 mL puff volume are too high for a ciga-like (which has high air resistance), while at an 8 puffs/minute pace a full day vaping journey (250 puffs) would take only 31 min, an extremely exhaustive and intense form of vaping that bears no connection to real life usage.

Melvin et al. (2020). This study [45] aims at the determination of the potential for the formation of α-dicarbonyl compounds, including diacetyl (DA), during the generation of aerosols from devices whose e-liquids contained no detectable DA or other α-dicarbonyl compounds. A model reaction system was set up to conduct mechanistic studies using a model microwave reaction system to identify key reaction precursors for DA. The same reference e-liquid (50:50 PG/VG + 2.5% (w/w) nicotine + 15% water (w/w)) from the method validation study was used for the subsequent evaluations of reactant combinations. The increase in DA content between the native e-liquid and the aerosol in all tested devices was indicative of its formation during aerosol generation potentially through a thermal degradation pathway.

The 8 commercial ciga-like devices that were tested were acquired in 2017 at local convenience stores, all contained rechargeable batteries with disposable e-liquid cartridges. However, the authors only identify two devices obtained internally: MarkTen XL Classic and MarkTen XL Menthol (products A and B, respectively). The puffing protocol was 55 mL puff volume, 5 s puff duration, and 30 s puff interval. The aerosol was collected using the standard methods, and 25 puffs were collected from each sample.

Concentrations of DA in the aerosols of the 8 tested tested devices were about 20–40 times lower than established occupational DA exposure limits of the American Conference of Governmental Industrial Hygienists (ACGIH): 0.04 mg/m^3 (0.01 ppm) and the recommended exposure limit (REL) National Institute of Occupational Safety and Health (NIOSH): 0.02 mg/m^3 (0.005 ppm). These outcomes lead to a daily exposure of 1/360 with respect to daily DA exposure from tobacco cigarette smoke (250 µg/cigarette).

The main shortcoming of this study is its choice of tested devices: old design ciga-likes of which the only two that were identified are of the Mark10 brand that is currently obsolete or of very marginal usage. Also, the study was published in 2020, 3 years after the acquisition of the devices in 2017, so that corrosion or leaching effects cannot be ruled out, as no information was supplied on their storage conditions. While the authors correctly claim that these results only apply to the ciga-likes they tested, these old design devices release higher levels of byproducts than more modern devices [11].

Jaegers et al. (2021) The authors [46] simulate an EC device by means of a single cavity using an in situ MAS NMR rotor containing e-liquid, gas, and metal solid samples (ZrO_2 and Cr_2O_3) to simulate coil materials. The rotor is transferred to a specially designed loading chamber where N_2 or O_2 is added at the specified pressures together with e-liquids to mimic the quantity of vapor evolved in an average puff ($\sim$10–50 mg). The purpose of the experiment is to monitor the transition of e-liquids in order to identify the decomposition products that might be present at low-temperatures (<200 °C) in EC emission pathways by controlling the oxygen availability and the temperature.

However, monitoring the detection of converted chemical species by natural abundance ^{13}C and ^{1}H NMR in the suggested low-temperature degradation pathway requires an extended time period (the MAS NMR spectra takes days to generate peaks at same temperature). Under the authors' experimental conditions, if sufficient oxygen is available, e-liquids liquids decompose at temperatures <200 °C forming byproducts (formic and acrylic acids) via an oxygen initiated radical-mediated mechanism.

While this study can be a valuable contribution to enhance current knowledge on the chemistry of degradation paths in EC emissions, its experimental setup bears no relation with the physics of EC operation. A loading chamber with the required oxygen supply necessary for the days long monitoring of e-liquid transitions at fixed target temperatures below 200 °C is a closed and highly controlled system, whereas an EC device is an open thermal system, with rapidly time and space varying temperatures and turbulent air fluxes (oxygen supply) as it is exchanging heat between its parts and with the environment, a large thermal bath (see Section 12). It is highly likely that these physical conditions might prevent the reaction pathways found by the authors to take place in EC devices, but this should be assessed by further experimental research.

10. Carbonyls and Nicotine Compensatory Behavior

We review two studies by the same group of researchers that illustrate how reduction of nicotine levels leads to a compensatory behavior characterized by an increase of device power and/or more intense puffing. These studies show that such compensatory behavior significantly increases the emission of toxic byproducts, in particular formaldehyde and acetaldehyde.

Dawkins et al. (2018). This observational study [47] was conducted during 4 weeks between September 2016 and February 2017, as a follow up of a previous study by the same group of researchers [76]. It is based on ad libitum vaping of 20 experienced vapers who received for the duration of the study the same device: an eVic Supreme (Joytech) endowed with adjustable voltage and recording the time for each puff, puff length (in seconds), atomizer resistance (1.6 Ω fixed), voltage and wattage. The eVic was fitted to a Nautilus Aspire tank. Participants received e-liquids with the two mentioned nicotine levels choosing flavors they sampled beforehand (tobacco, menthol, fruit and bakery).

This sample of users was used to examine the compensatory effects of nicotine levels and variability of power settings in a combination of 4 setups given by: high/low nicotine level (18 vs. 6 mg/mL) each with adjustable/fixed power settings, spending one week observation for each combination and looking at the interaction between them. The authors measured in this sample puffing parameters (daily puffs, puff duration, interpuff interval), e-liquid consumption, power settings (when not fixed), subjective effects (urge to vape), as well as metabolite biomarkers of nicotine (salivary cotinine), acrolein and formaldehyde (urinary 3-Hydroxypropyl mercapturic acid, 3-HPMA and formate). The study corroborates and provides further observational support to a previous pilot study (by same group) that examined compensatory effects in puffing habits when decreasing nicotine concentration in e-liquids (with analogous compensatory behavior in cigarette smoking).

The results displayed in the authors' Table 3 reveal an increase of about 12–18% in mean daily puffs for lower nicotine levels respect higher ones: 338 vs. 279 (fixed power) and 308 vs. 279 (variable power). Mean puff duration increased 20% from high to low nicotine levels (3.61 to 4.46 s), but only for fixed power, but e-liquid consumption increased for lower nicotine levels, 17% and 26% for variable and fixed power respectively. High nicotine levels decreased withdrawal symptoms. However, these compensatory effects on low nicotine concentrations are not sufficient to maintain a stable nicotine intake, as cotinine levels were higher in high nicotine 18 mg/mL concentration irrespective of fixed/variable power setting. While acrolein metabolite levels were insensitive to the setup combinations, formaldehyde metabolites showed a significant increase in lower nicotine levels in both power settings.

Kosmider et al. (2020). This study [48] is the upgrade and continuation of the previous study by the same research group [47], following a similar methodology and using exactly the same EC device, but now conducting laboratory tests whose puffing protocol was taken from the average puffing parameters observed in 19 experienced vapers in the 4 combination of: e-liquids with low/high nicotine levels (6 and 18 mg/mL) and fixed/variable power adjustments. The laboratory tests quantified daily exposure to carbonyl emissions by HPLC. The results further confirm those of [47]: significantly higher e-liquid consumption and thus higher exposure to formaldehyde and acetaldehyde were found when switching from higher to lower nicotine levels, regardless of power settings.

Table 2 of the study reveals statistically significant higher levels of daily nicotine intake for e-liquids with higher nicotine concentrations (mean ± SD, mg/day): 22.69 ± 15.16 vs. 13.22 ± 8.93 (fixed power) and 27.87 ± 16.86 vs. 15.23 ± 10.49 (adjustable power). However, low nicotine e-liquids produced significantly higher daily levels of aerosol yield (median, range, g/day): 2.26 (1.46–4.22) vs. 1.38 (0.7–3.01) (fixed power) and 2.64 (1.71–4.85) vs. 1.38 (0.7–3.01) (adjustable power); formaldehyde dose (µg/day, median range): 26.83 (11.99–56.11) vs. 13.69 (6.95–27.99) (fixed power) and 25.63 (15.82–70.74) vs. 20.23 (10.1–45.57) (adjustable power); acetaldehyde dose 19.91 (4.68–66.47) vs. 8.18 (3.42–34.03) (fixed power) and 20.17 (5.61–83.00) vs. 8.18 (3.42–34.03) (adjustable power). Following the methodology of Stephens, the authors also showed that the compensatory behavior of low nicotine levels contributes to a 1.98 fold increase (2.06 and 1.26 fold with fixed and adjustable voltage) of the Cancer Risk Index (CRO) associated with formaldehyde and acetaldehyde. The authors' assessments roughly agrees with the assessment of Stephens model estimating CRI from EC usage being 3–4 orders of magnitude below cigarette smoking.

11. Summary and Evaluation

On the grounds of the quality criteria presented in Section 4, we provide our evaluation of the revised studies listed in Table 1 in terms of the graphic codes displayed in Table 2: experimental consistency and reproducibility are graded with tickmark symbols: ✔,+/−, ✘, ? and toxicological confidence with a "traffic light" system ●, ●, ●, ●. Tables 3 and 4 display how each study rates according to these codes. This is a broad general evaluation, details are discussed extensively in the individual revision of each study on Sections 6–10 (Author names in the left columns of Tables 3 and 4 are hyperlinked to their review entries in these sections).

Table 2. Evaluation Codes. Toxicological Confidence (traphic lights) and Experimental Consistency (tickmark symbols)

Toxicological Confidence			
●	●	●	●
Fully Reliable	Restricted Reliability	Completely Unreliable	Missing Information
Experimental Consistency			
✔	+/−	✘	?
Fully Consistent	Restricted Consistency	Completely Inconsistent	Missing Information

A quick recount of the evaluation provided in Tables 3 and 4 reveals a significant pattern in 35 revised studies that quantified organic byproducts. The most frequent drawbacks were those marked as (1) and (2) in the "Comments" column in the extreme right of Tables 3 and 4: testing sub-ohm devices with a CORESTA or CORESTA-like protocol. This was found in 18 out of 35 studies, with:

- 10 testing them at too high power levels, thus almost certain overheating and most likely irrelevant to all end users (graded as ✘)
- 8 under recommended power levels, thus with likelihood of overheating with very restricted relevance limited to a small minority of users, see Sections 2, 3.1 and 12.1, (graded as +/−).

Regarding the traffic light toxicological confidence grading, 12 rated as unreliable (●), 12 as very restricted reliabilty (●), 11 as reliable (●), with a strong correlation between gradings ●/● and causes (1), (2). Therefore, this general evaluation clearly reveals frequent inappropriate testing of sub-ohm devices, with likely overestimation of health risks from these experiments, thus suggesting also the necessity to upgrade laboratory standards to address this frequent problem.

Table 3. Studies on carbonyls 2018–2022. Author names are hyperlinked to review entries in Section 6. The tickmark symbols and traffic light codes are given in Table 2: [✔,+/−,✘,?] and [●,●,●,●] are respectively [Fully Consistent, Restricted Consistency, Completely Inconsistent, Missing information] and [Fully Reliable, Restricted Reliability, Completely Unreliable, Missing information]. The number codes in the column "Comments" are: (1) sub-ohm device with CORESTA high powers, (2) sub-ohm device with CORESTA recommended powers, (3) other forms of inconsistent protocol, (4) incorrect computation of exposure, (5) outliers not properly identified, (6) devices not fully identified, (7) testing power not identified, (8) too frequent puffs, (9) too long puffs, (10) used old devices

First Author & Hyperlink	Experimental Consistency		Reproducibility		Toxicological Confidence	Comments
	Vaping Regime	Power Range	Emissions Generation	Trapping & Analysis		
			CARBONYLS			
			2018			
Vreeke [13]	+/−	+/−	✔	✔	●	(1)
Korzun [14]	✔	✔	✔	✔	●	(4)
El Hellani [15]	+/−	✔	✔	✔	●	(4)(5)(8)
			2019			
Beauval [16]	+/−	+/−	✔	✔	●	(2)
Ooi [17]	✘	✘	?	?	●	(1)(3)(4)(5)(6)
Balushkin [18]	+/−	+/−	✔	✔	●	(2)(10)
Reilly [19]	✔	✔	✔	✔	●	
			2020			
Son [21]	✔	+/−	✔	✔	●	(5)
Talih [22]	✘	+/−	✔	✔	●	(1)(5)
Zelinkova [23]	✘	✔	✔	✔	●	(2)
Uchiyama [24]	✘	✘	✔	✘	●	(1)(2)(6)
Cunningham [25]	✔	✔	✔	✔	●	
Noël [26]	✘	✘	?	✔	●	(1)(4)(6)
Mallock [27]	✔	✔	✔	✔	●	
			2021			
Chen [28]	✔	✔	✔	✔	●	
Crosswhite [29]	✔	✔	✔	✔	●	
Li [30]	+/−	✔	✔	✔	●	(2)(3)(4)
Yan [31]	✘	✘	✔	✔	●	(1)(3)(4)
Tehrani [32]	✘	✘	✔	✔	●	(1)(3)(4)(7)(8)
Cancelada [20]	+/−	+/−	✔	✔	●	(2)(3)
			2022			
Xu [33]	✔	✔	✔	✔	●	
Visser [34]	✔	✔	✔	✔	●	

Table 4. Studies on CO, ROS, degradation pathways and nicotine vs. carbonyls. Author names are hyperlinked to review entries in Sections 7–10. The traffic light codes are given in Table 2: [✔,+/−,✘,?] and [🔴,🟠,🟡,⚫] are respectively [Fully Consistent, Restricted Consistency, Completely Inconsistent, Missing information] and [Fully Reliable, Restricted Reliability, Completely Unreliable, Missing information]. The number codes in the column "Comments" are: (1) sub-ohm device with CORESTA high powers, (2) sub-ohm device with CORESTA recommended powers, (3) other forms of inconsistent protocol, (4) incorrect computation of exposure, (5) outliers not properly identified, (6) devices not fully identified, (7) testing power not identified, (8) too frequent puffs, (9) too long puffs, (10) used old devices. (NA) stands for "does not apply" (these studies only simulated an EC).

First Author & Hyperlink	Experimental Consistency		Reproducibility		Toxicological Confidence	Comments
	Vaping Regime	Power Range	Emissions Generation	Trapping & Analysis		
CO						
Casebolt [35]	✘	✘	+/−	✔	🟡	(1)(3)
El Hellani [36]	✘	✘	+/1	✔	🟡	(1)(3)(4)
Son [37]	+/−	✔	✔	✔	🟠	(2)(3)
ROS						
Bitzer (a) [38]	✘	+/−	✔	✔	🟡	(2)(3)
Bitzer (b) [39]	✘	✘	✔	✔	🟡	(2)(3)
Son [40]	✔	+/−	✔	✔	🟠	(3)(4)
Haddad [41]	✘	✘	+/−	✔	🟡	(1)(3)(9)
Degradation reactions & carbonyl formation						
Jensen [42]	✔	✔	✔	✔	🟠	(9)
Wang [43]	(NA)	+/−	+/−	✔	🟠	(3)
Li [44]	✔	✔	✔	✔	🟠	(8)(9)
Melvin [45]	✔	✔	+/−	✔	🟢	(6)(9)(10)
Jaegers [46]	(NA)	(NA)	✔	✔	(NA)	
Nicotine compensation vs. carbonyls						
Dawkins [47]	✔	✔	✔	✔	🟢	
Kosmider [48]	✔	✔	✔	✔	🟢	

12. Discussion

12.1. Testing Sub-Ohm Devices with Insufficient Airflow

Since the CORESTA protocol used in most of the revised literature was conceived for testing early ciga-like devices, its puffing parameters (airflow 1 L/min, puff volume 50–70 mL) are appropriate for testing the low powered recent device types (cartridge based and refillable pods, disposables) used by substantial numbers of vapers for MTL style, specially young adults [60,62,63]. The CORESTA or CORESTA-like puffing parameters might not be wholly appropriate for testing even those devices that are also meant for MTL vaping, but operate at power levels 10–30 W above recent pods and disposables. As shown in [49], it is very likely that these "intermediate" devices are fully compatible with airflows of up to 4 L/min larger than those specified by CORESTA or CORESTA-like protocols.

However, it is certain that puff volumes and airflows of CORESTA or CORESTA-like protocols are very problematic for testing sub-ohm devices that are mostly used for DTL vaping, as this vaping style involves much larger puff volumes and airflows (see Sections 3.1 and 3.2). As we show in Sections 6, 7 and 8 and summarized in Section 11, at least half (18 out of 35) of laboratory emission studies have tested sub-ohm devices with CORESTA or CORESTA-like protocols. Out of these 18 studies, 10 tested the devices also at too high powers levels [13,17,22,24,26,31,32,35,36,41], hence under almost certain overheating, which renders their outcomes and risk assessments from sub-ohm devices completely irrelevant for end users. The remaining 8 studies tested the devices at recommended power levels [16,18,20,23,24,30,37–39], hence overheating is possible but not certain. Evidently, only these latter 8 studies provide outcomes and risk assessments from sub-ohm devices that might be relevant for at least a minority niche of vapers. We estimate in this section that this minority constitutes around 5% of all vapers, roughly the proportion of vapers using high powered sub-ohm devices with MTL style.

As stated in Section 3.1, there is abundant anecdotal accounts of a very strong correlation between vaping styles and devices type from vaping forums and magazines, consumers and retailers. This correlation was also observed in the footage material examined in [54]: 80% of users of sub-ohm devices practice DTL and 98% of DTL vapers use sub-ohm devices, while 95% of users of low-powered supra-ohm devices practice MTL. Interestingly, the 20% minority of MTL vapers using sub-ohm devices take on average shorter puffs than the 80% DTL majority. Given the absence of insufficiently documented evidence, we can assume as a plausible working hypothesis the observed data in [54], with a vast majority (likely 80%) of high powered sub-ohm devices used for DTL vaping, with a minority of users (likely 20% or less) using them for the MTL style. thus, it is likely that outcomes of studies testing sub-ohm devices with CORESTA or CORESTA-like protocols might be relevant and realistic for this minority niche (which might not be a stable niche).

Since there is no direct demographic evidence, the distribution of MTL and DTL styles can be inferred indirectly (and very approximately) from demographic surveys in the US (2018–2020) [59], the UK (2022) [60] and Germany (2018) [61] that have inquired the type of device among vapers, showing that between 50–65% use "refillable tank models", with the rest using cartridge based and refillable pods. While all DTL vaping will necessarily correspond to tank models, not all tank models are sub-ohm devices meant for DTL. Since, as we argued in Section 3.1, usage of sub-ohm devices involves more expertise and maintenance than low powered devices, so it should occur typically among long time ex-smoking vapers. Since between 40–60% of vapers are now ex-smokers in the US and UK markets [59,60], it is reasonable to assume (as a working hypothesis) that sub-ohm devices are used by a large minority within the 40–60% of ex-smokers, which should roughly translate into 20%-25% of all vapers, with 75–80% using low powered devices (though demographic trends seem to show a steady evolution to low powered devices and even disposables [60,62,63]).

If the relevance of outcomes for testing sub-ohm devices with CORESTA or CORESTA-like protocols is restricted to those practicing MTL style with these devices. To estimate the proportion of this minority niche among all vapers, we assume as working hypothesis that (i) ∼25% of vapers use sub-ohm devices (likely an overestimation) and (ii) the observational data in [54] stating that ∼80% of these vapers practice DTL and ∼20% MTL. The proportion of vapers practicing MTL style in sub-ohm devices is then roughly ∼5% of all vapers (∼20% of ∼25%). Hence, outcomes and health risk assessments from testing sub-ohm devices with CORESTA or CORESTA-like protocols should be directly useful and relevant to a really small minority of vapers. Evidently, we have produced a very rough estimation of usage sub-ohm devices for MTL style, but even if this minority habit combination is larger than 5%, it is evident that these outcomes and risk assessments are not applicable to the substantial numbers of vapers using low powered devices (we discuss this issue further in Section 13).

12.2. Arbitrarily Fixing Power, Temperature and Puff Duration

Some of the revised studie considered ad hoc combination of varying/fixed parameters. Son et al. [37] varied power with fixed puff volume at 40 mL and airflow with fixed power at 50 Watts, Li et al. [30] varied the coil temperature under a CORESTA-like protocol with fixed airflow 1.186 LT/min and puff volume 55 mL. Cancelada et al. [20] varied airflow (opening the inlet venting holes in the atomizer) with fixed power, while Bitzer et al. [38] varied temperature with fixed power and power with fixed temperature, but at a fixed CORESTA-like airflow. While these studies present interesting results, their set of combinations of puffing parameters are disconnected with those of the vast majority of consumers, as usage of sub-ohm devices typically involves increasing puff volumes and airflows together with increasing power and temperature. Nevertheless, as shown in Table S9 of Son et al, the reported emitted mass of CO and all aldehydes are of the order of ng/puff for all tested puff flows, which is about 1 part in 10^7 of the aerosol mass of 84 ± 29.6 mg/puff (which should be close to the consumed e-liquid mass).

The fist problem with fixing the temperature is the lack of information on how it is evaluated by the device instrumentation. The second problem is the lack of experimental validation of temperature values, an important shortcoming because aerosol generation and vaping involve complex patterns of heat conduction that (in general) produce a time varying and inhomogeneous temperature. If the end user can determine a prior a fixed power or temperature to vape, this necessarily requires the user to control (i.e., to vary in a sequence of trials) the intensity of the inhalation (airflow, puff volume, puff duration) to levels that are adequate according to sensorial and taste criteria. In technical terms this process involves finding the appropriate puffing parameters (airflow, puff volume, puff duration) that allow for an efficient condensation (by forced convection in inhalation) of vaporized e-liquid that forms the aerosol in the optimal regime. Besides being wholly artificial and disconnected with realistic usage, testing sub-ohm devices with fixed airflows and puff volumes of CORESTA or CORESTA-like protocols for different (but fixed) power and temperature are not likely adequate for carrying on this condensation process efficiently and will more likely fail to comply with users' sensorial and good taste criteria (see Sections 2 and 3).

12.3. Physical Limitations on Chemical Processes

Chemical reactions can be studied and recreated in a wide range of temperatures that can be controlled in a laboratory, thus allowing for a better understanding of the different steps of degradation pathways. This approach can hardly be applied to a dynamic environment of an EC device in which it is extremely difficult to regulate correctly the temperature, which is not an extensive state variable that can be determined, fixed and supplied externally.

A chemical approach in a laboratory is very difficult to implement in an EC device, thus it is conceptually incorrect to present potential degradation reactions under the assumption that they will occur if testing an EC device by setting the temperature at a desired value from the device instruments. This conceptual error leads to the assumption that as power increases it leads proportionally to a more rapid evolution of the vaporization process through a higher heating temperature. In reality, e-liquid vaporization occurs through physical phenomena involving several regimes and limits which results in the ignition of different chemical degradations, it cannot be produced or induced by arbitrarily fixing the temperature to increasing constant values. This criticism applies to Li et al. [30], Bitzer et al. [38], Wang et al. [43] and Jaegers et al. [46].

The first main assumption is that an EC device is functional between specific powers (minimal and maximal powers) limiting an optimal regime of vaporization characterized by to nucleated boiling. Through this regime, e-liquid consumption linearly increases with icreasing the supplied power. However, these limits are obviously influenced by e-liquid composition and also by the vaping regime and to find them requires a consistent experimental verification.

The second main assumptions is a thermodynamic conceptual issue. Vaping products are open systems ventilated by fresh air induced by inhalation. This leads to the mixture of a gas at ambient conditions (pressure, moisture and temperature) to another formed by the vaporization of e-liquid (effects that cannot be reproduced in the simulated devices in [43,46]). It results in an aerosol at a temperature intermediate between the temperatures of each separated gas. Therefore, e-liquid constituents cannot be heated at temperatures above, at least, the boiling temperature of pure glycerol. Considering conditions above this assumption leads to experiments under overheating conditions.

Saliba et al. [104] in 2018 investigated the pyrolysis of PG using a quartz pyrolyric reaction in the presence and absence of a metallic coil available in vaping devices. The reactor was heated at 80, 256, 360, 460, 565 and 670 °C. With the exception of 80 °C, the remaining temperature conditions are above the boiling temperature of PG, which allows for exploring PG degradation in the gas phase. This is a typical example of an inappropriate in-lab experiment extrapolated to a vaping device. Indeed, PG has a boiling temperature of 188 °C. However, in a liquid solution, interactions with others compounds as glycerol can maintain PG in liquid phase at higher temperature as 256 °C. Therefore, only the conditions at 80 °C can be extrapolated to normal conditions of use of a vaping device.

These two fundamental assumptions highlight another chemically originated inconsistent approach. Some studies (Wang et al. [43] and Jaegers et al. [46]) conducted experiments with e-liquids in closed systems (an oven, a linear flow reactor) that allow for the heating of a controlled volume of a gas and/or a liquid sample. For many physical considerations, this type of experiments can lead to contradictory results or overestimation of risks from excess byproduct formation, but are irrelevant to the study of EC devices because of their incompatibility with the functionality of these devices as thermodynamically open systems.

13. Assessment of Risk Communication

Since EC emissions contain HPHCs, one of the main tasks of their testing in the laboratory is to provide objective guidelines to assess health risks that end users (and bystanders) would face if exposed to specific doses of these emissions. Most revised studies present assessments of health risks based on their experimental quantification of the abundance of potentially toxic byproducts, an abundance that must be compared with compound-specific toxicological markers. A substantial proportion of the risk assessments express serious concerns, some cast doubts on the safety of the devices and even recommend harsh regulatory restrictions [17,26,31,32].

However, the extensive revision of laboratory studies we have conducted shows that most of them have failed (in various degrees) to uphold the basic consistency criteria we described in Section 4. Therefore, we recommend due care and skepticism in evaluating most risk assessments, but question the objectivity of the most severe ones. We have evaluated the toxicological reliability of the risk assessments in 35 revised studies by a traffic light system in Tables 3 and 4 [●, ●, ●, ●], repectively corresponding to [reliable, limited reliability, unreliable, missing information].

From the extensive literature revision carried on in Sections 6 to 10, summarized in Tables 2, 3 and 4 of Section 11, the most frequent form of inconsistency is testing sub-ohm devices under CORESTA or CORESTA-like puffing protocols: 18 of 35 studies, marked with with (1) and (2) in the Comments column of Tables 3 and 4. From the outset, on the grounds of arguments of Sections 2 and 3, we can unequivocally state that risk assessments from these studies are:

- questionable and unrealistic for all users if coming from the outcomes of 10 studies that used high power settings with these protocols to test sub-ohm devices [17,22,24,26, 31,32,35,36,41]. The 10 studies are marked with red traffic light ● in Tables 3 and 4. It is practically certain that these testing conditions lead to overheating and possibly dry puffs, likely producing aerosols that could be repellent to end users (see Section 3.3).
- of very limited validity if coming from 8 studies that used these protocols to test sub-ohm devices, but at recommended power settings [13,16,18,20,23,24,30,37–39]. These assessments must be taken with skepticism, as they come from testing conditions that might involve overheating as a likelihood, but not as a near certainty (the corresponding traffic light is ●). As we argue in Sections 3.1 and 12.1, risk assessments from these testing conditions with recommended power settings are only relevant to a minority of consumers using these devices with an MTL vaping style, likely ∼20% of users of these devices and ∼5% of all users (since users of sub-ohm devices are very likely a minority of vapers).
- completely unaplicable and irrelevant for low powered pod and disposable devices used by a substantial proportion of vapers (at least 35–40% of vapers according to demographic surveys [59–63]).

Other problems in the experimental design (see Comments column of Tables 3 and 4) affect the reliability of risk assessments. Some studies miscalculated (overestimated) exposure in various ways [14,17,26,30–32,36,40]. Some risk assessment are based on ranges of outcomes that contain unrepresentative outlier values [15,21,37,40]. A number of studies failed to disclose important information to assess their results and open the possibility of replication [17,24,26,32,45]. Some studies tested devices under excessive puffing frequency [15,32,44]: multiple puffs one every 10 s or less, when demographic studies of vaping behavior (see Section 3.4) reveal that such bouts of up to 20 rapid puffs only occurs for short time periods, but is not representative of daily usage. Two studies tested old ciga-like devices and devices acquired years before testing without describing storage conditions [18,45], all of which makes it impossible to rule out corrosion or leaching effects. It is interesting to remark that the same inconsistencies were found in our review of laboratory studies that focused on metal contents in EC aerosol emissions [5].

The most frequent and abundant HPHCs reported in the revised literature are aldehydes, specially formaldehyde, acetaldehyde and acrolein, all formed from reactions of thermal degradation of the e-liquid solvents and whose toxic potential is well known. Less is known of the inhalation toxicity from the lesser yields of intermediate byproducts of these reactions, which as shown in [30,44] might play as important a role in PG and VG degradation as primary carbonyls. Free radicals, specially hydroxyl OHs, are also concerning. However, all HPHCs were found in negligible dose in comparison with tobacco smoke in all studies testing low powered devices without gross inconsistencies in their experimental design (as for example [17,32]). Evidently, the incorporation of vapers in the logistics of testing procedures would contribute to improve the objectivity of risks assessments, as suggested in the important review [11], something that (among all revised studies) only [21,40] attempted with a limited scope, but [34,53] have taken the first steps in a more thorough implementation. .

14. Conclusions

We have undertaken in this review an extensive critical revision of 36 laboratory studies published since 2018 on organic byproducts (carbonyls, CO and free radicals) in EC emissions. Details of the experiments, our criticism of their design and toxicological considerations are written in the extensive reviews in Sections 6–10 and summarized in Tables 1, 2 and 3 in Section 11. This summary is complemented by a thorough critical discussion on multiple aspects of the laboratory studies in Section 12. As in our previous review on metal contents [5], we have focused primarily on the consistency between aerosol generation by puffing protocols in the laboratory and an efficient aerosol generation fulfilling the physical constraints of the optimal regime (Section 2) in the tested devices and validated when they are operated by their end users, whose vaping habits and sensorial perceptions are discussed in detail in Section 3.

One of the main purposes of laboratory testing of emissions is to provide evidence of potential health risks from exposure to HPHCs in EC emissions. To fulfill this purpose efficiently, the studies must comply with minimal consistency conditions that we describe in Section 4. We evaluated in Section 11 these consistency conditions for all revised studies by a system of tick marks (experimental consistency) and traffic lights (toxicological confidence). As we stated in [5], we question the objectivity of negative health risk assessments and harsh policy recommendations that emerge from studies undertaken under severe experimental inconsistencies, including clear evident overheating conditions (rated with ✖ and ● in Tables 2 and 3). Studies with less severe inconsistencies, marked by +/− and ● in Tables 2 and 3, require to be carefully examined under a skeptical approach.

The revision of the literature we have undertaken further supports the available empiric evidence from self-consistent laboratory studies that vaping is a much safer option of nicotine consumption than smoking, thus motivating the support of its role in tobacco harm reduction. Nevertheless, EC emissions still involve residual health risks from inhalation and exposure to HPHC's, even if self consistent experiments find them in minute quantities in comparison with their presence in tobacco smoke. Long term risks (even if residual) are difficult to forecast, model and predict and the analysis and quantification of HPHCs in EC emissions is only the front line of a complex process of subsequent risk assessments to forecast, probe and test the biological and medical effects of the inhaled chemicals through studies of biomarkers, cytotoxicity, animal models, preclinical and clinical studies. However, for risk assessments from emission studies to be a useful component of this process and be of utility to stakeholders (users, bystanders, health professionals, manufacturers and regulators), these assessments must be solidly grounded on HPHC outcomes that have been quantified in well designed self consistent experiments testing the devices under conditions that best approach their realistic usage, otherwise these risk assessments can be fictitious and irrelevant.

Besides being the front line in estimating health risks from vaping, laboratory testing of emissions is essential for quality control, product comparison and technological development. While it is not expected that its standardized regimented procedures will reproduce real life user patterns, at least a minimal consistency with realistic usage must hold for the testing to have any relevance for end users. As in our previous review on metal studies, we have found in the literature on organic byproducts that most studies fail (in various degrees) to uphold this consistency, some studies often fail to do so even at the most basic levels.

The main methodological problem that we found (in 18 of 35 studies) is testing high powered "sub-ohm" devices whose aerosol emissions are generated with the puffing parameters of the CORESTA protocol (and/or with minor deviations), a protocol conceived and designed to be appropriate for testing early low-powered devices. Testing sub-ohm devices with these protocols is very likely unrealistic, as these devices are mostly used for the 'Direct to Lung' (DTL) style involving much higher airflows and puff volumes. Other serious methodological problems are: (i) failure to disclose important information on the devices, the puffing parameters, testing power ranges, the outcomes, making interpretation of results more difficult and future replication impossible; (ii) misleading health risk assessments, either from taking outlier outcomes as representative or simply miscalculation of exposures; (iii) testing old devices without disclosing their storage conditions and current status, (iv) excessively frequent puffing and/or too long duration puffs.

These methodological problems are not new, most were identified already in 2018 in the groundbreaking review by Farsalinos and Gillman [11] of 32 emissions studies published up to 2017 on carbonyls (see Section 5), which mostly tested fist and second generation low-powered ECs available at the time. After 5 years, with so many newer devices emerging constantly into the market, we found very similar inconsistencies in this review (see Section 11) and in our recently published review of studies focused on metal contents in EC emissions [5]. Looking back, it seems that the technological development of ECs has evolved much more rapidly than the methods and standards used to analyze the device emissions.

As we mentioned in [5] and after further extending the arguments in Section 2, the main root of these methodological problems stems from the lack of understanding of the thermal physics involved in aerosol formation in a vaping device, based on the equilibrium of various heat exchanges (specially between e-liquid vaporization by supplied power and forced convection to form aerosol by condensation), an equilibrium that leads (when broken) to abnormal overheating conditions and a dry puff phenomenon with pyrolysis of the wick. Understanding these phenomena makes it possible to determine in the laboratory (for each device and e-liquid) the experimental settings compatible with the physical conditions (power ranges, coils, e-liquids) that allow for vaping to proceed efficiently in an optimal regime according to this equilibrium.

As we explain in Section 2, testing powerful sub-ohm devices under the insufficient airflow and puff volumes of the CORESTA or CORESTA-like protocols (the most frequent problem we have found) reduces the power ranges for an optimal regime. Pending on the testing power ranges, this leads to either a higher likelihood or a certainty of overheating conditions (see Sections 3.1 and 12.1). Surprisingly, 10 of 18 revised studies that used CORESTA or CORESTA-like protocols to test these devices did so at high power settings above the optimal regime, under clear overheating conditions. Evidently, outcomes and risk assessments from these studies are irrelevant for end users. The remaining 8 studies tested the devices at power ranges within recommended values, leading to a high likelihood (but not certainty) of overheating conditions. However, as we show in Sections 12.1 and 13, even if avoiding overheating, the experimental outcomes and risk assessments from these 8 studies are only relevant for a small minority (∼20%) of users of these devices with the lower airflows of the 'Mouth to Lung' (MTL) vaping style, likely ∼5% of users in general. The outcomes and risk assessments of the 18 studies testing sub-ohm devices with CORESTA or CORESTA-like protocols are likely irrelevant for ∼95% of vapers (given the substantial proportion using low powered devices).

We also express again the urgent need to update and upgrade the current CORESTA testing standard, a standard created in the early days of vaping as an adaptation of the puffing protocols of tobacco cigarettes to the old ciga-likes that resembled them, but very insufficient for testing the wide variety of currently available devices. As shown in Section 2, probing the parameters of the optimal regime (power settings and mass of e-liquid vaporized) for specific devices and e-liquids, should be a requirement prior to performing laboratory testing under conditions that avoid overheating.

Most of the studies we revised have conducted experiments without or with very insufficient input from the habits and needs of consumers and the evolution and trends in the market of vaping products. As pointed out and emphasized by Farsalinos and Gillman in [11], it should be a priority to complement laboratory testing by incorporating recruited vapers to assist in the logistics of experiments, as end users can perceive sensorially the effects (hot aerosol, foul taste) associated with a break down of an efficient vaping. It is also necessary to study in more detail how vapers vape, for example conducting research focused on

- Creating a data base of optimal regime laboratory testing for large samples of devices, e-liquids and coils, as described in Section 2 and [8,9]. This data basis can contribute to identify power ranges that avoid overheating.
- Cohort longitudinal studies for updating the scientific knowledge on the puffing behavior of EC users for all currently available devices.
- The development of inbuilt safety features, as user alerting systems, on EC devices that will at least notify users that the device is operating beyond its optimal regime with thermodynamic efficiency.
- Guidelines to inform and regulate the market of old age EC devices and their maintenance and storage conditions.

The present review shows that laboratory testing requires a much more flexible standard, not only providing appropriate technical guidelines, but facilitating the incorporation of end users to complement laboratory logistics. As future research we are planing an experimental replication of various emission studies that we revised in this review and in [5].

Author Contributions: Conceptualization, R.A.S. and S.S.; methodology, R.A.S. and S.S.; software, R.A.S. and S.S.; validation, R.A.S. and S.S.; formal analysis, R.A.S. and S.S.; investigation, R.A.S. and S.S.; resources, R.A.S. and S.S.; writing—original draft preparation, R.A.S. and S.S.; writing—review and editing, R.A.S. and S.S.; visualization, R.A.S. and S.S.; supervision, R.A.S and S.S. All authors have read and agreed to the published version of the manuscript.

Funding: R.A.S. received no external funding. S.S. is employed by Ingésciences. Ingésciences had received funding from région Nouvelle Aquitaine. Ingésciences has never received funding from the tobacco industry and its third parties.

Institutional Review Board Statement: Not applicable.

Informed Consent Statement: Not applicable.

Data Availability Statement: Not applicable.

Conflicts of Interest: R.A.S. declares no conflict of interest. S.S. declares that Ingésciences is completely independent of the tobacco industry and its third parties.

Abbreviations

The following abbreviations are broadly used in this manuscript (other abbreviations are fully described where defined):

EC	Electronic Cigarette
HPHC	Harmful and Potentially Harmful Compounds
CO	Carbon Monoxide
ROS	Reactive Oxygen Species
CORESTA	Cooperation Centre for Scientific Research Relative to Tobacco
CORESTA-like	Minor modifications of CORESTA protocols
MTL	Mouth to Lung
DTL	Direct to Lung
MEV	Mass of E-liquid Vaporized
PG	Propylene glycol
VG	Vegetable glycerine (glycerol)
DNPH	2,4-dinitrophenyl hydrazine (2,4-DNPH)
LC	Liquid Chromatography
GC	Gas Chromatography
MS	Mass Spectrometry
HP	High Performance
HR	High Resolution
UV	Ultraviolet
EPR	Electron Paramagnetic Resonance
NMR	Nuclear Magnetic Resonance
ICP	Inductively Coupled Plasma
C	degrees centigrades
pg	picogram
ng	nanogram
µg	microgram
g	gram
mg	milligram
mL	milliliter
L	Litter
cm	centimeter
m	meter
s	secondsr
min	minutes
h	hour
W	watts
V	Volts
Ω	ohms

References

1. Amos, A.; Arnott, D.; Aveyard, P.; Bauld, L.; Bogdanovica, I.; Britton, J.; Chenoweth, M.; Collin, J.; Dockrell, M.; Hajek, P.; et al. *Nicotine without Smoke: Tobacco Harm Reduction*; Royal College of Physicians: London, UK, 2016.
2. Daynard, R. Public health consequences of e-cigarettes: A consensus study report of the National Academies of Sciences, Engineering, and Medicine. *J. Public Health Policy* **2018**, *39*, 379–381. [CrossRef]
3. McNeill, A.; Brose, L.S.; Calder, R.; Bauld, L.; Robson, D. *Evidence Review of E-Cigarettes and Heated Tobacco Products 2018*; A Report Commissioned by Public Health England; Public Health England: London, UK, 2018.
4. Pisinger, C.; Døssing, M. A systematic review of health effects of electronic cigarettes. *Prev. Med.* **2014**, *69*, 248–260. [CrossRef]
5. Soulet, S.; Sussman, R.A. A Critical Review of Recent Literature on Metal Contents in E-Cigarette Aerosol. *Toxics* **2022**, *10*, 510. [CrossRef]

6. CORESTA Recommended Method No 81, 2017. Collaborative Study for Determination of Glycerin, Propylene Glycol, Water and Nicotine in Collected Aerosol of E-Cigarettes. Available online: https://www.coresta.org/2015-collaborative-study-determination-glycerin-propylene-glycol-water-and-nicotine-collected-30486 (accessed on 14 October 2022)
7. EVAP. Available online: https://www.coresta.org/groups/e-vapour (accessed on 14 October 2022)
8. Soulet, S.; Duquesne, M.; Toutain, J.; Pairaud, C.; Mercury, M. Impact of vaping regimens on electronic cigarette efficiency. *Int. J. Environ. Res. Public Health* **2019**, *16*, 4753. [CrossRef] [PubMed]
9. Soulet, S.; Duquesne, M.; Toutain, J.; Pairaud, C.; Lalo, H. Influence of coil power ranges on the e-liquid consumption in vaping devices. *Int. J. Environ. Res. Public Health* **2018**, *15*, 1853. [CrossRef]
10. Wadkin, R.; Allen, C.; Fearon, I.M. E-Cigarette Puffing Topography: The Importance of Assessing User Behaviour to Inform Emissions Testing. *Drug Test. Anal.* **2022**, *online ahead of print*. [CrossRef]
11. Farsalinos, K.E.; Gillman, G. Carbonyl emissions in e-cigarette aerosol: A systematic review and methodological considerations. *Front. Physiol.* **2018**, *8*, 1119. [CrossRef]
12. Ward, A.M.; Yaman, R.; Ebbert, J.O. Electronic nicotine delivery system design and aerosol toxicants: A systematic review. *PLoS ONE* **2020**, *15*, e0234189. [CrossRef]
13. Vreeke, S.; Peyton, D.H.; Strongin, R.M. Triacetin enhances levels of acrolein, formaldehyde hemiacetals, and acetaldehyde in electronic cigarette aerosols. *ACS Omega* **2018**, *3*, 7165–7170. [CrossRef]
14. Korzun, T.; Lazurko, M.; Munhenzva, I.; Barsanti, K.C.; Huang, Y.; Jensen, R.P.; Escobedo, J.O.; Luo, W.; Peyton, D.H.; Strongin, R.M. E-cigarette airflow rate modulates toxicant profiles and can lead to concerning levels of solvent consumption. *ACS Omega* **2018**, *3*, 30–36. [CrossRef]
15. El-Hellani, A.; Salman, R.; El-Hage, R.; Talih, S.; Malek, N.; Baalbaki, R.; Karaoghlanian, N.; Nakkash, R.; Shihadeh, A.; Saliba, N.A. Nicotine and carbonyl emissions from popular electronic cigarette products: Correlation to liquid composition and design characteristics. *Nicotine Tob. Res.* **2018**, *20*, 215–223. [CrossRef] [PubMed]
16. Beauval, N.; Verriele, M.; Garat, A.; Fronval, I.; Dusautoir, R.; Anthérieu, S.; Garçon, G.; Lo-Guidice, J.M.; Allorge, D.; Locoge, N. Influence of puffing conditions on the carbonyl composition of e-cigarette aerosols. *Int. J. Hyg. Environ. Health* **2019**, *222*, 136–146. [CrossRef] [PubMed]
17. Ooi, B.G.; Dutta, D.; Kazipeta, K.; Chong, N.S. Influence of the e-cigarette emission profile by the ratio of glycerol to propylene glycol in e-liquid composition. *ACS Omega* **2019**, *4*, 13338–13348. [CrossRef]
18. Belushkin, M.; Tafin Djoko, D.; Esposito, M.; Korneliou, A.; Jeannet, C.; Lazzerini, M.; Jaccard, G. Selected harmful and potentially harmful constituents levels in commercial e-cigarettes. *Chem. Res. Toxicol.* **2019**, *33*, 657–668. [CrossRef]
19. Reilly, S.M.; Bitzer, Z.T.; Goel, R.; Trushin, N.; Richie, J.P., Jr. Free radical, carbonyl, and nicotine levels produced by Juul electronic cigarettes. *Nicotine Tob. Res.* **2019**, *21*, 1274–1278. [CrossRef] [PubMed]
20. Cancelada, L.; Tang, X.; Russell, M.L.; Maddalena, R.L.; Litter, M.I.; Gundel, L.A.; Destaillats, H. Volatile aldehyde emissions from "sub-ohm" vaping devices. *Environ. Res.* **2021**, *197*, 111188. [CrossRef]
21. Son, Y.; Weisel, C.; Wackowski, O.; Schwander, S.; Delnevo, C.; Meng, Q. The impact of device settings, use patterns, and flavorings on carbonyl emissions from electronic cigarettes. *Int. J. Environ. Res. Public Health* **2020**, *17*, 5650. [CrossRef]
22. Talih, S.; Salman, R.; Karam, E.; El-Hourani, M.; El-Hage, R.; Karaoghlanian, N.; El-Hellani, A.; Saliba, N.; Shihadeh, A. Hot Wires and Film Boiling: Another Look at Carbonyl Formation in Electronic Cigarettes. *Chem. Res. Toxicol.* **2020**, *33*, 2172–2180. [CrossRef]
23. Zelinkova, Z.; Wenzl, T. Influence of battery power setting on carbonyl emissions from electronic cigarettes. *Tob. Induc. Dis.* **2020**, *18*, 77. [CrossRef]
24. Uchiyama, S.; Noguchi, M.; Sato, A.; Ishitsuka, M.; Inaba, Y.; Kunugita, N. Determination of thermal decomposition products generated from E-cigarettes. *Chem. Res. Toxicol.* **2020**, *33*, 576–583. [CrossRef]
25. Cunningham, A.; McAdam, K.; Thissen, J.; Digard, H. The evolving e-cigarette: Comparative chemical analyses of e-cigarette vapor and cigarette smoke. *Front. Toxicol.* **2020**, *2*, 586674. [CrossRef] [PubMed]
26. Noël, A.; Hossain, E.; Perveen, Z.; Zaman, H.; Penn, A.L. Sub-ohm vaping increases the levels of carbonyls, is cytotoxic, and alters gene expression in human bronchial epithelial cells exposed at the air–liquid interface. *Respir. Res.* **2020**, *21*, 305. [CrossRef]
27. Mallock, N.; Trieu, H.L.; Macziol, M.; Malke, S.; Katz, A.; Laux, P.; Henkler-Stephani, F.; Hahn, J.; Hutzler, C.; Luch, A. Trendy e-cigarettes enter Europe: Chemical characterization of JUUL pods and its aerosols. *Arch. Toxicol.* **2020**, *94*, 1985–1994. [CrossRef] [PubMed]
28. Chen, X.; Bailey, P.C.; Yang, C.; Hiraki, B.; Oldham, M.J.; Gillman, I.G. Targeted characterization of the chemical composition of juul systems aerosol and comparison with 3r4f reference cigarettes and iqos heat sticks. *Separations* **2021**, *8*, 168. [CrossRef]
29. Crosswhite, M.R.; Bailey, P.C.; Jeong, L.N.; Lioubomirov, A.; Yang, C.; Ozvald, A.; Jameson, J.B.; Gillman, I.G. Non-targeted chemical characterization of Juul Virginia tobacco flavored aerosols using liquid and gas chromatography. *Separations* **2021**, *8*, 130. [CrossRef]
30. Li, Y.; Burns, A.E.; Tran, L.N.; Abellar, K.A.; Poindexter, M.; Li, X.; Madl, A.K.; Pinkerton, K.E.; Nguyen, T.B. Impact of e-Liquid Composition, Coil Temperature, and Puff Topography on the Aerosol Chemistry of Electronic Cigarettes. *Chem. Res. Toxicol.* **2021**, *34*, 1640–1654. [CrossRef] [PubMed]

31. Yan, B.; Zagorevski, D.; Ilievski, V.; Kleiman, N.J.; Re, D.B.; Navas-Acien, A.; Hilpert, M. Identification of newly formed toxic chemicals in E-cigarette aerosols with Orbitrap mass spectrometry and implications on E-cigarette control. *Eur. J. Mass Spectrom.* **2021**, *27*, 141–148. [CrossRef]
32. Tehrani, M.W.; Newmeyer, M.N.; Rule, A.M.; Prasse, C. Characterizing the chemical landscape in commercial e-cigarette liquids and aerosols by liquid chromatography–high-resolution mass spectrometry. *Chem. Res. Toxicol.* **2021**, *34*, 2216–2226. [CrossRef]
33. Xu, T.; Niu, Z.Y.; Xu, J.; Li, X.D.; Luo, Q.; Luo, A.; Huang, Y.L.; Jiang, X.T.; Wu, Z.H. Chemical analysis of selected harmful and potentially harmful constituents and in vitro toxicological evaluation of leading flavoured e-cigarette aerosols in the Chinese market. *Drug Test. Anal.* **2022**, *online ahead of print*. [CrossRef]
34. Visser, W.F.; Krüsemann, E.J.; Klerx, W.N.; Boer, K.; Weibolt, N.; Talhout, R. Improving the analysis of e-cigarette emissions: Detecting human "dry puff" conditions in a laboratory as validated by a panel of experienced vapers. *Int. J. Environ. Res. Public Health* **2021**, *18*, 11520. [CrossRef]
35. Casebolt, R.; Cook, S.J.; Islas, A.; Brown, A.; Castle, K.; Dutcher, D.D. Carbon monoxide concentration in mainstream E-cigarette emissions measured with diode laser spectroscopy. *Tob. Control* **2022**, *29*, 652–655. [CrossRef]
36. El-Hellani, A.; Al-Moussawi, S.; El-Hage, R.; Talih, S.; Salman, R.; Shihadeh, A.; Saliba, N.A. Carbon Monoxide and Small Hydrocarbon Emissions from Sub-ohm Electronic Cigarettes. *Chem. Res. Toxicol.* **2019**, *32*, 312. [CrossRef] [PubMed]
37. Son, Y.; Bhattarai, C.; Samburova, V.; Khlystov, A. Carbonyls and carbon monoxide emissions from electronic cigarettes affected by device type and use patterns. *Int. J. Environ. Res. Public Health* **2020**, *17*, 2767. [CrossRef]
38. Bitzer, Z.T.; Goel, R.; Reilly, S.M.; Foulds, J.; Muscat, J.; Elias, R.J.; Richie, J.P., Jr. Effects of solvent and temperature on free radical formation in electronic cigarette aerosols. *Chem. Res. Toxicol.* **2018**, *31*, 4–12. [CrossRef] [PubMed]
39. Bitzer, Z.T.; Goel, R.; Reilly, S.M.; Elias, R.J.; Silakov, A.; Foulds, J.; Muscat, J.; Richie, J.P., Jr. Effect of flavoring chemicals on free radical formation in electronic cigarette aerosols. *Free Radic. Biol. Med.* **2018**, *120*, 72–79. [CrossRef] [PubMed]
40. Son, Y.; Mishin, V.; Laskin, J.D.; Mainelis, G.; Wackowski, O.A.; Delnevo, C.; Schwander, S.; Khlystov, A.; Samburova, V.; Meng, Q. Hydroxyl radicals in e-cigarette vapor and e-vapor oxidative potentials under different vaping patterns. *Chem. Res. Toxicol.* **2019**, *32*, 1087–1095. [CrossRef]
41. Haddad, C.; Salman, R.; El-Hellani, A.; Talih, S.; Shihadeh, A.; Saliba, N.A. Reactive oxygen species emissions from supra-and sub-ohm electronic cigarettes. *J. Anal. Toxicol.* **2019**, *43*, 45–50. [CrossRef]
42. Jensen, R.P.; Strongin, R.M.; Peyton, D.H. Solvent chemistry in the electronic cigarette reaction vessel. *Sci. Rep.* **2017**, *7*, 42549. [CrossRef]
43. Wang, P.; Chen, W.; Liao, J.; Matsuo, T.; Ito, K.; Fowles, J.; Shusterman, D.; Mendell, M.; Kumagai, K. A device-independent evaluation of carbonyl emissions from heated electronic cigarette solvents. *PLoS ONE* **2017**, *12*, e0169811. [CrossRef]
44. Li, Y.; Burns, A.E.; Burke, G.J.; Poindexter, M.E.; Madl, A.K.; Pinkerton, K.E.; Nguyen, T.B. Application of high-resolution mass spectrometry and a theoretical model to the quantification of multifunctional carbonyls and organic acids in e-cigarette aerosol. *Environ. Sci. Technol.* **2020**, *54*, 5640–5650. [CrossRef]
45. Melvin, M.S.; Avery, K.C.; Ballentine, R.M.; Flora, J.W.; Gardner, W.; Karles, G.D.; Pithawalla, Y.B.; Smith, D.C.; Ehman, K.D.; Wagner, K.A. Formation of Diacetyl and Other α-Dicarbonyl Compounds during the Generation of E-Vapor Product Aerosols. *ACS Omega* **2020**, *5*, 17565–17575. [CrossRef] [PubMed]
46. Jaegers, N.R.; Hu, W.; Weber, T.J.; Hu, J.Z. Low-temperature (<200 C) degradation of electronic nicotine delivery system liquids generates toxic aldehydes. *Sci. Rep.* **2021**, *11*, 7800.
47. Dawkins, L.; Cox, S.; Goniewicz, M.; McRobbie, H.; Kimber, C.; Doig, M.; Kośmider, L. 'Real-world' compensatory behaviour with low nicotine concentration e-liquid: Subjective effects and nicotine, acrolein and formaldehyde exposure. *Addiction* **2018**, *113*, 1874–1882. [CrossRef] [PubMed]
48. Kosmider, L.; Cox, S.; Zaciera, M.; Kurek, J.; Goniewicz, M.L.; McRobbie, H.; Kimber, C.; Dawkins, L. Daily exposure to formaldehyde and acetaldehyde and potential health risk associated with use of high and low nicotine e-liquid concentrations. *Sci. Rep.* **2020**, *10*, 6546. [CrossRef] [PubMed]
49. Soulet, S.; Duquesne, M.; Pairaud, C.; Toutain, J. Highlighting Specific Features to Reduce Chemical and Thermal Risks of Electronic Cigarette Use through a Technical Classification of Devices. *Appl. Sci.* **2021**, *11*, 5254. [CrossRef]
50. Soulet, S.; Casile, C. Thermodynamic behaviour of an e-cigarette: Investigation of nicotine delivery consistency using nicotine yield. *Therm. Sci. Eng. Prog.* **2022**, *35*, 101452. [CrossRef]
51. Gillman, I.; Kistler, K.; Stewart, E.; Paolantonio, A. Effect of variable power levels on the yield of total aerosol mass and formation of aldehydes in e-cigarette aerosols. *Regul. Toxicol. Pharmacol.* **2016**, *75*, 58–65. [CrossRef]
52. Floyd, E.; Greenlee, S.; Oni, T.; Sadhasivam, B.; Queimado, L. The Effect of Flow Rate on a Third-Generation Sub-Ohm Tank Electronic Nicotine Delivery System, Comparison of CORESTA Flow Rates to More Realistic Flow Rates. *Int. J. Environ. Res. Public Health* **2021**, *18*, 7535. [CrossRef]
53. DiPiazza, J.; Caponnetto, P.; Askin, G.; Christos, P.; Maglia, M.L.P.; Gautam, R.; Roche, S.; Polosa, R. Sensory experiences and cues among E-cigarette users. *Harm Reduct. J.* **2020**, *17*, 75. [CrossRef]
54. McAdam, K.; Warrington, A.; Hughes, A.; Adams, D.; Margham, J.; Vas, C.; Davis, P.; Costigan, S.; Proctor, C. Use of social media to establish vapers puffing behaviour: Findings and implications for laboratory evaluation of e-cigarette emissions. *Regul. Toxicol. Pharmacol.* **2019**, *107*, 104423. [CrossRef]

55. Ecigclick. Mouth to Lung (MTL) VS Direct to Lung (DTL) Vaping: What's the Difference? 2022. Available online: https://www.ecigclick.co.uk/mouth-to-lung-vs-direct-to-lung/ (accessed on 8 November 2022)
56. Vaping 360. Mouth to Lung (MTL) VS Direct to Lung (DTL) Vaping: What's the Difference? 2022. Available online: https://vaping360.com/learn/what-is-vaping-how-to-vape/ (accessed on 8 November 2022)
57. Tobin, M.J.; Schneider, A.W.; Sackner, M.A. Breathing pattern during and after smoking cigarettes. *Clin. Sci.* **1982**, *63*, 473. [CrossRef]
58. Marian, C.; O'Connor, R.J.; Djordjevic, M.V.; Rees, V.W.; Hatrukami, D.K.; Shields, P.G. Reconciling human smoking behavior and machine smoking patterns: Implications for understanding smoking behavior and the impact on laboratory studies. *Cancer Epidemiol. Biomarkers Prev.* **2009**, *18*, 3305. [CrossRef] [PubMed]
59. Gravely, S.; Meng, G.; Hammond, D.; Reid, J.; Seo, Y.; Hyland, A.; Cummings, M.; Rivard, C.; Fong, G.; Kasza, K. Electronic nicotine delivery systems (ENDS) flavours and devices used by adults before and after the 2020 US FDA ENDS enforcement priority: Findings from the 2018 and 2020 US ITC Smoking and Vaping Surveys. *Tob. Control* **2022**, *31* (Suppl. S3), s167.
60. Action on Smoking and Health (ASH). Fact Sheet: Use of E-Cigarettes (Vapes) among Adults in Great Britain. 2022. Available online: https://ash.org.uk/resources/view/use-of-e-cigarettes-among-adults-in-great-britain-2021 (accessed on 8 November 2022)
61. Kotz, D.; Böckmann, M.; Kastaun, S. The use of tobacco, e-cigarettes, and methods to quit smoking in Germany: A representative study using 6 waves of data over 12 months (the DEBRA study). *Dtsch. Ärzteblatt Int.* **2018**, *115*, 235.
62. Leventhal, A.M.; Dai, H.; Barrington-Trimis, J.L.; Tackett, A.; Pedersen, E.R.; Tran, E.D. Use of social media to establish vapers puffing behaviour: Disposable e-cigarette use prevalence, correlates, and associations with previous tobacco product use in young adults. *Nicotine Tob. Res.* **2022**, *24*, 372. [CrossRef] [PubMed]
63. Tattan-Birch, H.; Jackson, S.E.; Kock, L.; Dockrell, M.; Brown, J. Rapid growth in disposable e-cigarette vaping among young adults in Great Britain from 2021 to 2022: A repeat cross-sectional survey. *medRxiv*, 2022, online ahead of print. [CrossRef]
64. Rana, S.S.; Kharabanda, O.P.; Agarwal, B. Influence of tongue volume, oral cavity volume and their ratio on upper airway: A cone beam computed tomography study. *J. Oral Biol. Craniofacial Res.* **2020**, *10*, 110. [CrossRef]
65. Havermans, A.; Krüsemann, E.J.Z.; Pennings, J.; Graaf, K.D.; Boesveldt, S.; Talhout, R. Nearly 20,000 e-liquids and 250 unique flavour descriptions: An overview of the Dutch market based on information from manufacturers. *Tob. Control* **2021**, *30*, 57–62. [CrossRef]
66. Zhang, C.; Chao, L.; Zhang, Z.; Zhang, L.; Li, Q.; Fan, H.; Zhang, S.; Liu, Q.; Qiao, Y.; Tian, Y.; et al. Pyrolysis of cellulose: Evolution of functionalities and structure of bio-char versus temperature. *Renew. Sustain. Energy Rev.* **2021**, *135*, 110416. [CrossRef]
67. Zhao, C.; Jiang, E.; Chen, A. Volatile production from pyrolysis of cellulose, hemicellulose and lignin. *J. Energy Inst.* **2017**, *90*, 902–913. [CrossRef]
68. Collard, F.X.; Blin, J. A review on pyrolysis of biomass constituents: Mechanisms and composition of the products obtained from the conversion of cellulose, hemicelluloses and lignin. *Renew. Sustain. Energy Rev.* **2014**, *38*, 594–608. [CrossRef]
69. Bouzalakou-Butel, L.A.; Provatidis, P.; Sturrock, K.; Fiore, A. Primary Investigation into the Occurrence of Hydroxymethylfurfural (HMF) in a Range of Smoked Products. *J. Chem.* **2018**, *2018*, e5942081. [CrossRef]
70. Cadwallader, K.R. Wood Smoke Flavor. In *Handbook of Meat, Poultry and Seafood Quality*; John Wiley & Sons, Ltd.: Hoboken, NJ, USA, 2007; pp. 201–210. [CrossRef]
71. McGrath, T.E.; Chan, W.G.; Hajaligol, M.R. Low temperature mechanism for the formation of polycyclic aromatic hydrocarbons from the pyrolysis of cellulose. *J. Anal. Appl. Pyrolysis* **2003**, *66*, 51–70. [CrossRef]
72. Prasad, K. A review of electronic cigarette use behaviour studies. *Beitr. Tab. Int. Contrib. Tob. Res.* **2018**, *28*, 81–92.
73. Robinson, R.; Hensel, E.; Morabito, P.; Roundtree, K. Electronic cigarette topography in the natural environment. *PLoS ONE* **2015**, *10*, e0129296. [CrossRef]
74. Dautzenberg, B.; Bricard, D. Real-time characterization of e-cigarettes use: The 1 million puffs study. *J. Addict. Res. Ther* **2015**, *6*, 4172. [CrossRef]
75. Robinson, R.; Hensel, E.; Roundtree, K.; Difrancesco, A.; Nonnemaker, J.; Lee, Y. Week long topography study of young adults using electronic cigarettes in their natural environment. *PLoS ONE* **2016**, *11*, e0164038. [CrossRef]
76. Cox, S.; Kośmider, L.; McRobbie, H.; Goniewicz, M.; Kimber, C.; Doig, M.; Dawkins, L. E-cigarette puffing patterns associated with high and low nicotine e-liquid strength: Effects on toxicant and carcinogen exposure. *BMC Public Health* **2016**, *16*, 999. [CrossRef]
77. Cox, S.; Goniewicz, M.L.; Kosmider, L.; McRobbie, H.; Kimber, C.; Dawkins, L. The time course of compensatory puffing with an electronic cigarette: Secondary analysis of real-world puffing data with high and low nicotine concentration under fixed and adjustable power settings. *Nicotine Tob. Res.* **2021**, *23*, 1153–1159. [CrossRef]
78. Kośmider, L.; Jackson, A.; Leigh, N.; O'connor, R.; Goniewicz, M.L. Circadian puffing behavior and topography among e-cigarette users. *Tob. Regul. Sci.* **2018**, *4*, 41–49. [CrossRef]
79. Williams, M.; Luo, W.; McWhirter, K.; Ikegbu, O.; Talbot, P. Chemical Elements, Flavor Chemicals, and Nicotine in Unused and Used Electronic Cigarettes Aged 5–10 Years and Effects of pH. *ChemRxiv* **2022**. Available online: https://chemrxiv.org/engage/chemrxiv/article-details/635cb36faca19892ffe9ebc4 (accessed on 8 November 2022)
80. Farsalinos, K.E.; Voudris, V.; Poulas, K. E-cigarettes generate high levels of aldehydes only in 'dry puff' conditions. *Addiction* **2015**, *110*, 1352–1356. [CrossRef] [PubMed]

81. Jensen, R.P.; Wental, L.; Pankow, J.F.; Strongin, R.M.; Peyton, D.H. Hidden Formaldehyde in E-Cigarette Aerosols. *N. Engl. J. Med.* **2015**, *372*, 392–394. [CrossRef] [PubMed]
82. Sleiman, M.; Logue, J.M.; Montesinos, V.N.; Russell, M.L.; Litter, M.I.; Gundel, L.A.; Destaillats, H. Emissions from electronic cigarettes: Key parameters affecting the release of harmful chemicals. *Environ. Sci. Technol.* **2016**, *50*, 9644–9651. [CrossRef] [PubMed]
83. Farsalinos, K.E.; Voudris, V.; Spyrou, A.; Poulas, K. E-cigarettes emit very high formaldehyde levels only in conditions that are aversive to users: A replication study under verified realistic use conditions. *Food Chem. Toxicol.* **2017**, *109*, 90–94. [CrossRef]
84. Bates, C.D.; Farsalinos, K.E. Research letter on e-cigarette cancer risk was so misleading it should be retracted. *Addiction* **2015**, *110*, 1686–1687. [CrossRef]
85. Pankow, J.F.; Strongin, R.M.; Peyton, D.H. Formaldehyde From E-Cigarettes-It's Not as Simple as Some Suggest. *Addiction* **2015**, *110*, 1687–1688. [CrossRef]
86. Bates, C.D.; Farsalinos, K.E. E-cigarettes need to be tested for safety under realistic conditions. *Addiction* **2015**, *110*, 1688–1689. [CrossRef]
87. Farsalinos, K.E.; Kistler, K.A.; Pennington, A.; Spyrou, A.; Kouretas, D.; Gillman, G. Aldehyde levels in e-cigarette aerosol: Findings from a replication study and from use of a new-generation device. *Food Chem. Toxicol.* **2018**, *111*, 64–70. [CrossRef]
88. Khlystov, A.; Samburova, V. Flavoring compounds dominate toxic aldehyde production during e-cigarette vaping. *Environ. Sci. Technol.* **2016**, *50*, 13080–13085. [CrossRef]
89. Farsalinos, K.; Gillman, G.; Kistler, K.; Yannovits, N. Comment on "flavoring compounds dominate toxic aldehyde Production during E Cigarette vaping". *Environ. Sci. Technol.* **2017**, *51*, 2491–2492. [CrossRef]
90. Khlystov, A.; Samburova, V. Response to Comment on "Flavoring Compounds Dominate Toxic Aldehyde Production during E Cigarette Vaping". *Environ. Sci. Technol.* **2017**, *51*, 2493–2494. [CrossRef] [PubMed]
91. Farsalinos, K. Measuring aldehyde emissions in e-cigarettes and the contribution of flavors: A response to Khlystov and Samburova. *Food Chem. Toxicol.* **2018**, *120*, 726–728. [CrossRef] [PubMed]
92. Gillman, I.G.; Pennington, A.S.; Humphries, K.E.; Oldham, M.J. Determining the impact of flavored e-liquids on aldehyde production during Vaping. *Regul. Toxicol. Pharmacol.* **2020**, *112*, 104588. [CrossRef] [PubMed]
93. Ting, C.Y.; Ahmad Sabri, N.A.; Tiong, L.L.; Zailani, H.; Wong, L.P.; Agha Mohammadi, N.; Anchah, L. Heavy metals (Cr, Pb, Cd, Ni) in aerosols emitted from electronic cigarettes sold in Malaysia. *J. Environ. Sci. Health Part A* **2020**, *55*, 55–62. [CrossRef]
94. Dalton, P.; Soreth, B.; Maute, C.; Novaleski, C.; Banton, M. Lack of respiratory and ocular effects following acute propylene glycol exposure in healthy humans. *Inhal. Toxicol.* **2018**, *30*, 124–132. [CrossRef]
95. Son, Y.; Wackowski, O.; Weisel, C.; Schwander, S.; Mainelis, G.; Delnevo, C.; Meng, Q. Evaluation of e-vapor nicotine and nicotyrine concentrations under various e-liquid compositions, device settings, and vaping topographies. *Chem. Res. Toxicol.* **2018**, *31*, 861–868. [CrossRef]
96. Zhao, D.; Navas-Acien, A.; Ilievski, V.; Slavkovich, V.; Olmedo, P.; Adria-Mora, B.; Domingo-Relloso, A.; Aherrera, A.; Kleiman, N.J.; Rule, A.M.; et al. Metal concentrations in electronic cigarette aerosol: Effect of open-system and closed-system devices and power settings. *Environ. Res.* **2019**, *174*, 125–134. [CrossRef]
97. Stein, Y.S.; Antal, M.J.; Jones, M. A study of the gas-phase pyrolysis of glycerol. *J. Anal. Appl. Pyrolysis* **1983**, *4*, 283–296. [CrossRef]
98. Shen, D.K.; Gu, S. The mechanism for thermal decomposition of cellulose and its main products. *Bioresour. Technol.* **2009**, *100*, 6496–6504. [CrossRef]
99. Wang, Q.; Song, H.; Pan, S.; Dong, N.; Wang, X.; Sun, S. Initial pyrolysis mechanism and product formation of cellulose: An Experimental and Density functional theory(DFT) study. *Sci. Rep.* **2020**, *10*, 3626. [CrossRef]
100. Goel, R.; Durand, E.; Trushin, N.; Prokopczyk, B.; Foulds, J.; Elias, R.J.; Richie, J.P., Jr. Highly reactive free radicals in electronic cigarette aerosols. *Chem. Res. Toxicol.* **2015**, *28*, 1675–1677. [CrossRef] [PubMed]
101. Zhao, J.; Zhang, Y.; Sisler, J.D.; Shaffer, J.; Leonard, S.S.; Morris, A.M.; Qian, Y.; Bello, D.; Demokritou, P. Assessment of reactive oxygen species generated by electronic cigarettes using acellular and cellular approaches. *J. Hazard. Mater.* **2018**, *344*, 549–557. [CrossRef] [PubMed]
102. Gonzalez, D.H.; Kuang, X.M.; Scott, J.A.; Rocha, G.O.; Paulson, S.E. Terephthalate Probe for Hydroxyl Radicals: Yield of 2-Hydroxyterephthalic Acid and Transition Metal Interference. *Anal. Lett.* **2018**, *51*, 2488–2497. [CrossRef]
103. Talih, S.; Balhas, Z.; Eissenberg, T.; Salman, R.; Karaoghlanian, N.; El Hellani, A.; Baalbaki, R.; Saliba, N.; Shihadeh, A. Effects of user puff topography, device voltage, and liquid nicotine concentration on electronic cigarette nicotine yield: Measurements and model predictions. *Nicotine Tob. Res.* **2015**, *17*, 150–157. [CrossRef] [PubMed]
104. Saliba, N.A.; El Hellani, A.; Honein, E.; Salman, R.; Talih, S.; Zeaiter, J.; Shihadeh, A. Surface chemistry of electronic cigarette electrical heating coils: Effects of metal type on propylene glycol thermal decomposition. *J. Anal. Appl. Pyrolysis* **2018**, *134*, 520. [CrossRef] [PubMed]

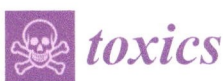

Review

A Critical Review of Recent Literature on Metal Contents in E-Cigarette Aerosol

Sebastien Soulet [1,†] and Roberto A. Sussman [2,*,†]

1 Ingesciences, 2 Chemin des Arestieux, 33610 Cestas, France
2 Institute of Nuclear Sciences, National Autonomous University of Mexico, Mexico City 04510, Mexico
* Correspondence: sussman@nucleares.unam.mx
† These authors contributed equally to this work.

Abstract: The inhalation of metallic compounds in e-cigarette (EC) aerosol emissions presents legitimate concerns of potential harms for users. We provide a critical review of laboratory studies published after 2017 on metal contents in EC aerosol, focusing on the consistency between their experimental design, real life device usage and appropriate evaluation of exposure risks. All experiments reporting levels above toxicological markers for some metals (e.g., nickel, lead, copper, manganese) exhibited the following experimental flaws: (i) high powered sub-ohm tank devices tested by means of puffing protocols whose airflows and puff volumes are conceived and appropriate for low powered devices; this testing necessarily involves overheating conditions that favor the production of toxicants and generate aerosols that are likely repellent to human users; (ii) miscalculation of exposure levels from experimental outcomes; (iii) pods and tank devices acquired months and years before the experiments, so that corrosion effects cannot be ruled out; (iv) failure to disclose important information on the characteristics of pods and tank devices, on the experimental methodology and on the resulting outcomes, thus hindering the interpretation of results and the possibility of replication. In general, low powered devices tested without these shortcomings produced metal exposure levels well below strict reference toxicological markers. We believe this review provides useful guidelines for a more objective risk assessment of EC aerosol emissions and signals the necessity to upgrade current laboratory testing standards.

Keywords: e-cigarettes; vaping; aerosol emissions; puffing protocols; metals

Citation: Soulet, S.; Sussman, R.A. A Critical Review of Recent Literature on Metal Contents in E-Cigarette Aerosol. *Toxics* **2022**, *10*, 510. https://doi.org/10.3390/toxics10090510

Academic Editors: Andrzej Sobczak, Leon Kośmider and Irfan Rahman

Received: 5 July 2022
Accepted: 26 August 2022
Published: 29 August 2022

Publisher's Note: MDPI stays neutral with regard to jurisdictional claims in published maps and institutional affiliations.

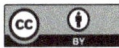

Copyright: © 2022 by the authors. Licensee MDPI, Basel, Switzerland. This article is an open access article distributed under the terms and conditions of the Creative Commons Attribution (CC BY) license (https://creativecommons.org/licenses/by/4.0/).

1. Introduction

There is a broad consensus that "vapers" (users of electronic cigarettes (ECs)) inhale substantially lower content of toxic and carcinogenic compounds in comparison with tobacco smoke [1–3] (see [4] for a diverging opinion). This fact has motivated large numbers of smokers to adopt "vaping" (usage of ECs) as a significantly less risky alternative to smoking within the framework of tobacco harm reduction.

However, vapers are still exposed to the inhalation of harmful or potentially harmful compounds (HPHCs), particularly carbonyls, nitrosamines, metallic compounds and possibly carbon monoxide (CO) and Reactive Oxygen Species (ROS). Detection of metals in the chemical analysis of e-cigarette emissions is not surprising, as metallic compounds are already present in e-liquids at trace levels [5,6] and e-cigarette parts are made of various metallic alloys. Given their high level of toxicity and carcinogenic effects [7,8], it is a public health priority to provide vapers and smokers with an accurate analysis and evaluation of the involved risks of inhaling metallic content in adopting EC usage.

There is an extensive literature of laboratory studies analyzing metallic contents of e-liquids and EC aerosol (see descriptive review of experimental methodology in [9]). We provide in the present paper a critical examination of the more recent body of this literature consisting of 12 articles published after 2017 [10–21]. We will not deal with (i) studies on metal contents only in e-liquids and (ii) articles published before 2017, as older studies tested devices that are now obsolete [22–26]. Our emphasis is to examine the compatibility between puffing protocols, realistic usage and risk evaluation through comparison with toxicological references.

Aerosol collection techniques in the revised literature are diverse and a variety of devices have been tested, chemical analysis mostly relies in Gas Chromatography and Mass Spectrometry. However, there is a common generic feature in this literature: EC aerosols are artificially generated by puffing machines through regimented experimental protocols based on the ISO 20768 standard with puffing parameters defined by the the Cooperation Centre for Scientific Research Relative to Tobacco (CORESTA) protocol recommended method 81 [27]. This standard, which emerged as a natural adaptation to early vaping "ciga-like" devices of the standards used for laboratory testing of tobacco cigarettes [28], is followed (exactly or roughly) by almost all current laboratory testing of vaping devices. We will denote as CORESTA-like the puffing protocols that approximate the CORESTA protocol.

The puffing parameters of the CORESTA and CORESTA-like protocols are appropriate for vaping devices whose airflows and puff volumes are close to those of cigarettes [29], namely, low powered devices such as second generation clearomizers, tank equipped starter kits or pods, used with the 'Mouth to Lung' (MTL) vaping style with coil resistances above 1 Ω and power outputs typically below 20–25 W. However, CORESTA and CORESTA-like protocols are completely inappropriate to test high powered tank devices with coil resistances below 1 Ω (sub-ohm devices) designed to operate with much larger airflows, puff volumes and power outputs, used for the 'Direct to Lung' (DTL) vaping style (see [30] for comprehensive discussion on the relation between airflow and coil resistance).

It is not surprising that some of the studies testing sub-ohm devices with CORESTA-like puffing protocols found high levels of various metal elements that can even surpass toxicological markers (see for example [11,12,16]), but even if these markers are not surpassed (as in [10,18,19]) the obtained metal levels represent unrealistic exposures. The problem with these studies is not only usage of airflows and puff volumes that fall short of those for which sub-ohm devices were designed for their real life usage in DTL vaping, but also because this inadequacy very likely leads (even at relatively low power) to overheating conditions (see Soulet et al. [31,32] and Floyd et al. [33]), which for sufficiently high power might lead also to a 'dry puff' with depleted e-liquid and the coil pyrolyzing the wick [34,35]. Overheating conditions that increase coil temperature are known to correlate with sharp increases of the abundance of carbonyls in aerosol emissions [36] (see also [34,35,37–40]).

A useful way to determine experimentally, for any given combination of device and e-liquid, the parameters that should lead to the emergence of overheating (thus distinguishing normal vs abnormal operation modes) is the optimal regime defined by a linear relation between the mass of vaporized e-liquid (MEV) and supplied power that holds in a specific power range, with an overheating regime taking place above this power range where this relation becomes non-linear. As shown by Soulet et al. [31,32] the above mentioned relation between MEV and power is connected with the thermodynamical efficiency of the vaporization of the e-liquid prior to the formation of the aerosol.

Since ECs are aimed at real life consumers, it is important to bear in mind the limitations of laboratory testing, as there is evidence that regimented puffing by itself might produce (pending on the device and the puffing protocol) an increase of coil [37] and mouthpiece [38] temperatures that could be uncomfortable to end users (see example in [37]), thus suggesting to bear into consideration the specifications recommended by the manufacturer design, as well as users' sensorial experiences.

Evidently, consultation or cooperation with human vapers in the testing procedure should be very helpful to determine testing parameters (see a welcome development on this issue in [41]). However, as far as we are aware, none of the studies on metal content that we have revised have done so. Disregarding these issues can lead to misleading emission outcomes from an artificial aerosol that is too hot and most likely repellent to end users, while the vaping machines (which do not taste nor feel) continue operating. Risk assessments under these conditions are of little utility for the end user (even under correct trapping and analytic techniques).

The revised literature exhibits other experimental flaws besides inappropriate puffing protocols for sub-ohm devices. In some studies tested devices were acquired months or years before the experiments without providing information on storage conditions: [14–16,18], thus raising the possibility of metallic components subjected to corrosion or degradation (this was recognized in [14,15,18]). Actual exposure from experimental outcomes was miscalculated in [10,11,13,16,18]. Important information on the device characteristics, aerosol collection and experimental outcomes was omitted in [12,13,15,16,18], making it very difficult to understand and evaluate the relevance and scope of their results (and to replicate the experiments). In particular, it is impossible to rule out testing of defective devices and cartridges in [14,15,18] that would probably be repellent to human users.

Most of the revised articles reported significant health risks and recommendations of strict EC regulation on the grounds of their laboratory outcomes. However, our findings in this review suggests that such conclusions are questionable, not only because they emerge from experiments with the methodological flaws that we have commented, but because even under the best possible experimental conditions the regimented puffing of laboratory testing provides at best an approximate proxy of human exposure. In this context, it is interesting to remark that studies on metal biomarkers in urine and plasma [42–44] do not seem to indicate serious short term health risks for human vapers (who most likely inhaled vaping aerosol under normal conditions, as opposed to a machine generated aerosol).

Laboratory testing is very useful for developing quality control standards, product comparison and technological development, but its capacity to asses health risks is limited. At best, laboratory outcomes might provide a reasonable inference of potential health risks from users' inhalation of HPHCs as long as the experimental design is appropriate and puffing parameters (puff duration, puff volume, airflow) are roughly consistent with those of real life usage of the tested devices (information that can be gathered from consumer reports or manufacturer specifications).

Our section by section plan is as follows. Section 2 provides a description of real life vaping: vaping styles in Section 2.1 MTL and DTL vaping and habits of vapers in natural settings in Section 2.2, with reference values of various toxicological markers given in Section 2.3 presents. In Section 3, we examine the physical processes associated with EC aerosol generation and puffing parameters, while in Section 4, we revise the outcomes of the reviewed studies, offering a detailed discussion on their comparison with toxicological markers and a critique of their experimental methodology. In Section 5, we provide a comprehensive discussion on the findings of the previous section. A critique of risk communication in the reviewed literature is given in Section 6, while our conclusions are stated in Section 7. We also provide a supplementary file to explain the conversion of aerosol condensate concentrations into mass per puff values.

2. Realistic Usage Conditions and Toxicological Markers

2.1. Vaping Styles

The so called "Mouth to Lung" (MTL) vaping style is the most frequent one among vapers and currently remains typical of initiating users, most of them ex-smokers or current smokers. It involves mouth cavity retention followed by lung inhalation, a puffing mechanics roughly similar to that of cigarette smoking, thus being well suited for the design of early generation vaping devices (cigalikes, clearomizer models) and currently it is practiced in pods and tank models used as starter kits.

The "Direct to Lung" (DTL) style that avoids the mouth retention of MTL is typically practiced by more experimented and younger vapers. It involves a much deeper inhalation than MTL, which translates into more intense puffing parameters: airflow rates of 200 mL/s, puff volumes of 500 mL (or even more [15]), as well as longer puff times, resulting in much larger mass of inhaled aerosol. As opposed to the MTL style, DTL style bears no resemblance to tobacco cigarette puffing (as opposed to vapers, smokers tend to avoid a DTL style because tobacco smoke is a strong irritant [46]). Evidently, the heating element of vaping devices appropriate for this puffing regime must be able to deliver much higher power (combined with lower electric resistance) to generate the needed larger aerosol mass for a usage characterized by larger airflows for its inhalation. CORESTA and CORESTA-like puffing protocols are completely inappropriate and totally unrelated to consumer usage of sub-ohm devices intended for DTL vaping. Unfortunately, there is still no recognized standardized protocol to test devices intended for DTL usage.

2.2. Puffing Habits of Vapers in Natural Settings

In order to place laboratory studies in their proper context, it is important to examine the available information on the immense individual and circadian time variability of real life vaping. The best estimation of typical vaping behavior follows from observational studies of vapers under natural conditions carried on for extended periods (see review up to 2017 in [47]). Table 1 displays the main puffing parameters of 5 of such observational studies with information on daily puff numbers.

As shown in Table 1, the studies by Robinson et al. [48,49], Dautzenberg and Bricard [50] and Kosmider [51] report around 156–225 average daily puffs numbers for first and second generation devices, which are today obsolete or of marginal usage and whose nicotine delivery was much less efficient than that of more modern devices. In contrast, average daily puff numbers are in the range 272–338 in the more recent study by Dawkins et al. [52] involving more experienced vapers using modern devices (second and third generation) in which they can modify power settings and nicotine levels.

Table 1. Puffing topography under natural conditions. The table displays the main puffing parameters in 5 studies on vapers in natural conditions for extended periods. Numbers are averages with the symbol ± denoting standard deviation, the letters CL, 2G, 3G stand for closed, second generation (cartomizer) and third generation (tank) devices. In Dautzenberg and Bricard the symbols denote: single isolated puff (a), 2–5 clustered puffs (b), 5–15 clustered puffs (c) and more than 15 clustered puffs (d). In Dawkins et al.: low nicotine level fixed power (1), low nicotine level variable power (2), high nicotine level fixed power (3), high nicotine level variable power (4), with 6 mg/mL and 18 mg/mL for low and high nicotine level. Notice that puff numbers and e-liquid consumption increase with devices operating at fixed power and with low nicotine concentration.

	Robinson 2015 [48]	Robinson 2016 [49]	Kosmider 2018 [51]	Dautzenberg & Bricard 2015 [50]	Dawkins 2018 [52]
Device	CL	CL	2G	CL & 2G	60% 2G 40% 3G
Follow up	24 h	1 week	24 h	116 days	4 weeks
puffs/day	225 ± 59	162 ± 78 (14–275)	156.2 ± 95.3	163 ± 138 (1–1265)	(1) 338 ± 161 (2) 308 ± 135 (3) 279 ± 127 (4) 272 ± 128
puff duration (s)	3.5 ± 1.8 (0.7–6.9)	2.0 ± 0.6 (1–3)	3.0 ± 1.2	(a) 4.57 ± 2.24 (b) 4.07 ± 1.94 (c) 3.73 ± 1.77 (d) 3.20 ± 1.61	(1) 4.46 ± 1.22 (2) 3.81 ± 1.11 (3) 3.61 ± 0.97 (4) 3.91 ± 1.44
inter-puff interval (s)	47.7 ± 12.1 (10–150)		15.4 ± 22.0	(a) >60 (b) 19.26 ± 15.12 (c) 16.77 ± 13.23 (d) 13.68 ± 11.53	(1) 34.22 ± 20.08 (2) 39.32 ± 26.8 (3) 41.22 ± 26.23 (4) 37.32 ± 27.18

Table 1. Cont.

	Robinson 2015 [48]	Robinson 2016 [49]	Kosmider 2018 [51]	Dautzenberg & Bricard 2015 [50]	Dawkins 2018 [52]
puff volume (mL)	133 ± 90 (9–388)	65.4 ± 24.8 (24–114)	73.9 ± 51.5		
airflow (mL/s)	37 ± 16 (23–102)	30.4 ± 9.2 (19–60)	24.7 ± 10.2		
e-liquid per day (mL)					6.19 ± 3.74 4.63 ± 2.13 5.79 ± 3.63 4.79 ± 2.35

In the follow up study by Cox et al. [53] (see also [54]) larger daily puff numbers (308–338) and puff duration occurred when experienced vapers were asked to vape with fixed power settings and variable nicotine concentration. For the combination of low nicotine concentration and controllable power settings in third generation devices average daily puff numbers are around 272–279. As expected, inter-puff lapses under natural conditions listed in Table 1 are longer than those of laboratory studies.

Putting together the information described above and the data summarized in Table 1 and bearing in mind that both closed and open systems are currently in use, we believe that it is reasonable to assume 250 daily puffs as a rough but representative average value for real life daily vaping. In the following sections, we will use this value of 250 daily puffs to evaluate a daily inhaled dose of each metal element reported in laboratory studies in terms of various concentrations that will be converted to ng per puff.

2.3. Toxicological References

As mentioned in the introduction, laboratory testing does not reproduce real life vaping, but if puffing parameters used to generate the aerosol are appropriate for the tested devices, outcomes from laboratory testing can serve as valuable approximate proxies of human vaping to evaluate potential health risks in comparison with toxicological reference values. We consider the following three toxicological references:

- PDE-ICH: The International Council for Harmonization of Technical Requirements for Pharmaceuticals for Human Use (ICH [55]) provides the Permissible Daily Exposure (PDE) to inhalational medication, as a reference to manufacturing quality AFNOR-XP-D90-300 part 3 standard (page 15 of [56]). The ICH-PDE is endorsed by The US Department of Health and Human Services.
- ATSDR-MRL: The Minimal Risk Level (MRL) defined by the Agency for Toxic Substances Disease Registry (ATSDR) [57] as a safety limit for the general population of continuous daily environmental air concentrations (in $\mu g/m^3$) that can be of daily, intermediate (14 to 365 days) or chronic (over 365 days) duration.
- REL or PEL NIOSH-REL: Recommended Exposure Limits (REL) or Permissible Exposure Level (PEL) of the National Institute for Occupational Safety and Health (NIOSH) [58]. These are exposure limits that should be protective of worker lifetime safety to hazardous substances or conditions in the workplace.

Available values of these references for each metal element are listed in Table 2. We give priority to the PDE-ICH values, as these are strict protective and applicable to the general population, as well as already specified as a daily exposure referring explicitly to inhalation of medicines. While ECs are not medication, it is still useful to evaluate them under pharmaceutical standards. The ATSDR-MRL is also strict and applicable to the general population, given as a concentration defined to encompass safe continuous environmental exposure. The REL-NIOSH and PEL NIOSH specifically refer to workplace exposure in terms of time weighed averages (TWA) working shift in 40 h weekly journeys. For metals without PDE-ICH we consider the MRL-ATSDR evaluated for a volume of 20 m^3 of inhaled air of average adults engaged in moderated activity. If there is no PDE-ICH nor MRL-ATSDR, we will use the PEL-NIOSH for a volume of $20/3 = 6.67$ m^3 of inhaled air during an 8 h work journey of average adults engaged in moderated activity.

Table 2. Toxicological References. The table displays the minimal recommended values to avoid noticeable harm. The daily values for the MRL-ATSDR and REL-NIOSH are, respectively, computed for 24 and 8 h. The asterisks denote short term exposures (* daily, ** 15 days) and chronic exposure *** (more than 360 days).

Metal	PDE ICH µg/day	ATSDR MRL µg/m^3	Daily Value µg	NIOSH REL mg/m^3	Daily Value mg
Aluminum (Al)				5	33.3
Arsenic (As)	2				
Cadmium (Cd)	3	0.03 *	0.6	0.005	0.03
Chromium (Cr)	3			0.5	3.3
Cobalt (Co)	3	0.1	2.0		
Copper (Cu)	30			1.0	6.7
Iron (Fe)				5.0	33.3
Manganese (Mn)		0.3 ***	6.0	1.0	6.7
Nickel (Ni)	6	0.2 ** / 0.09 ***	4.0 / 1.8	0.015	0.1
Lead (Pb)	5			0.03	0.2
Antimony (Sb)	20	1.0	20		
Silicon (Si)				5.0	33.3
Tin (Sn)	60	300 *	6000	2.0	13.3
Zinc (Zn)				5.0	33.3

For the comparison of toxicological references in Table 2 with detected metal content in laboratory studies we evaluate a potential daily exposure in µg by multiplying the ng/puff = 0.001 µg/puff values in Tables 4, 5, 8, 10 and 11 times 250 daily puffs for average vapers that arise from studies of vaping patterns in natural settings discussed in Section 2.2 (for the REL-NIOSH we assume 83 puffs, one third of 250 daily puffs).

3. Optimal Regime, Power Ranges and Airflows

Efficient operation of ECs requires specific ranges of supplied power, temperature, coil resistance, inhalation airflow and puff volume. In particular, an optimal performance requires an appropriate airflow to efficiently generate an aerosol by condensation of the vapor generated by the supplied power. As mentioned in the introduction, all revised laboratory studies that looked at metal content in the aerosol generated by high powered sub-ohm devices [10–13,16,18,19] failed to fulfill this basic efficiency condition by testing the devices under inappropriate puffing protocols, specially low airflows and puff volumes (which also lead to enhanced production of carbonyls [36]). We discuss below the physical principles behind this issue.

ECs use as a heating element a wire or a mesh to heat and vaporise an e-liquid. They function between two typical powers: minimal and maximal, representing physical limits between three functioning regimes that are characterized at a first level using the Mass of E-liquid Vaporised (MEV) or e-liquid consumption expressed in mg by puff [31]. Below the minimal power no e-liquid is vaporized (MEV = 0) and no aerosol is generated (under-heating Regime). Between the two powers, MEV increases linearly with respect to the supplied power. This linearity denotes an optimal regime energetically efficient process of vaporisation under almost thermodynamic equilibrium conditions (this linearity followed by a non-linear behavior at higher power can be observed in Figure 4 of Floyd et al. [33]).

It is well known [32,59] that airflow rate [40,60,61] and e-liquid composition influence the power limits that define the optimal regime. A pure propylene glycol (PG) liquid has closer limits than a pure glycerol (VG) one. Adding a low concentration of ethanol and/or water in an e-liquid with a fixed PG/VG ratio slightly modifies the values. Then, testing the devices at a high airflow rate increases the power range between minimal and maximal values that define the optimal regime. This experimental observation is specially important for high powered sub-ohm devices used for DTL vaping, as testing these devices at a low airflow significantly reduces the power range of the optimal regime, with the overheating regime appearing at lower wattage.

Besides its influence in setting up the functionality limits of the optimal regime, airflow rate is the basic cooling process (through forced convection) during aerosol formation. The mixture of a hot and a cold gas is a fast process during which an important energy transfer occurs between air and vapor until they reach an equilibrium. This mixture leads to the formation of a "particle" phase in the form of liquid droplets whose composition is very close to that of the e-liquid. In fact, the higher is the airflow compared to the vaporized flow, the lower is the temperature of the mixture. This is supported by empiric evidence: for fixed power an increase of airflow tends to decrease coil temperatures and total particulate mass [60,61] and (at least) keeps the production of toxic byproducts (carbonyls) stable [40].

The right airflow depends on the supplied power. Since powerful devices vaporize a large amount of e-liquid, a large airflow is needed for the cooling through forced convection of the vapor to facilitate aerosol generation by condensation. A small airflow operating a powerful device will not carry on cooling through forced convection efficiently, leaving the atomizer full of hot vapor. In laboratory experiments characterized by a regimented repetition of puffs, the atomizer keeps accumulating heat even without e-liquid depletion (dry hit), increasing the temperature of the whole device (by conduction). While the vaping machines can continue operating, a human user would find first a very hot aerosol to inhale and later a device too hot to handle and most likely a repellent taste. In either case, testing a device under these conditions is completely unrealistic and misleading.

Once supplied power exceeds the maximal value of the optimal regime the relation MEV vs power becomes non-linear, marking the outset of an overheating regime characterized by different physical conditions under which the devices operate. This was discussed in a recent publication [62], suggesting that boiling processes are dominant in the optimal regime, with maximal power linked to critical heat flux. Following this assumption, boiling in an optimal regime would be through bubbles formed on the wire (nucleate boiling) whereas in overheating conditions, the wire would be surrounded by a film of gas, with vaporization taking place on the liquid–gas interface. Their results illustrate that under an overheating regime above maximal power, wire temperature increases significantly and carbonyls (specially formaldehyde) are produced in higher quantities, whereas in the optimal regime relatively small (even negligible) quantities of aldehydes are produced. This is consistent with the known relation between supplied power and carbonyl production [34–36,39,40].

Production of high levels of HPHCs (including metals) in the aerosol emissions from sub-ohm high powered devices might occur even at relatively low power when these devices are laboratory tested with a low intensity airflow (such as CORESTA or CORESTA-like protocols). This should be connected to the fact that the power threshold marking the outset of the overheating regime is lower when tested under such airflows in comparison with testing them with an intense protocol that fits the DTL parameters [32,59]. This suggests that a wider power range of the optimal regime in real life usage for DTL vaping should produce lesser levels of HPHCs.

Finally, it is important to mention that, regarding the puffing parameters, a regimented puffing regime can produce by itself a gradual temperature increase in the various components of the devices, even if the applied airflow is consistent with the device characteristics and the vaping machines keep the testing under the optimal regime. This temperature increase has been experimentally tested at the mouthpiece [38] and at the coil [37] (by thermography). While temperature increases reported by these references might not be accurate, this increase is plausible because the inter-puff time might not be sufficiently long to allow for the device temperature to decay to its initial value after each puff in frequent puffing testing, and thus as frequent puffs accumulate (with same supplied power) the devices can become too hot to handle for human vapers (or could have a repellent taste for them), but puffing machines operate normally.

4. Laboratory Studies: Outcomes, Toxicological Evaluation and Methodological Critique

We review, in this section, 12 articles published after 2017 [10–21] and listed in Table 3. For further discussion and comments see Section 5. There is in this literature a significant variation in aerosol collecting techniques, with Inductively Coupled Plasma Mass Spectroscopy (ICP-MS)) the preferred analytic technique (see descriptive review in [9]).

Table 3. Laboratory studies on metal content in aerosol emissions published after 2017. The puffing parameters appear in this order: puff duration, inter-puff interval, puff volume, airflow rate. All studies have used puffing flow rates and volumes similar to the CORESTA 81 protocol. Aerosol collection (see Section 5.6) and analytic techniques are summarized in the text. We do not consider studies before 2017 because they involve devices that are either obsolete or of marginal usage.

Study	Device and Properties	Puffing Parameters	Analytic Technique
	Third Generation Tank Models		
Zhao et al., 2019 & 2022 [11,12]	Smok, 6–220 W, 0.6 Ω Istick, 0–85 W, 0.2 Ω	4 s, 26 s, 66 mL, 16.67 mL/s 15–120 puffs 15–120 puffs	ICP-MS
Kapiamba et al., 2022 [16]	Voopoo, 5–60 W Unspecified resistance	2 s, 60 s, 35 mL, 16.67 mL/s 30 puffs	ICP-MS
Liu et al., 2020 [13]	Unspecified 3rd Generation Tank Model	4 s, 30 s, 66 mL, 16.67 mL/s Unspecified puff number	ICP-MS Arsenic Species
Williams et al., 2019 [18]	Smok Alien, sub-ohm iPV6X, Tsunami 2.4 RDA + Nemesis Clone RDA	4.3 s, 60 s, 30.1 mL, 7 mL/s 60 puffs	ICP-OES
Olmedo et al., 2018 [10]	56 assorted tank devices	4 s, 30 s, 66 mL, 16.67 mL/s 30–50 puffs	ICP-MS
Halstead et al., 2019 [14]	Joyetech eGO 2016 Model	3 s, 30 s, 55 mL, 16.67 mL/s 50 puffs	ICP-MS
Kim et al., 2018 [19]	Aspire Cleito, 0.2 Ω Kanthal coil, cotton wick	4 s, 18 s, 50 mL, ~20 mL/s 150 puffs	GC-MS
	Pods		
Kapiamba et al., 2022 [16]	Vapor4Life	2 s, 60 s, 35 mL, 16.67 mL/s 30 puffs	ICP-MS
	Juul	2 s, 60 s, 35 mL, 16.67 mL/s 30 puffs	ICP-MS
Chen et al., 2021 [17]	Juul (not intense)	4 s, 30 s, 55/70 mL, 16.67 mL/s 3 blocks of 100 puffs	ICP-MS
	Juul (intense)	6, 30 s, 110 mL, not specified 3 blocks of 100 puffs	ICP-MS
Zhao et al., 2019 & 2022 [11,12]	myblu	4 s, 11 s, 66 mL, 16.67 mL/s 50–100 puffs	ICP-MS
	Juul	4 s, 11 s, 66 mL, 16.67 mL/s 290–330 puffs	ICP-MS

Table 3. Cont.

Study	Device and Properties	Puffing Parameters	Analytic Technique
Grey et al., 2020 [15]	Juul myblu Vuse Alto	3 s, 30 s, 55 mL, 16.67 mL/s 50 puffs	ICP-MS
Halstead et al., 2019 [14]	Juul Blu Vuse Obsolete disposables	3 s, 30 s, 55 mL, 16.67 mL/s 75 puffs	ICP-MS
Second Generation			
Beauval et al., 2017 [20]	Lounge	3 s, 30 s, 55 mL, 16.67 mL/s 96 puffs	various techniques
Palazzolo et al., 2017 [21]	eGO	5 s, 10 s, 6.67 mL/s 45 puffs	Scanned microscopy
Williams et al., 2019 [18]	EgoC Twist Protank EgoX Twist Nautilus iTaste MVP Kanger	4.3 s, 60 s, 17–81 mL, 4–19 mL/s 60 puffs: continuous & 10 min clusters	ICP-OES ICP-OES ICP-OES

As mentioned in the introduction, a common feature is aerosol generated by puffing parameters based on the CORESTA Recommended Method 81 [27] or with parameters that approach it (CORESTA-like). Typically laboratory studies assume puff duration 3–4 s, inter-puff lapse 30–60 s, flow rate below 20 mL/s (1 L/min) and puff volume below 70 mL.

4.1. The Olmedo-Zhao Group

A group of researchers, originally from the Johns Hopkins School of Public Health, have published since their first article in 2016 [63] a series of articles on metal content associated with ECs, in e-liquids [42,64], on biomarkers in urine and serum samples of vapers [44] and on non-metallic contents in emissions from high powered devices [65]. The study by Olmedo et al. [10] in 2018 was continued by two more studies in collaboration with Zhao in 2019 and 2022: [11,12] and a review [9]. We examine below these studies.

The experimental method of the three papers [10–12] is specified in the 2016 article [63] with slight modifications: aerosol is generated by puffing e-cigarettes by a peristaltic pump, collection is done by direct condensation into a system of pipettes and tubes into a glass flask. The analytical technique is ICP-MS and the puffing parameters are listed in Table 3. The same experimental methodology was followed in more recent papers [13,65]. Since in the three studies [10–12] aerosol analysis by ICP-MS is performed on a liquid sample diluted from a condensed liquid aerosol of specified volume range in mL, it is straightforward to transform the interquartile values of µg/kg = ng/g concentrations into a range of ng/puff values listed in Tables 4 and 5 (tank models) and 8 (pods), obtained from estimating of the mass of vaporized aerosol from the collected and retained aerosol and from the puff numbers needed to obtain the condensed aerosol under their puffing protocol (see details in our supplementary file). Comparison with toxicological reference markers is displayed in Tables 4, 6 and 9.

Table 4. First rows are outcomes of metal elements reported by Olmedo et al. [10] given as ng/puff values converted from their µg/kg concentrations (see supplementary file). The second rows are daily exposures form 250 daily puffs and third rows are toxicological reference markers from Table 2. Minimal values in the range of $O \sim 10^{-3}$ µg are not displayed.

Metal	Al	Cd	Cr	Cu	Fe	Mn
ng/puff	0.07–0.52	<0.01	0.002–1.02	0.03–1.19	0.002–1.65	0.001–5.5
daily exp. (µg)	0.0175–0.13	<0.0025	<0.255	0.0075–0.298	<0.4125	<1.375
Tox. Ref. (µg)	33,300 NIOSH	3 PDE	3 PDE	30 PDE	33,300 NIOSH	6 ATSDR
Metal	Ni	Pb	Sb	Sn	Zn	
ng/puff	0.03–6.74	0.02–0.86	<0.45	0.01–0.45	1.28–18.88	
daily exp. (µg)	0.0075–1.685	<0.215	<0.1125	<0.1125	0.32–4.72	
Tox. Ref (µg)	6 PDE	5 PDE	20 PDE	60 PDE	33,300 NIOSH	

Table 5. Range of mass (in ng) per puff of each metal element for the sub-ohm tank devices OD1 and OD2 tested by Zhao et al. in their 2019 study [11] at three power levels (the numbers are rounded up to two decimals). These values were computed from the range of concentrations in µg/kg = ng/g reported in Table 2 of Zhao et al. and the information provided by Zhao et al. on aerosol collection (see Supplemental file).

M	OD1 20 W	OD1 40 W	OD1 80 W	OD2 40 W	OD2 120 W	OD2 200 W
Al	0.02–0.04	0.04–0.14	0.09–0.61	0.04–0.14	0.10–0.42	0.2–2.50
As	$<10^{-3}$	0.01–0.04	0.02–0.10	0.005–0.01	0.006–0.045	0.05–0.58
Cd	$<10^{-3}$	0.0003–0.03	0.004–0.028	$<10^{-2}$	$<10^{-2}$	0.02–0.14
Cr	$<10^{-3}$	0.01–0.06	0.04–0.18	0.001–0.24	0.14–0.80	0.006–3.06
Cu	0.02–0.51	0.32–5.64	3.72–13.84	2.85–12.51	4.21–22.27	18.14–184.01
Fe	0.015–0.03	0.45–2.43	0.07–1.96	0.01–5.45	1.31–2.99	0.09–20.77
Mn	0.0002–0.03	0.11–0.27	0.36–2.11	0.02–0.65	0.53–2.00	0.13–6.94
Ni	0.02–1.55	4.27–13.69	3.94–34.64	2.95–18.20	0.29–56.95	12.93–147.17
Pb	0.01–0.27	0.59–1.61	7.91–39.31	1.41–28.99	4.62–14.09	11.06–198.80
Sb	$<10^{-2}$	0.02–0.15	0.03–0.20	0.01–0.22	0.02–0.08	0.11–1.08
Sn	0.002–0.054	1.85–7.01	0.32–2.16	0.11–1.92	0.22–0.73	0.55–11.37
Zn	1.06–4.79	15.28–48.04	87.07–344.87	6.99–145.86	8.89–26.61	53.48–1510.26

Table 6. Comparison of daily exposure of those metals from sub-ohm devices tested by the 2019 article Zhao et al. [11] whose daily exposure (in µg) surpass toxicological reference values (displayed in red). The meaning of PDE and REL is explained in Table 2 and in the text of this section. Daily exposures for the remaining metals are below available toxicological reference, including zinc and iron whose contents are large. We assumed 250 as the average number of daily puffs for typical vapers to evaluate daily exposure to potential users.

Device	Cu	Mn	Ni	Pb
OD1 20	0.005–0.12	$<10^{-2}$	0.005–0.39	0.002–0.07
OD1 40	0.08–1.41	0.027–0.067	1.07–3.44	0.15–0.40
OD2 40	0.71–3.12	0.005–0.16	0.737–4.55	0.35–7.24
OD1 80	0.93–3.46	0.09–0.52	0.985–8.66	1.98–9.83
OD2 120	1.05–5.57	0.13–0.50	0.07–14.24	1.15–3.52
OD2 200	4.53–46.0	0.03–1.73	3.23–36.79	2.76–49.7
Reference	30 (PDE)	0.3 (MRL)	6 (PDE)	5 (PDE)

4.1.1. Olmedo et al. [10]

Emissions. The authors tested 56 devices and their e-liquids collected from recruited vapers for analysis. Besides studying metal contents in aerosol emissions, they provide valuable results by comparing metal content in e-liquids in dispensers and in tanks, before and after aerosol generation. Outcomes of metal elements in units µg/kg = ng/g were obtained in terms of self reported usage classification: voltage ranges (<4.02, 4.02–4.2, >4.2 V), coil alloy (kanthal and stainless steel and frequency of coil replacement). Since the information contained in these classifications is too vague (given the lack of data on individual devices), the most useful values of metal element content in aerosol emission is given in their third interquartile values listed in their Table 2 (middle column, second number in parentheses). With the information provided on their experimental procedures we transform their µg/kg = ng/g concentrations values into a range of values in ng/puff for each metal (see details in the supplementary file). The outcomes for each metal are listed in Table 4.

The authors also provide at the end of their discussion section (for comparison with tobacco cigarettes assuming a smoked cigarette to be equivalent to 15 puffs) a median and a range of values based on their average puff volumes of ng per 15 puffs for six important metals (As, Cr, Mn, Ni. Pb, and Zn) in the emissions of the tested devices. Dividing by 15 the values they provide yields in ng/puff the following ranges and median values: <0.067 (0.01), As; <2.0 (0.0057), Cr; <0.093 (0.0013), Mn; <7.33 (0.029), Ni; <1.8 (0.007), Pb; <4.4 (0.299), and Zn. Save for Zn, these ranges are of roughly the same magnitude as the values we estimated in Table 4, but we will not consider them any further as there is no information on which specific tests these values were taken.

Toxicological evaluation. Olmedo et al. [10] claimed that 50% or more of the samples for Cr, Mn, Ni, and Pb exceeded toxicological reference values. However, as shown by Farsalinos and Rodu [66], they miscalculated in their Equation (1) the daily intake of these metals, as their conversion of µg/kg concentrations from chemical analysis into air density concentrations in mg/m^3 (for comparison with the environmental ATSDR reference value) is mistaken (see our Section 5.4). They assume for their experimental airflow $Q = 1$ L/min and $t = 4$ s puff duration that for each puff the collected aerosol would dilute in an air volume $V_{air} = Q \times t = 66.67$ mL, which is their experimental puff volume. Their estimations representing overexposures by at least a factor 12, since in real life usage the aerosol dilutes in a tidal volume of about 800 mL (assuming MTL vaping), about 30% larger than the rest tidal volume of ~500 mL (this is because the lungs require extra volume to generate suction [45]) However, as we explain in Section 5.4, it is necessary to bear in mind that vaping represents an intermittent exposure, thus special care to incorporate exposure times must be exerted when comparing inhaled concentrations in users (from aerosol condensate concentrations) with time weighed toxicological markers (such as ATSDR or NIOSH). We find it more useful to compute the total dose for each metal per puff. We estimated (see supplementary file) an absolute range for these doses displayed in Table 4 given the uncertainty in the puff numbers needed (30–50) to collect a volume of aerosol (0.2–0.5 mL).

As shown in Table 4, none of metal elements examined by the authors of [10] produce a daily exposure that surpass the toxicological reference values. The metal that most approaches these values in Table 2 is nickel (a fraction about $1.685/6 \approx 1/3.5 \approx 28\%$ of the reference value). For nickel to reach the PDE of daily intake of 6 μg a vaper would have to do 875 daily puffs. While some vapers might do this amount of daily puffs, demographic evidence displayed in Table 1 shows that such puffing frequency is an extreme outlier. It might be argued that the MRL-ATSDR values in Table 2 for nickel should be used because they are more strict than the PDE. In this case, assuming 20 m^3 of daily inhaled air by average adults we have: 4 μg for the intermediate MRL (14–365 days of exposure) and 1.8 μg for the chronic MRL (over 365 days of exposure). However, the daily exposure of 1.685 μg, computed for 250 daily puffs, is still below these strict thresholds, though the intermediate one is more realistic, as the the chronic one is a valid comparative reference only if one assumes a daily exposure to vaping that lasts at least a full year, which would indicate an abnormally and extremely intensive form of vaping.

Methodological critique. The authors did not provide complete information and characteristics of the individual 56 devices that were analyzed: coil resistance, power settings and PG/VG mixtures in e-liquids constitute important information to assess their results. The authors examined metal outcomes in terms of three self declared voltage categories: <4.02, 4.02–4.2, >4.2 V. However, the lack of information on coil resistance and power makes it impossible to determine if the tested devices were sub-ohm or operated for resistances >1 Ω. This is important information (see discussion in [30]) because the puffing protocol used in this laboratory study is inappropriate for sub-ohm devices used for DTL vaping that requires much larger airflows and puff volumes. Some of the missing information was supplied by Zhao et al. [11] who explicitly mention that 18% of the devices tested by the authors were the same sub-ohm devices they tested. This information is useful to interpret their statistical data: looking at aerosol emissions in the middle column of their Table 2 and the low wattage values (<4.2 Volts) in their Table 5 reveals a skewed distribution with a large interquartile dispersion and medians much closer to the lowest bound (first interquartile) than to the upper bound (third interquartile). This skewed distribution suggests that the possible 18% minority of tested sub-ohm devices produced unrepresentative ranges in the third quartiles, hiding the likely fact that for most of the devices the concentrations were closer to the lower bound given by the first interquartile.

4.1.2. Zhao et al., 2019 and 2022 (Sub-Ohm Devices)

Emissions. Zhao et al. [11] published a study in 2019 following the same aerosol collection technique as Olmedo et al. [10] (with slight modifications), testing two sub-ohm devices of recent manufacture: OD1: Istick 25 (Eleaf Electronics) with power range 0–85 W and OD2: Smok (Smoktech) with power range 6–220 W, both with sub-ohm coil resistances. These devices were tested at three power settings: 20, 40, 80 W for OD1 and 40, 120, 200 W for OD2.

The authors published a paper in 2022 [12] to examine the effects on metal element content in aerosol emissions from varying flavorings (fruity, tobacco and menthol), nicotine concentrations (0, 6 and 24 mg/mL) and puff duration (2 s, 4 s and 6 s), utilizing exactly the same devices and aerosol collection technique as the 2019 paper, with fixed power for each tank device: 40 W for OD1 and 120 W for OD2. However, their reported outcomes lump together OD1 and OD2 in a single category "OD".

Since the 2019 paper of Zhao et al. [11] followed the same experimental methodology and used same units as Olmedo et al. [10], we proceed as we did with the data supplied by the latter authors (see a detailed account of this conversion of units in the supplementary file). The range of ng/puff values we obtained for the sub-ohm devices tested by Zhao et al. in the 2019 study [11] appear in Table 5. We did not convert the metal elements in μg/kg = ng/g concentrations from their 2022 article [12] into ranges of ng/puff, since they did not provide in that study concentrations for individual devices, presenting only statistical data on concentrations corresponding to the various flavorings, nicotine concentrations and puff duration values lumping together the outcomes the devices OD1 and OD2 in the same category "OD". However, their reported μg/kg = ng/g concentrations are qualitatively similar to those of their 2019 paper.

Toxicological evaluation. From the ng/puff values in Table 5 and considering an average of 250 daily puffs, we obtain daily exposure values for the open tank devices OD1 and OD2 for all metals and power ranges examined by Zhao et al. in their 2019 paper [11]. These daily exposure values only become comparable (or surpass) toxicological reference values listed in Table 2 for Cr, Cu, Mn, Ni and Pb and only in the highest power ranges of the devices. Daily exposure values for these metals and a comparative toxicological reference are listed in Table 6. For the pod devices CD1 (myblu) and CD2 (Juul), daily exposures are orders of magnitude below these references (see Table 8).

Zhao et al. [11] obtained from their Equation (1) and their μg/kg aerosol concentrations the following values for daily average exposure: 0.62 μg (Mn) and 0.14 μg (Ni), placed in their Table 4, but it is not clear how these values were obtained from their Equation (1), though they mention having followed the same exposure computation as Olmedo et al. [10], which (as we argued in Section 4.1.1) was shown to be incorrect by Farsalinos and Rodu [66] and might be conceptually problematic (see Section 5.4).

The values displayed in red in Table 6 correspond to daily exposure values of four metals (Cu, Mn, Ni, Pb) that surpass toxicological references by both devices in the high end of the power range of tests (80 to 200 W). Notice that for the device OD2 (SMOK) at its highest tested power (200 W), toxicological references are surpassed by 2 orders of magnitude in these metals. For the remaining metals daily exposure is at least an order of magnitude below toxicological references, even for iron and zinc which produced abundant content (but their available reference, the REL of NIOSH, is 1–2 orders of magnitude above). We do not offer a toxicological comparison of the outcomes of their 2022 paper because they lumped together data from both devices (OD1 and OD2).

Methodological critique. The 2019 study by Zhao et al. [11] is valuable for showing that all metal contents sharply increase with increasing supplied power (beyond manufacturers recommendations) while keeping the puffing parameters fixed but varying puff numbers. However, the authors' assessment of health risks to end users by comparison with toxicological references is questionable. As we argue in Section 3, the excessively high outcomes reported by Zhao et al. [11] of Cu, Mn, Ni and Pb in their higher power settings (Table 5), with daily exposures surpassing toxicological references (Table 6), are linked to their testing of powerful sub-ohm devices (operating up to 200 W) by means of CORESTA-like puffing parameters (see Table 3) that fail short of the much larger values of the real life usage of these devices for DTL vaping (which is also the usage recommended by the manufacturers, in particular the manufacturer recommended power ranges of the OD2 device are between 20–50 W with best performance in the range 30–40 W [67]) (see Methodological critique in Section 4.7). Although lower power settings at 20–40 W of the sub-ohm devices are within the manufacturers recommended values and metal levels were below toxicological markers, the testing with inappropriate airflow and puff volumes render these outcomes unrealistic and likely overestimations with respect to real life usage.

The experimental design of Zhao et al. [11] required a large number of consecutive regimented puffs (120) to collect sufficient aerosol for the condensed 0.3–0.6 mL sample to be analyzed. Since the temperature of the heating element does not decay between puff to puff to the initial value, this long sequence of regimented puffs can easily produce a gradual heating of the atomizer to temperatures that gradually become too uncomfortable for the user to handle the device (besides the fact that users do not puff 120 regimented puffs every 30 s). This gradual temperature rise is a likely explanation of the large difference between the first and third quartiles in the concentrations C_i for both sub-ohm devices in their lowest power settings (extreme left column in Table 2 of Zhao et al.): for example for nickel at 20 W in the Istik device there is a large interquartile range $(C_{Ni}^{(1)}, C_{Ni}^{(3)}) = (5.89 - 222)$ ng/g, with median value $\bar{C}_{Ni} = 8.0$ ng/g, thus indicating a likely distribution of tests results clustered around the median value with large outlier values possibly at later puffs already with the device possibly too hot for a user to handle. The same phenomenon occurs for the Smok device at 40 W.

4.2. Zhao et al. (Pod Devices)

Zhao et al. also tested in their 2019 and 2022 papers [11,12] two pod "closed" devices: myblu (Imperial Brands) and Juul (Juul Labs), respectively, denoted CD1 and CD2, at their fixed power settings (the authors only identified CD1 as "BLU" but reading between lines it is evident that the device is a myblu). Separate outcomes for each one of the two devices were given only in [11], with both devices lumped together as "CD" in [12]. As we did with sub-ohm devices, we converted the µg/kg = ng/g interquartile concentrations they reported in Table 3 of their 2019 paper [11] for Cr, Cu, Ni, Pb, Sn, Zn into the ranges of ng/puff displayed in Table S8 (see the supplementary file). Considering the average of 250 daily puffs, the daily exposure for these two devices is 1–2 orders of magnitude below their corresponding reference toxicological marker, even for the relatively high concentrations values of Al and Cu.

It is interesting to consider nickel as an example. From the interquartile values in Table 3 of Zhao et al. we have the following ranges, for the myblu device $C_{Ni} = 1.32\,(0.39, 3.35)$ ng/g and for the Juul $C_{Ni} = 11.9\,(10.7, 22.7)$. From these values, we obtain from Equations (3a) and (3b) of the supplementary file a nickel mass range of $M_{Ni} = 0.0016 - 0.056$ ng/puff for the myblu, while for the Juul we have $M_{Ni} = 0.014 - 0.066$ ng/puff. The range of daily nickel exposure (250 daily puffs) is then 0.0005–0.016 µg for the myblu and 0.0042–0.02 µg for the Juul, both ranges 2–4 orders of magnitude below the PDE of 6 µg for nickel. Notice that for the Juul device collecting the 0.3–0.6 mL of condensed aerosol sample required many puffs (290–330) taken at short inter-puff periods of 11 s. It is evident that even this small daily metal mass is likely an overestimation considering that such intense puffing regime is completely divorced from normal usage of this device.

In their 2022 study [12], Zhao et al. examined the effect of nicotine concentration and flavors on metal contents in emissions, but they report a joint outcome for CD1 and CD2 in a single category "CD". This is problematic because each individual closed pod (besides operating at different powers) utilizes different type of nicotine in different concentrations: salts formed with benzoic acid (Juul, 59 mg/mL) and base (myblu, 24 mg/mL). Nicotine chemistry plays a role in the phase partition of the aerosol [68], with the less volatile protonated acidic nicotine (salts) tending to concentrate in the particulate phase and unprotonated (base) evaporating into the gas phase. While the implication of nicotine differences on metal content is not known, conflating both types of nicotine into a single statistic does not seem to be a correct approach.

4.3. Chen et al.

Chen et al. [17] conducted a comprehensive targeted study of chemicals in the emissions of the four Juul devices available in the US market in 2021: nicotine concentrations of 35 and 59 mg/mL in two favors: Virginia Tobacco (VT) and Menthol (Me), thus making four product combinations: VT5, VT3, Me5, Me3. The targeted analytes were divided in two groups (I and II) based on FDA USA guidance for vaping devices in its Pre Market

Tobacco Authorization (PMTA) process. Each group was tested with different analytic methods, all validated according to ICH guidelines and standard ISO protocols. Depending on the analytic method aerosol collection method was by an impinger containing a trapping solvent or (for heavy metals) a glass fiber pad. Aerosol was collected for two puffing intensity regimes: "non-intense" (NI) with puff duration and inter-puff interval of 3 and 30 s, respectively, puff volumes 55 and 70 mL for group I and II, and "intense" (Int) with 6 s puff duration (the maximum allowed by Juul) and 110 mL puff volumes (other parameters unchanged).

Most of the analytes were below the limit of detection (BLOD) or below limit of quantification (BLOQ), though a thorough background subtraction was carried air blank measurements, with measurements for some analytes deemed not different from blank (NDFB) values. Six metals were targeted: Cd, Cr, Cu, Ni, Pb (group I) and Au (group II), with the numerical mass outcomes normalized with nicotine given for VT5 and Me5 in their Table 2 (quantifiable analytes) and averaging for the beginning, middle and end sequential puffing blocks we obtain the mass of these metals in ng per puff. These values are listed in Table 7.

Table 7. Mass in ng per puff for Juul devices tested by Chen et al. [17], for 50 mg/mL nicotine concentration and Menthol and Virginia Tobacco flavors (Me5, VT5) and non-intense and intense regime (NI, Int). NDFB stands for Not Different From Blank.

			Me5			
Metal	Au	Cd	Cr	Cu	Ni	Pb
NI	0.0123	0.009	NDFB	0.015	0.798	0.004
Int	0.022	0.08	NDFB	0.019	0.827	0.005
			VT5			
Metal	Au	Cd	Cr	Cu	Ni	Pb
NI	0.0126	0.008	NDFB	0.245	0.698	0.036
Int	0.0156	0.005	NDFB	0.067	0.108	0.045

As the authors comment, mass outcomes of these six metals are negligible and below BLOQ: Cd and Au were BLOD, chromium was NDFB and copper, nickel, and lead were alternately BLOD or BLOQ for all flavors, nicotine concentrations and puff blocks.

4.4. Liu et al.

The study by Liu et al. [13] specifically targeted arsenic species in e-liquids and in EC aerosol. The tested devices are not properly identified, only referred to as "*rechargeable USB-like devices ... chosen based on their high market shares*" and "*tank type devices from two popular stores in Toronto, Canada*". Aerosol collection resulted in 0.2–1 mL of aerosol condensate and 89–100% recovery, following the methods of the first 2016 paper by Olmedo et al. [63], with a button mechanism to activate the tank devices. The puffing topography was allegedly taken from [69] but the parameters do not correspond to that reference, but to the puffing parameters of the 2018 paper of Olmedo et al. [10]: 4 s and 30 s for puff duration and inter-puf interval, with airflow 1 L/min = 16.66 mL/s, using 40 puffs. The resulting arsenic species aerosol condensate concentrations in μg/kg are summarized in their Table 2.

Besides the lack of information on the devices and their characteristics and the problematic usage of a CORESTA-like puffing protocol for a sub-ohm tank device, Liu et al [13] also incurred in the same miscalculation of Olmedo et al. [10] on the "air concentrations" in mg/m^3 to compare in their Section 2.3 with the occupational toxicological NIOSH marker (equivalent to the PEL OSHA) for arsenic and inorganic arsenic species in an 8 h work journey. As we comment in Section 4.1.1, Olmedo et al. [10] overestimated exposures by a factor of at least 12 (inhaled aerosol dilutes in a tidal volume of 800 mL for MTL vaping [45]), but also comparisons with time weighted toxicological references need to be carefully examined (see Section 5.4). However, even with this overestimation the detected concentrations found by Liu et al. [13] are below the PEL OSHA (same as NIOSH) of 10 µg/m^3. Assuming a user vaping with MTL style with tidal volume of 800 mL and correcting the overestimation by a factor of 12, the maximal reported value of arsenic concentration mentioned in [13] (4 µg/m^3) becomes ~0.33 µg/m^3, which is much smaller than the PEL NIOSH. This low value for arsenic species in EC aerosol is consistent with the fact that no other study looking at arsenic has found significant presence of this metal in aerosol emissions (for example, see for comparison ng/puff values in Table 5). As a consequence, the estimated cancer risk form arsenic inhalation evaluated in Section 2.4 of Liu et al. [13] is questionable.

4.5. Kapiamba et al.

The study by Kapiamba et al. published in 2022 [16] tested three devices, two low powered pod systems: a Juul (Juul Labs) and a Vapor4Life (XL pen EC, AUTO VAPOR ZEUS KIT, Vapor4Life Inc. Northbrook, IL, USA, ended sales in July 2021) and tank system VOOPOO (Drag X, Shenzhen Woody Vapes Technology Co., Shenzhen, China), all purchased in 2019. They do not use the standard CORESTA protocol, but the standard puff profile for tobacco cigarette aerosol measurements (ISO 3308:2000): 30 puffs with 2 s duration, 60 s inter-puff interval, 35 mL puff volumes and 1.05 lT/min = 16.67 mL/s. Aerosol collection through teflon filters and unspecified tubing. They conduct separate tests on aerosol metal contents to examine seven "tasks" (see Table 1 of [16]): (1) differences between devices, (2) flavors, (3) nicotine concentrations, (4) device power, (5) puff duration, (6) aging, as well as (7) environmental emissions through a respiratory model.

The article reveals a problematic lack of key information to understand its outcomes and several inconsistencies, for example:

- All devices were acquired in 2019, at least 2 years before the experiments and were possibly subjected to corrosion or leaching of metal alloys. The authors provide no information on their storage conditions.
- Their Table 1 states that zero nicotine and no flavor were assumed in tasks (1), (5) and (6), but these tasks involve a Juul and a Vapor4Life, devices that lack a zero nicotine option and are not flavorless (by "flavorless" we understand an e-liquid containing only solvents and possibly nicotine). It seems that the voopoo was tested with such an e-liquid, but the authors provide no information on the e-liquids used in its testing this tank device and the Vapor4Life.
- The authors provide in the abstract the following outcomes on ng per 10 puffs for chromium and nickel

	Juul	Voopoo	Vapor4Life
Cr	117 ± 54	124 ± 77	33 ± 10
Ni	50 ± 24	219 ± 203	27 ± 2

which do not appear in the remaining of the article and there is no description in the abstract or in the body of the article on how they were obtained.
- In their Section 3, dealing with task (1), the only one involving the three devices, the authors report the following average ng per 10 puffs outcomes for nickel: 2.9 ± 3.2 (Vapor4Life), 240.1 ± 234.9 (voopoo), 50.3 ± 24.9 (Juul), which are different from those given in the abstract. No explanation is given (were there different tests?).
- For the Juul device, the ng per 10 puffs range of values for chromium in the three favors of task (5): 73.24 ± 44.2 (Menthol), 76.36 ± 47 (Virginia Tobacco) and 107 ± 83.5 (Classical Tobacco), significantly differ from the values for chromium in task (1) and with those mentioned in the abstract. This is strange because the unspecified Juul flavor in the test of task (1) should coincide with at least one of the flavor tests in task (5) and thus the outcomes should not differ much, as it should be the same testing protocol applied to the same device with same flavor. The authors provide no explanation on this difference.

The authors found high chromium levels for the Juul, comparable to those of the voopoo (a tank device). This is strange, not only because it is at odds with other laboratory studies [11,14,15,17], but because the Juul has an inbuilt control of the coil temperature that prevents operation under overheating conditions [17]. In addition, it is very odd that increasing supplied power (from 5 to 60 Watts) to the voopoo does not produce a significant increase in metal levels (as it clearly happens for example in [11]). It is possible that this odd outlier result emerges from corrosion effects in devices acquired 2 years before the experiments.

Kapiamba et al. also miscalculate their risk evaluation along the reasoning of Olmedo et al. [10] (see Section 4.1.1), but even in a more problematic manner. They assume a rest tidal volume of inhalation (450 mL) and compute the amount of breathed air in 10 puffs ($4.5\,\text{LT} = 4.5 \times 10^{-3}\,\text{m}^3$), multiplying this quantity times the mg/m^3 concentrations of PEL of NIOSH for every metal, comparing this product with their ng per 10 puffs outcomes. However, as we argue in Section 5.4, this risk evaluation is conceptually mistaken, the PEL NIOSH is an occupational reference value obtained by time weight averaging of 8 h work shifts in 40 h week journeys, so it does not make any sense to compute it for the short time lapse of 10 puffs (besides the fact that PELs in general are higher for short term exposures). Kapiamba et al. also invoke (without providing a reference) the European Medicines Agency (EMA) to quote inhalation toxicological thresholds of 10 and 100 ng per day, respectively, for chromium and nickel. However, the EMA does not mention these values [55], it provides the PDE ICH of daily exposure for these metals that we have listed in Table 2 (3 and 6 µg for chromium and nickel, not 10 and 100 ng).

Contrary to the claims of Kapiamba et al., they did not examine environmental emissions (task (7)), but a sort of lung deposition model. Environmental emissions cannot be simulated by vaping machines because users retain a large percentage (∼90%) of the components of inhaled aerosol [70]. This is a confusing article, full of missing information and inconsistencies.

4.6. The CDC Group

Researchers from the CDC published two articles, the first one by Halstead et al. [14] and the follow up by Gray et al. [15], on metal contents in aerosol emissions following strictly the CORESTA 81 puffing protocol: 3 s puff duration, inter-puff lapse of 30 s, 55 mL puff volume and flow rate of 16.67 mL/s, using 75 puffs in [14] and 50 puffs in [15]. The experimental methodology (specially aerosol collection) and validation techniques are described in full detail in the fist paper: collection by fluoropolymer condensation trap built with high purity fluoropolymer to prevent metal leaching contaminating the samples, analytic analysis by ICP-MS. Using "spiked" e-liquids (i.e., inseminated with known metal content) they showed a very low rate of direct transfer of metal particles into the aerosol (between less than 1% to 4.7%).

The third paper by Pappas et al. [71] analyzed metallic particulate matter through single particle inductively coupled plasma–mass spectrometry (SP-ICP-MS) and dynamic light scattering (DLS), performing both single and dual element analyses to determine if particles are composed by individual or multiple metal oxides, with calibration and validation techniques that they describe in detail. Pappas et al. [71] tested the same type of devices as Gray et al. [15] and found similar anomalous outcomes as these authors did for elementary metal content. We discuss these results below.

Emissions. Halstead et al. [14] tested twelve devices, all acquired years before the experiments (2016–2018). The devices and acquisition date are: Vuse Menthol (2014 and 2017), Vuse Original (2014 and 2017), Njoy King Menthol (2016 and 2017), Blu Classic Tobacco single use (2014 and 2017), Logic Platinium (2014 and 2017), 21st Century Menthol, Regular, and Zero Nicotine (2014 and 2016), Joyeteck eGO tank device (2017), Juul (2018). They provide the outcomes of metal contents in their Table V as ng per 10 puffs, which we list as ng/puff for the Joyetech model in Table 11 and for the cartridge pods: Juul, blu and Vuse in Table 8 (together with pod devices examined by Zhao et al. [11]). We omit the values for the various cigalikes models that are no longer in use today (in fact, Vuse and blu devices acquired in 2017 are likely also discontinued).

Table 8. Mass per puff for pods devices tested by the CDC group ([14,15]) and Zhao et al. [11]. The values displayed in red correspond to the testing of the Vuse Alto (V. Alto) and myblu devices with Menthol flavor. Notice that nickel, lead, manganese and zinc outputs per puff from these particular cartridges are comparable to those found in the highest power settings of sub-ohm devices tested by Zhao et al. [11] listed in Table 5, thus suggesting an anomalous situation.

Study	Device	Cr	Cu	Ni	Pb	Sn	Zn
Halstead, 2019 [14]	Juul	< LOD	< LOD	< LOD	< LOD	< LOD	< LOD
	V. Alto M	0.05–0.17	< LOD	0.44–0.48	< LOD	< LOD	< LOD
	V. Alto T	0.03	0.05–0.21	0.11–0.27	< LOD	< LOD	< LOD
Gray et al., 2020 [15]	V. Alto M	0.89–2.99	1.71–20.9	15.8–37.3	9.65–46.3	0.98–4.41	86.7–458.0
	V. Alto T	0.01–0.18	0.1–1.46	0.05–9.79	0.09–1.63	0.01–0.03	1.0–4.05
	myblu M	0.06–0.07	14.6–17.4	3.1–10.8	0.05–0.17	8.12–12.7	<1.0
	myblu T	<0.05	4.61–5.32	0.015–0.13	0.05–0.29	0.94–5.1	<1.0
	Juul M	<0.05	0.1–1.6	0.05–0.2	0.06–0.08	0.01–0.06	0.5–1.78
	Juul T	<0.05	0.02–0.36	0.05–0.28	<0.05	0.01–0.05	<1.0
Zhao et al., 2019 [11]	myblu	< 0.012	0.076–1.13	<0.06	0.015–0.26	<0.013	3.23–41.29
	Juul	$<10^{-2}$	<0.022	0.01–0.06	$<10^{-2}$	$<10^{-2}$	0.76–2.50

The second paper by Gray et al. [15] tested three current usage pods acquired in 2019: Juul (Juul Labs), myblu (Imperial Brands) and Vuse Alto (R.J. Reynolds Vapor Company), with the following cartridge flavors: Mint and Classical Tobacco (Juul), (Intense Mint-sation and Tobacco Chill (myblu) and Menthol and Rich Tobacco (Vuse Alto). As with Halstead at al. [14], we report in Table 8 their outcomes (their Table II but in ng/puff) for seven metals (Cd, Cr, Cu, Ni, Pb, Sn, and Zn) for each device and flavor.

Toxicological evaluation. The devices tested by Halstead et al. [14] were all acquired well before the experiment: pods in 2017, the Juul in 2018 and the Joyeteck eGO in 2016 (though updated forms of the latter devices are still used). Even if there is a risk of corrosion (a possibility the authors acknowledge), it is evident from the ng/puff values listed in Table 8 that daily exposure is below toxicological references given in Table 2 for all metals they tested.

The second paper by Gray et al. [15] tested contents of same metals in aerosols of more recent cartridge pod devices: Juul, myblu and Vuse Alto, under the same experimental methodology as [14], each with tobacco-like and menthol-like flavors and high nicotine concentrations. The metal analysis found consistently low mass contents of all targeted metals in aerosol from the Juul devices, but surprisingly enormous variation of values were reported for the Vuse Alto device with Mint-sation cartridge (less in the tobacco flavor cartridge of the Vuse Alto and in both flavors of the myblu). It is not expected that cartridge based devices powered by 8 W can produce aerosol emissions with contents of Cu, Ni, Pb, Sn and Zn comparable to those of high powered sub-ohm devices tested by Zhao et al. in [11], but as shown in Table 9 this is what happens: copper content emitted by the Vuse Alto is higher than that of devices tested at 80–120 W (though it is still below the toxicological reference PDE of 30 μg in Table 2), while for nickel, lead and zinc the daily emission from the Vuse Alto are comparable to those emitted by the same sub-ohm devices tested at the same range 80–120 W, which surpass toxicological references.

Table 9. Daily exposure (in µg) of the Vuse Alto and myblu Menthol favors examined by Gray et al. [15]. A comparison (higher levels in red) is offered with daily exposure from same metals tested by Zhao et al. [11] on high power sub-ohm devices. The daily exposure was computed assuming 250 daily puffs.

	Vuse Alto Menthol	myblu Menthol	OD1 80 W	OD2 120 W	OD2 200 W	Toxicological Reference
Cr	0.22–2.24	0.015–0.017	0.01–0.04	0.02–0.2	0.001–0.77	3 PDE
Cu	0.43–15.67	3.65–4.35	0.93–4.35	1.05–5.57	4.53–46.0	30 PDE
Ni	3.45–9.32	0.78–2.7	0.98–8.66	0.07–14.24	3.23–36.79	6 PDE
Pb	2.41–11.57	0.01–0.04	1.98–9.83	1.15–3.52	2.76–49.7	5 PDE
Sn	0.24–1.1	2.03–3.17	0.08–0.54	0.05–0.18	0.14–2.84	60 PDE
Zn	21.67–114.5	<0.25	21.76–82.2	2.22–6.65	13.37–377.5	33,000 REL

Methodological critique. Halstead et al. [14] provide a valuable comprehensive discussion on trapping methods and validating techniques that were used in the follow up paper by Gray et al. [15]. They acknowledge the likelihood that their experimental outcomes have been affected by metal corrosion and degradation, as the devices were necessarily stored between 1 and 3 years before testing (most of them are no longer in use).

Gray et al. [15] also tested e-liquids from the pod cartridges, reporting specially high levels (in µg/g) of Cu, Sn and Ni in the myblu cartridges with flavor Intense Tobacco Chill (elevated but much lesser values were reported for Ni in the Vuse Alto cartridges of both flavors). As commented before, surprisingly high values also occurred in aerosol emissions only for one the Vuse Alto device with the flavor Mint-sation cartridge. These are outcomes restricted to a single combination of device and cartridge and thus require a proper explanation, as it is a clear signal of some special anomalous outlier situation affecting the tested cartridges, but not the pods, since significant lower outcomes occur with the same pod device and the other flavor cartridges. It is extremely unlikely that aerosol emissions from thousands of commercially sold Vuse Alto devices would exhibit, only for the Mint-sation flavor cartridges, such high metal levels (comparable to those of sub-ohm devices running at 80–120 W), without consumers having noticed this phenomenon likely in a foul testing aerosol (and consumer reports do note the existence of defective cartridges and pods).

Unfortunately, Gray et al. [15] provide very insufficient information on the tested devices and cartridges. It is impossible to know from the information they supply how many of the Mint-sation cartridges they tested produced such high metal outcomes (probably by being defective) or how large or representative is the sample they tested. This information should be accessible by placing it in a supplementary file, but the authors only provide minimal and maximal range of values in their test outcomes, not a median or average or any minimal descriptive statistics.

It would be very useful for consumers and regulators to know if the finding of high metal content in the Mint-sation cartridges was generic, as it would point out to a deficient quality control by manufacturers, but since the authors do not provide sufficient information on the samples, it is impossible to rule out that they acquired and tested a batch of unrepresentative defective cartridges. Another important information vacuum is on the precise test timing and conditions of storage in the 4 months time lapse they report between purchase and analysis of the devices and cartridges. They mention that the devices and cartridges had no manufacture or expiration dates, but this information can be supplied by the manufacturers. The authors do not report requesting such information and/or that it was denied. This lack of information hinders the understanding (and possibility of replication) of the authors' results.

Although 4 months is a shorter period than the years between purchase and analysis in [14], it is a still a sufficiently large time to suspect a high likelihood of leaching and corrosion effects. While the authors do recognize this likelihood, they remark that it is an uncertain possibility and offer alternatively explanations deemed to be just as plausible: "pod-to-pod variability" or heating of internal components. However, we believe that such alternative explanations are very unlikely, given the large storage time and the fact that excessively high metal contents only appeared in one combination of pod and cartridges. The authors could have avoided this uncertainty (made more problematic by the lack of information) by involving end users in tasting the aerosol from pods with specific cartridges, as this would have signaled them whether the tested cartridges were defective or not.

The laboratory studies by Gray et al. [15] and Kapiamba et al. [16]were the only two among the 12 reviewed studies that found in low powered devices high levels of metal content in aerosol emissions (surpassing toxicological markers), though as we have argued above and in Section 4.5, neither one of these two studies supplied sufficient information to determine if these findings are representative of the products. Therefore, the authors's conclusion in [15] that recent pod devices pose increasing health risks to users can hardly be sustained by their experimental outcomes.

The third study of the same group [71] by Pappas et al. estimated the number of nano-particles containing metallic oxides in the aerosol generated on (apparently) the same devices of Grey et al. [15] and resulting in analogous anomalies: consistently few particle numbers (less than 10,000) of all metallic oxides for the Juul device, higher but uneven numbers for both flavors of the mylu and tobacco flavor of the Vuse Alto, but extremely high number of particles of lead oxide (222,000) and huge variation for the Vuse Alto with tobacco flavor (nickel nano-particles per 10 puffs range between 630–190,000). As in [15], the authors do not provide a coherent explanation for these odd results, vaguely alluding to a high variability among devices and e-liquids, without any descriptive statistical analysis of samples (just ranges of values).

4.7. The Williams-Talbot Group

A number of studies has been undertaken by researchers of the University of California [18,22–24,72,73], providing useful assessments on the design of metallic parts and alloys in the coils, wires, solders and batteries of a large number of devices [22,72], the effects of aerosol collection techniques and puffing protocols the detected metal concentrations [18], as well as the evolution of these features with the introduction of newer devices [23,72].

Experimental methods and exposures. Three of the studies cited above [18,22,24] also obtained experimental results on metal contents in aerosol emissions, using either the CORESTA protocol or similar protocols and the analysis through induced coupled plasma optical emissions spectroscopy (ICP-OES) (the three papers refer their experimental methodology to [24]). We will not consider outcomes from earlier studies by this group [22,24] because the devices tested are no longer in use.

In a more recent study [18], the group tested several second generation cartomizer models: EgoC Twist mod with KangerTech Protank and Nautilus atomizers and iTaste MVP 2.0 with Kanger T3S atomizer (all acquired in 2014), a sub-ohm high power third generation kit model with commercial resistance (SMOK Alien) and two tank models Nemesis and iPV6X with reconstructed resistances (acquired in 2017). Their aims were to probe experimentally how two collection methods (impingers and cold trap) affect detected metal contents in aerosols emissions (the first laboratory study undertaking such comparison), to identify and quantify the transfer of metals into the aerosols produced by tank-style devices (they include cartomizers in this category), and to evaluate the effect of varying puffing topography. All devices were tested for "continuous" puffing (60 puffs of 4.3 s duration every 60 s) and "interval" puffing (clusters of 10 continuous puffs separated by 5 min brake).

Gathering all the information supplied by Williams et al. in [18] together with plausible assumptions based on the specifications of the devices manufacturers, we converted the µg/L concentrations into ng/puff values considering the maximal values for every metal reported in their supplementary files (see our supplementary file). These ng/puff values are listed in Table 10. Notice that silicon is abundant in all models dated 2014 (the three clearomizer models and the Nemesis Clone), something also reported in their previous paper [74] and likely related to wicks made of silica. It is worth remarking that the ng/puff values for their SMOK device are close to those reported by Zhao et al. in [11] for the tested open devices OD1 and OD2 in the 40 Watt power range (see Table 5).

Toxicological evaluation. In an early 2013 study [24] Williams et al. found silica and metal nano-particles and metal concentrations in the aerosol of cigalike devices. Farsalinos and colleagues [74] showed this metal content to be below occupational toxicological markers. In a 2015 study metal content in the aerosol of cigalikes and cartomizer devices was heavily dominated by silicon [22], likely generated from the silicon content of the wick/sheath of the tested devices or by leaching from the vessels of aerosol collection (see [18]), all other metals were detected in practically negligible concentrations. Since these studies looked at old devices that are now obsolete, we will not consider them any further.

Although Williams et al. did consider in their 2019 paper [18] combinations of various puffing parameters ("high/low" voltage HV/LV and flow rate HF/LF), these parameters do not deviate much from those of the CORESTA protocol and thus remain inappropriate for high powered devices used for DTL vaping. Still, for all metals and devices they tested the daily exposures are below PDE-ICH toxicological references. This can be easily appreciated by comparing the relevant toxicological reference in Table 2 with the product of each the ng/puff values in Table 10 times 250 daily puffs and converting to µg. In fact, the highest outcome in the study of Williams et al. is 14.44 ng/puff for nickel produced by their SMOK Alien device, leading to a daily exposure of 3.61 µg, which is below the PDE-ICH of 6 µg for nickel (it is even below the nickel intermediate MRL-ATSDR of 4 µg).

Table 10. Mass (ng) per puff for devices tested by Williams et al. in their 2019 study [18]. These values were obtained from the concentrations reported in their supplementary file (See unit conversion in our supplementary file). All metal levels are below toxicological markers given in Table 2.

Device	EgoC T Protank	EgoC T Nautilus	iTaste MVP Kanger	Nemesis Clone	iPV6X Tsunami	Smok Alien
Al	0.08–0.11	0.03–0.05	0.09–0.14	0.16–0.2		0.27–0.36
Bo	0.52–0.75	0.18–0.26			0.32–0.40	
Ca	3.84–5.49	5.82–8.32	5.66–8.08	18.5–23.12	22.5–28.12	
Cd		0.002–0.003	0.002–0.003	0.006–0.007		
Cr		0.01–0.02	0.007–0.01		0.66–0.82	0.48–0.64
Cu	1.05–1.50	1.13–1.62	1.4–2.0		0.10–0.12	1.02–1.36
Fe				2.9–3.62	7.40–9.25	4.65–6.20
Ka	1.49–2.13	1.22–1.75	0.80–1.14	2.36–2.95		
Mg	0.09–0.13	0.3–0.4	0.08–0.12	1.76–2.20	1.70–2.12	
Na	0.60–0.87	2.17–3.11		9.4–11.75		
Ni	0.14–0.20	0.03–0.04	0.2–0.3	0.04–0.05	0.64–0.80	10.83–14.44
Pb	5.79–8.27	2.67-3.81	7.43–11.33	0.12–0.15	0.64–0.8	1.65–2.20
Si	23.0–32.8	24.5–35.0	15.39–21.98	23.28–29.10	2.12–2.65	1.74–2.32
Sn	1.78–2.54	1.03–1.47	2,42–3.45	0.60–0.75	3.64–4.55	1.8–2.4
Zn	0.64–0.99	3.16–4.52	0.88–1.26	0.5–0.62	8.7–10.87	23.67–31.56

Methodological critique. The most innovative feature of the 2019 study by Williams et al. [18] is the experimental comparison of the effect of two aerosol collection methods, cold trap and impinger, on aerosol emissions, recommending the latter method for better performance (see further discussion in Section 5.6).

While the authors advice to minimize the amount of storage time before analysis, it is not evident that they followed this advice, since a major drawback of the study [18] is the fact that most devices were acquired in 2014, at least 4 years before the experiments, while the SMOK and iPVeX are dated at 2017. Unfortunately, the authors do not provide information on the storage of these devices and their parts. Another major drawback is testing devices with reconstructible resistances (RDA), as these are typically operated in very varied "do it yourself" manner, requiring constant wetting of the wick. In fact, it is not clear how did they machine puffed devices of this type and, evidently, such experiments cannot be reproduced.

Williams et al. [18] claim that concentrations of chromium, copper, lead, nickel, zinc in their own 2019 study exceed the OSHA PEL. As an example, they stress that the concentration of chromium from the tank-style device (Tsunami 2.4, a RDA model) reported in their supplementary file 5×10^7 ng/m^3 far exceeds (by 4 orders of magnitude) 3.3×10^3 ng/m^3, the OSHA PEL value for chromium. However, these comparisons are completely mistaken, as they are based on a mere comparison of concentrations from aerosol collection analyzed by an ICP-OES instrument and air concentrations disregarding the actual inhalation volumes. It is easy to prove this wrong. The chromium outcome that results from their Tsunami 2.4 device is 0.66–0.82 ng/puff (see Table 10), which multiplied times 250 daily puffs yields a daily exposure to chromium of 0.165–0.205 µg, which is between one and two orders of magnitude below the PDE ICH of 3 µg for chromium.

Both, Wiliams et al. [18] and Zhao et al. [11] al used the Istick 25 and a SMOK power units recommended for, respectively, 1–85 W and 6–220 W. For both devices they conducted the laboratory experiments outside these power ranges of best performance recommended by the manufacturers (besides using puffing protocols that do not correspond to real life usage of the devices for DTL vaping). There is also a vacuum of information: the mere commercial brand names do not identify a unique atomizer among the range offered by the manufacturers. Since the resistance value and coil metal alloy are reported to be Kanthal with 0.2 Ω for Istick and Stainless Steel with 0.6 Ω for SMOK, an internet search reveals that the Istick brand could be the Istick Pico 25 atomizers from Eleaf that have a power unit with a maximal electrical power of 85 W. The HW-N/M2/N2 coils equipped with the Ello atomizer could have been used, with recommended power range between 40 and 90 W with the optimal power in the range 65–75 W according to tests by Eleaf factory. Regarding the SMOK device, the Alien Kit with TFV8 baby atomizer has a power unit that could reach 220 Watts, while the TFV8-Q2 coil is built with stainless steel and resistance 0.6 Ω. Its recommended operation range is 20–50 W with best performance in the range 30–40 W. Both atomizers are recommended for DTL vaping.

In [18] Wiliams et al. tested 5 atomizers reporting their commercial name: Kangertech Protank, Aspire Nautilus, Kangertech T3S, SMOK alien kit (TVF8 Baby atomiser), Clone RDA and Tsunami 2.4 RDA without any additional specification. Two of the devices are rebuildable dripping atomizers that (as mentioned before) require a personalized "do it yourself" handmade coil building and are not designed for the usage of typical vapers, but rather for experimented *aficionado* type of vaper in a framework based on many trial and error repetitions to find the right power set-up for a desired sensorial feeling during vaping. Additionally, these devices require manual wetting of the cotton wick following changing patterns of the user subjective perception.

Evidently, testing this type of specialized devices requires a detailed dedicated study that takes into account their peculiarities, in particular the extreme difficulty to introduce any standardized procedure. Testing this type of RDA devices is clearly out of place in a publication based on regimented puffing patterns (all this besides the fact that applied airflow rates do not correspond to realistic usage by being the same or below the ISO:20768 requirements or CORESTA method 81). These devices have low air resistance leading to an inhalation close to natural breathing. Reaching the required airflow to be applied needs a physical restriction to increase lung pressure (i.e., mouth closing). It is quite uncomfortable and is consequently not representative of real use.

4.8. Other Laboratory Studies Detecting Metal Content
4.8.1. Kim et al.

The authors examined changes in cariogenic potential in tooth surfaces exposed to e-cigarette aerosols generated by a sub-ohm tank device (0.2 Ω) running at 40 W, with atomizers filled with e-liquids (80/20 PG/VG percent mixture) with sweet flavors and nicotine concentration of 10 mg/mL [19].

E-cigarettes were puffed by a Universal Electronic-Cigarette Testing Machine (UECTM) developed by the American Dental Association (ADA), using a commercial sub-ohm tank (Aspire Cleito: 0.2 O Kanthal coil with cotton wick). Aerosols were generated at a power setting of 3.14 V (total of 49.2 W based on $W = V^2/\Omega$) determined by the manufacturer's manual (capable up to 55–70 W). Each atomizer was used for 750 puffs (approximately 5 days usage) and replaced thereafter, taking care to replace atomizers performing abnormally. As puffing topography the authors considered what they describe as "published physiological human e-cigarette puffing topography": 50 mL puff volume in 4 s puff duration every 18 s, justifying these parameters by their reference [46] (Behar et al.). They defined 10 puffs as one vaping session and 150 puffs as one-day use.

However, the puffing protocol used by the authors was that used by Behar et al. to test cigalike devices, collecting aerosols by a syringe and unspecified tubes, a completely inappropriate experimental methodology for testing a sub-ohm device at 49 W. As a consequence, their outcomes on cariogenic potential in tooth surfaces does not apply to real life vapers using such device. Nevertheless, the metal concentrations detected by their ICP-OES instruments were listed in their Table 3 for Ca, Cu, Fe, Mn and Si, remaining metals were either non-targeted of below LOD, all of them are well below the Threshold Limit Value of the National Institute for Occupational Safety and Health (TLV-NIOSH). We transformed their mg/LT into ng/puff in Table 11.

Table 11. Metal elements in other studies (outputs converted in ng/puff). Kim et al. [19] tested a third generation sub-ohm tank device, the rest tested second generation devices. The values for Beauval et al. [20] are in picograms.

	Halstead 2019 [14]	Kim 2018 [19]	Beauval 2017 [20]	Palazzolo 2017 [21]
Al				35.55
As				1.11
Ca		81.8		
Cd			0.14 ± 0.3 (pg)	0.97
Cr			3.4 ± 0.6 (pg)	
Cu	0.747 ± 0.67	2.2		0.42
Fe		1.02		
Mn		3.4		0.02
Ni	0.495 ± 0.19			0.53
Pb	1.14 ± 0.4			0.13
Sb			0.47 ± 0.3 (pg)	
Si		33.3		
Sn	0.04 ± 0.01			
Zn	3.34			3.77

4.8.2. Beauval et al.

The authors [20] used various analytic techniques (gas chromatography, high and ultra performance liquid chromatography and inductively coupled plasma with mass spectrometry or ultraviolet flame ionization detection) in order to identify the main e-liquid and its vapor constituents (PG, VG, nicotine), as well as potentially harmful compounds, all of which were found at negligible low levels: trace elements, including metals ($\leq$3.4 pg/mL puff), pesticides (below quantifiable levels LOQ), polycyclic aromatic hydrocarbons ($\leq$4.1 pg/mL puff), carbonyls ($\leq$2.11 ng/mL puff). As a comparison these compounds in cigarette smoke, respectively, appeared as 45.0, 8.7, 560.8 and 1540 (in the same units). The device tested was a second generation Lounge with resistance 2.8 Ω at 3.6 V ($\sim$8 W). The e-liquids had 65% PG, 35% VG, with the rest made of several and no flavorings, with zero and 16 mg/ml nicotine levels. Aerosol was produced through the CORESTA protocol: 55 mL puff volume, 96 puffs of 3 s duration every 30 s. Blank collection was conducted for all experiments. Most metals in aerosol emissions were found below LOQ, quantified concentrations were found of Al, Co, Mn No, Pb, likely from contaminations as they were comparable to those of the blank samples. Only Cd, Cr and Sb were present in some aerosol collections up to 0.14, 2.3 and 0.47 pg/mL per puff (as a comparison, As, Cd, Pb and Ti were quantified in the 3R4F cigarette smoke from 1.02 pg/mL for Ti to 44.98 pg/mL per puff for Cd).

4.8.3. Palazzolo et al.

These authors [21] used as aerosol collecting method mixed ester celullose membranes and scanned electron microscopy as analytic technique. They examined metal contents of a second generation eGO Twist device in comparison with cigarette smoke (their control state). All metal element contents were reported below toxicological references.

5. Discussion

The previous section presented an extensive—article by article—review of 12 studies on metal content in EC aerosol published after 2017. We provide in this section further discussion and a summary that is itemized by shortcomings shared by various articles and other features.

5.1. High Powered Sub-Ohm Devices

All studies testing high powered sub-ohm devices [10–13,16,18,19] (mostly used and recommended for DTL vaping) did so by means of CORESTA or CORESTA-like puffing protocols that are appropriate for low powered devices used for MTL vaping, but not for DTL vaping that requires much larger airflows and puff volumes. While Olmedo et al. [10] claimed that 5 metals (Cr, Mn, Ni, and Pb) produced exposures above toxicological markers, their computation of these exposures was mistaken (see Section 5.4), their outcomes lead to exposures to all metals below toxicological markers (see Table 4). Outcomes of Liu et al. [13] (arsenic species), Williams et al., 2019 [18] and Kim et al., 2018 [19] also produced exposures below toxicological markers for all metals (see Tables 10 and 11). Exposures surpassed toxicological markers in three studies: Zhao et al., 2019 and 2022 [11,12] (nickel, copper, lead and manganese, see Table 6) and Kapiamba et al., 2022 [16] (nickel and chromium). As we have argued in Section 3, these high levels of metals occur under testing conditions most likely affected by overheating outside the optimal regime. However, this testing of sub-ohm devices is unrealistic by failing to achieve even a minimal approximation to the real life usage of the devices. It is thus of little relevance to end users.

5.2. Pod Devices

All metal contents in pod devices were detected in negligible quantities well below toxicological markers in three out of five studies: Zhao et al. [11,12], Halstead et al. [14] and Chen et al. [17], with metal outcomes in the latter study being below quantification limit. However, outcomes for copper, nickel and lead where surprisingly higher than these markers (comparable to those found by Zhao et al. in [11], see Table 9), but only in Mint-sation flavor cartridges of the Vuse Alto device examined by Grey et al., 2019 [15]. As we argued in Section 4.6, a device operating below 10 W producing comparable metal output as sub-ohm devices tested at 80 and 120 W is a strange outlier result that raises suspicion of a defective cartridge subjected to leaching or corrosion that could have been repellent to users, Unfortunately, the authors do not provide sufficient information on their tested samples to verify or rule out these possibilities. Kapiamba et al. [16] also found high metal levels in the two pods they tested (Juul and Vapor4Life), but these are not reliable outcomes given the numerous inconsistencies of their study (see Section 4.5).

5.3. Testing Old Devices: Corrosion

Some of the studies (Williams et al. [18], Halstead et al. [14] and Kapiamba et al. [16]) tested devices that were acquired years before their laboratory testing (4 months lapse in Gray et al. [15]). None of the authors describes storage conditions, but [14,15] do recognize the risk of corrosion in testing such devices. The aim of these studies was not looking at the effects of corrosion or metal degradation from the aging of the devices and all authors are employed in public institutions in the US, where new devices can be easily bought in vape shops, thus it is hard to understand why they tested aged devices stored so much time before their testing.

Halstead et al. [14] examined the concentrations of metals in cartridges and pods of old devices. In all cases the older cartridges showed higher metal levels, thus indicating that longer storage time makes corrosion and leaching extremely likely. The 4 months between purchase and analysis in the devices and cartridges tested by Gray et al. [15], together with finding very high metal levels only in a single combination of pod/cartridge (Vuse Alto flavor Mint-sation), clearly favors corrosion effects over the alternative explanations suggested by the authors (product variability, heating effects, PH of e-liquids).

It is possible that leaching and corrosion might be more prevalent in closed systems because their cartridges are more likely to undergo longer storage time between their manufacturing and usage. Open devices are not stored with e-liquid and the delay between purchase, e-liquid filling and its vaporization for usage is typically shorter (below one or two days), thus reducing the likelihood of leaching and corrosion. While long time stored cartridges can be valuable in laboratory experiments to understand leaching, corrosion and degradation phenomena, it is irrelevant for most users typically consuming these products within the next few days after their purchase (though lack of proper maintenance by users might also cause these problems).

5.4. Comparison with Toxicological References

Olmedo et al. [10] claimed that exposure from their experimental outcomes was above the MRL-ATSDR toxicological markers for Cr, Mn, Ni and Pb. Liu et al. [13] and Kapiamba et al. [16] made similar claims in comparison with the PEL-OSHA, while Williams et al. [18] claimed that chromium levels in a sub-ohm device were orders of magnitude above the PEL OSHA by erroneously comparing concentrations in aerosol condensate and those of this occupational marker.

We can easily identify two basic mistakes in these exposure estimations: First, Olmedo et al. [10] (and Liu et al. [13] following suite) assumed that the inhaled aerosol dilutes in a puff volume (66.67 mL) generated by vaping machines or pumps, when it actually dilutes in a much larger tidal volume of 800 mL [45] (a fact that was noticed by Farsalinos and Rodu [66], though these authors assumed a resting tidal volume of 500 mL). Second, vapers are only exposed to EC aerosol while vaping (not continuously), but puffs are intermittent events lasting few seconds each and adding up to a reduced time lapse in a day of inhalation. Assuming 250 puffs of 3 s duration leads to a total of 12.5 min during the 480 min of an 8 h working shift inhalation (if using the PEL-NIOSH) or 1440 min (if using a daily value), which amounts to (respectively) 2.6% and 0.9% of the total times of exposure. It is important to bear this in mind, since toxicological references markers (PDF-ICH, MRL

ATSDR and PEL-NIOSH) have been conceived and obtained for very specific exposure timeframes (see Section 2.3).

Comparison of concentrations while disregarding exposure times can be misleading. To look at an extreme case, consider the most worrying metal level we have estimated in our revision of metal studies: 0.147 µg of nickel per puff for the OD2 device tested by Zhao et al. [11] at 200 Watts (see Table 5). Assuming a puff diluted in 800 mL of tidal volume (not the puff volume of 66.67 mL from the vaping machine considered by Olmedo et al. in [10]) this leads to a concentration of 184 µg/m^3 for a single puff. This concentration seems enormous compared with the occupational concentration of the PEL-NIOSH: $C_{\text{NIOSH}} = 15$ µg/m^3. However, once we take into consideration vaping exposure times within the 8 h timeframe of the PEL-NIOSH and the highest seasonal nickel concentration in Mexico City (to choose an extreme value in a polluted urban area: $C_{\text{air}} = 0.01953$ µg/m^3, see Table 4 of [75]), we obtain a concentration that is about one third of the PEL-NIOSH concentration (C_{NIOSH}):

$$C = \frac{\Delta t_{\text{puff}}}{t_{\text{tot}}} \times N_p \times C_{\text{vap}} + \left(1 - \frac{\Delta t_{\text{puff}}}{t_{\text{tot}}} \times N_p\right) \times C_{\text{air}} = 4.803 \frac{\mu g}{m^3} < 15 \frac{\mu g}{m^3}, \quad (1)$$

where we assumed equal time ($\Delta t_{\text{puff}} = 3$ s) and equal aerosol concentration ($C_{\text{vap}} = 184$ µg/m^3) for each puff and even put the daily $N_p = 250$ puffs in these 8 h ($= t_{\text{tot}}$). This concentration is still way above the daily MRL-ATSDR value for nickel (0.2 µg/m^3 for the intermediate timeframe, see Table 2). Moreover, the MRL-ATSDR marker is expected to be much lower than the PEL-NIOSH, as it is a toxicological threshold for the general population subjected to continuous longer time environmental exposure [57]. It is obtained from (typically) extrapolating from animal models to humans a NOAEL (No Observed Adverse Effect Level), a more strict toxicological criterion than the PEL. The longer the exposure timeframe the lower the MRL-ATSDR threshold becomes and the exposure assumptions are also more strict. The PDE-ICH is also a much stricter threshold than the PEL-NIOSH, it is also based on a NOAEL and can be also computed for continuous long term dosing [55].

The exposure comparison can also be accomplished in terms of mass doses. Intake of air diluted aerosol for the PEL-NIOSH concentration (6.67 m^3 for 8 h) leads to an upper limit of nickel intake of 100.05 µg, which is 2.7 times larger than than the daily intake of 36.79 µg from the OD2 device (see Table 6) for 250 puffs taken in 8 h. However, as expected, daily exposure dose with the MRL-ATSDR leads (for 20 m^3 daily inhaled air) to 4 µg of nickel intake which is much less than the daily intake of 36.70 µg from the OD2 device at 200 W.

To avoid problematic comparisons between concentrations of environmental toxicological markers and air diluted aerosol (which are problematic to evaluate and exhibit huge individual and time/space variation), we have preferred to incorporate the discrete intermittent nature of the puffing time exposure of vaping by going directly to comparison of intake doses, that is, by estimating the inhaled mass of a given metal per puff (from the experimental outcomes) and multiplying it by our estimate of 250 daily puffs to get a daily dose to compare it with the daily values of the PDE-ICH or the MRL-ATSDR, using the PEL-NIOSH with 83 puffs in 8 h only when the other two references are unavailable.

It is important to emphasize that we are comparing experimental outcomes with very strict toxicological markers that are applicable to the general population. As we showed above, even for the most worryingly high measured nickel levels (the OD2 device at 200 W) these levels are below the PEL-NIOSH occupational marker, while as shown in the tables of Section 4 those outcomes that surpass the more strict toxicological markers (MRL-ATSDR and PDE-ICH) do not correspond to real life usage and/or exhibit methodological flaws and (extremely likely) overheating conditions. Nevertheless, as we argue in Section 6, the occupational PEL-NIOSH can also be an appropriate toxicological marker for vaping, as a voluntary activity that is not aimed at the general population, but at adult smokers.

5.5. Information Vacuum

Failure to provide sufficient information on the devices, puffing protocols and outcomes hinders the evaluation of the quality and utility of laboratory studies. Several of the revised studies omitted valuable information. Olmedo et al. [10] tested 56 tank devices, without providing a list of individual devices (something they could easily have done in their supplementary material). They classified the devices in terms of voltage ranges, coil alloy and frequency of coil replacement, but not in terms of their resistance, which makes it impossible to determine their power range, thus analyzing together (what could be) very different tank devices: powerful sub-ohm and low powered tank ones. Since this distinction is technically very important [30], failure to provide this information hinders the evaluation of their results, as coil resistance and power are the main factors behind the increase of metal content (specially nickel, copper and lead) in EC aerosol emissions, as it was shown in the continuing paper by Zhao et al. [11] (though the CORESTA-like protocol used by both papers is inappropriate for sub-ohm devices).

In their 2022 study [12], Zhao et al. used the same devices as in their 2019 paper [11], but lumped together into a single statistic the outcomes of the two sub-ohm devices operating at two distinct powers (40 and 80 W) and the two pod devices (Juul and myblue). At least for the pods, these conflalatted outcomes do not seem to be reliable because the Juul uses nicotine salts (59 mg/mL) and the myblu basic nicotine (24 mg/mL), a fact that must bear influence on the aerosol phase partition and on its emissions (see comments in Section 4.2).

Liu et al. [13] just identified the tested devices as "USB-like" pods and a tank model, without specifying their characteristic parameters. Kapiamba et al. [16] (among many other irregularities) did not specify the coil resistance of the tested tank model. Williams et al. [18] also failed to provide an accurate description of the devices they tested (including one with a reconstructible coil), some of whom were purchased as far back as 2014. Grey et al. [15] did identify the pod models they tested, but did not provide sufficient information to analyze their outcomes, as the latter were given only in terms of mass ranges (in ng per 10 puffs) without a minimal descriptive statistics to understand their distribution (with high likelihood to mix frequent and outlier values).

5.6. Aerosol Collection

A critical examination of aerosol collection methods is essential in the evaluation of emission studies, as element leaching from various materials and vessels: glassware and plasticware (in tubings), ceramic containers and glass and quartz fiber filters, is a potential source of contaminants that can affect the outcomes of metal elements detected in EC aerosol. This leaching can be quantified by suitable acid presoaking of vessels and it must be taken into consideration to avoid detecting metal outcomes that can be overestimations.

There is no standard method for EC aerosol collection, so the studies on metals we have reviewed have utilized different methods: pipette tips and narrow tubing ([10,11,13]), syringe and unspecified tubing ([19]), high purity fluoropolymer tubing ([14,15]), tubing with teflon filters ([16]), Millipore Mixed Cellulose Ester membrane ([21]), cold trap ([18]), quartz pad extracted with 10% high purity nitric acid ([17]) and impingers ([18,20]). However, only two of the studies discussed in detail the possible contamination of metal outcomes by the materials of the collection method they used: Williams et al. [18] and Halstead et al. [14].

The detailed experimental comparison in [18] between the cold trap and impinger methods shows that, on average, the cold trap method yields higher metal contents than the impinger, but metal outcomes in each method depend on specific metals: some metals are only detected by the impinger method, which the authors showed to be more effective in collecting heavy metals, while the cold trap method was better with alkali, earth metals and metalloids. Though, the efficiency between collection methods also depended on the devices and on puffing topography through mechanisms that are still uncertain. For better accuracy, the authors of [18] recommend the impinger method that best avoids leaching from contact with large surfaces of tubing, acid soaking glass surfaces for increasing times (in day lapses) and avoiding large time storage after collection to prevent leaching from storage vessels (though it is not clear that they followed this advice in their study, see Section 4.7).

The authors of [14] also discussed the possible contamination by leaching from trapping systems, recommending the avoidance of EC aerosol collection by low purity quartz material and glass fiber filters, as well as aerosol trapping by electrostatic precipitation in high purity, fused silica quartz tubes, the preferred aerosol trapping technique of mainstream cigarette smoke. This is consistent with the large variability of metal outcomes when trapping EC aerosol through quartz filters [76]. They suggest aerosol collection by means of high purity fluoropolymer tubing, with the tubes characteristics found by appropriate validating techniques.

It is possible that some of the reviewed studies might have reported overestimations of metal outcomes from contamination from aerosol collection methods and materials, though it is beyond the scope of the present review to verify this possibility.

5.7. Metal Biomarkers

As opposed to metal content from machine generated aerosol in a laboratory, metal biomarkers are measured on body fluids of human vapers, whom we can safely assume carried on with normal usage of their devices, meaning without overheating and repellent flavor (most likely within the optimal regime). Metal biomarkers are then a more direct indicator of health effects based systemic absorption of vaping emissions by actual human subjects (as opposed to artificially generated aerosols). Three studies on metal biomarkers [42–44] found no statistically significant difference between vapers and non-users, thus suggesting that inhaled metal content under normal vaping conditions does not seem be of concern at least for acute exposure.

5.8. Comparison with Tobacco Smoke

All reviewed studies provide some comparison of their experimental outcomes with content of same metals in tobacco smoke, as ECs are conceived as harm reduction products providing a safer alternative to tobacco cigarettes. Several of the studies emphasize that nickel appears in comparable or larger mass content as in tobacco smoke (see for example Palazzolo et al. [21]). However, this comparison must be carefully examined, since metals in tobacco smoke and EC aerosol originate from different processes and involve larger content for different metals: the usually most abundant ones in EC aerosol (nickel and zinc) are often found in practically negligible amounts in tobacco smoke, while the most abundant metals in tobacco smoke [77] are either found in minute amounts (cadmium) or not detected (mercury) in EC aerosol.

6. Assessment of the Risk Communication

Most of the reviewed metal studies ([10–13,15–19]) have reported alarmingly high risks of health hazards from their experimental outcomes, even if (as we have shown in Sections 4 and 5) in most of these studies such outcomes are below the reference toxicological markers listed in Table 2 and all studies detecting such high metal levels exhibit serious methodological flaws. Further, most of the revised metal papers take their risk assessments to suggest policy recommendations for stricter EC regulation.

On the grounds of our findings in the present review, we believe we need to question this risk communication, as it is based on laboratory outcomes often obtained when vaping machines operate with inappropriate puffing protocols that disregard real life usage, as well as other methodological flaws that we have described in Section 4 and further discussed in Section 5. For the same reasons stated before, we believe we need to question the conclusions on health hazards from metal content in vaping emissions found in the reviews by Zhao et al. [9] and Gaur et al. [78], as well as in the cancer risk assessment by Fowles et al. [79], as they are based on considering large metal levels that were obtained in laboratory studies whose shortcomings we have reported.

We also criticize a form of risk communication that emphasizes the comparable or higher levels of metal content with respect to tobacco smoke as a signal of EC toxicity, disregarding the fact that metals form merely a tiny fraction of the set of toxic and carcinogenic compounds found in tobacco smoke, while they are among the few trace toxic byproducts found in EC aerosol. As an example of this risk miscommunication, a 2013 study by Williams et al. [24] remarked that nickel was detected in amounts 200 times those of tobacco smoke, though these concentrations in EC aerosol were already negligible and well below toxicological markers (see Farsalinos et al. [74]).

Some of the reviewed studies recognize that laboratory testing does not reproduce human vaping, attempting to provide real life connection to their outcomes to justify their health risks assessments. In their 2019 study, Zhao et al. [11] allude to a "sensitivity analysis" stating that their outcomes are not affected by increasing the puff numbers from those of a session to real life daily puff numbers (which they assume to be 120, arguing that they might be reporting an underestimation of actual risks). This reasoning is incorrect, since the disconnection from real life usage in sub-ohm device testing in [11] is not a matter of counting puff numbers and comparing them with the surveys listed in Table 1, but of inappropriate puff volumes and puffing airflow required by the optimal operation of powerful sub-ohm devices used for DTL vaping. Other revised studies [10,12,13,15,16] have incurred in similar mistakes.

We have compared experimental outcomes of metal content of the 12 revised studies with various reference toxicological markers for 14 metal elements, giving preference to the PDE-ICH, a strict safety threshold applicable to the general population as a maximal daily intake of impurities in inhaled medication [55]. We have also placed for reference another strict safety threshold applicable to the general population: the environmental MRL-ATSDR [57]. It is worth mentioning that in all cases the experimental outcomes that produced exposures surpassing these strict toxicological markers were plagued by methodological flaws: testing sub-ohm devices in extreme power ranges disconnected with real life vaping [12], failure to provide sufficient information on tested samples to rule out testing unrepresentative defective cartridges [15], as well as a number of shortcomings discussed in detail in Sections 4 and 5. For devices tested under appropriate conditions (and even those under inappropriate conditions but not at maximal power) the experimental outcomes lead to exposures below these strict markers.

We also refereed to the occupational toxicological references: PEL-NIOSH or REL-OSHA (see Section 2.3), whose application as safety thresholds to vaping has been criticized for "not being sufficiently protective" to the general population, or as stated by Williams et al. [18] (when discussing Potential health effects of EC elements/metals) because they are not " recreational" safety thresholds. In this context, it is interesting to see the critique by Hubbs et al. [80] to occupational safety thresholds and the response by Farsalinos et al. [81]. While we prioritize a stricter reference such as the PDE-ICH to be on the side of more stringent precaution and do recognize the limitations of occupational thresholds, we believe that Farsalinos et al. are right in responding to this criticism and arguing the case for using occupational markers: vaping is not recommended for the general population or vulnerable individuals (infants, pregnant women or individuals with ill health), but for voluntary usage by adult smokers aiming at significantly reducing their exposure to the toxicity of tobacco smoke, a usage condition that is not much different from voluntary occupational exposure. Since "recreational" safety thresholds for vaping do not exist, other existing toxicological markers (occupational, environmental and medicinal) are perfectly applicable under their own limitations, together with the inherent limitation of laboratory testing that is (at best) a proxy to assess human exposure.

Finally, perhaps the over precautionary approach often expressed on the safety of vaping, demanding that it must be determined only by the strictest possible protective standards, comes from its mistaken association with smoking, which does require such strict level of protection. However, EC aerosol emissions are chemically and physically distinct from tobacco smoke and thus require completely different (and risk proportionate) safety and regulatory evaluation standards.

7. Conclusions

We have provided in this review an extensive critical revision of 12 laboratory studies looking at metal element content in EC aerosols published after 2017 (see Sections 4 and 5). Nine of these studies are authored by researchers from academic and government institutions in the US, one from China (Liu et al. [13]) and one from France (Beuval et al. [20]). Only one study (Chen et al. [17]) is industry funded.

Our review mostly focused on the outcomes of metal elements, their comparison with reference toxicological markers and a methodological critique based on self-consistency and compatibility between puffing protocols and the characteristics and real life of the tested devices and compatibility with absence of overheating conditions that do not (necessarily) involve a "dry hit" condition associated with e-liquid depletion. We argue that this compatibility can also be associated to an optimal regime that can be tested in the laboratory (see Soulet et al. [31,32] and Floyd et al. [33]). As with other technologies, different ECs are suitable for different consumers and modes of usage that determine specific parameter ranges. Testing EC emissions must be compatible with these requirements.

Since all the 12 revised studies on metal contents (and likely most laboratory studies on non-metallic content) have relied on CORESTA or CORESTA-like puffing protocols, incompatible with the large airflows and high power input of sub-ohm devices, it is not surprising that high levels of certain metals (nickel, lead, copper, manganese) were found, specially at highest device power, surpassing strict toxicological references applicable to the general population (PDE-ICH and MRL-ATSDR). However, even if metal levels did not surpass these toxicological references, these outcomes are not realistic for coming out of experiments whose protocols are incompatible with real life usage of the devices. As a contrast, metal levels in the emissions of low powered devices (mostly pods, starting kits and second generation devices) were well below the strict toxicological markers in all self consistent laboratory testing, an expected and consistent finding given the fact that CORESTA or CORESTA-like protocols are still appropriate for testing such devices. High metal levels above toxicological markers were found in low powered devices in [15,16], but these are not reliable outcomes because these two studies are plagued by methodological irregularities (see Sections 4.5 and 4.6).

We emphasize once more that laboratory testing is valuable for product comparison, quality control and technological advancement, but it does not reproduce human vaping experience (even under the best experimental conditions, regimented puffing might involve uncomfortable or repellent sensations for human users). While laboratory testing under extreme conditions divorced from real life usage might be of theoretical and practical interest in itself, it is irrelevant to assess health risks in users. However, well conducted experiments (appropriate puffing protocols and operating within manufacturer recommendations) may be useful to assess approximately the potential of health risks. Evidently, the full information that defines the device characteristics and puffing parameters must be fully and explicitly supplied in the materials and methods sections or in the supplementary files of the studies to render them valuable for consumers, public health officials and regulators. Studies conducted outside of these consistency parameter limits must explicitly notify the readership that the testing involves abnormal usage conditions (likely involving overheating or corrosion).

Unfortunately, most of the revised studies did not provide full information on key physical parameters (coil resistance, full specification of the device, manufacturer recommendation on power/voltage ranges and their experimental outcomes). None of the 12 revised studies relied on human subjects to confirm that testing conditions would (at least) minimally relate to users' sensorial experience. However, it would be very useful for researchers on vaping emissions to involve human vapers (as done in [41]) and consult the information provided by manufacturers of the devices, as well as information contained in vaping magazines containing consumer opinions and experiences on recommendation of power, voltage and resistance, as well as the appropriate vaping behavior. This information is very useful, not only for comprehending the parameters associated with a safe and pleasant usage, but also for concrete technical advice on the experimental design to undertake realistic testing of the devices, contributing to improve the standards of EC testing in a laboratory. By ignoring this data researchers run the risk of conducting unrealistic experiments whose outcome would be an aerosol that real life users could find too hot and repellent. Such laboratory studies do not contribute to a public health benefit to the end user.

Our findings in this review point out to the pressing necessity to upgrade current laboratory standards, created for early devices and clearly inappropriate for efficiently testing the wide diversity of presently available devices. An upgraded standard needs to comply with real life usage of the devices and manufacturer specifications, as demanded by the Tobacco Product Directive (TPD) [82] of the European Union. Besides considering the appropriate puffing protocols that accommodate the diversity consumer usage as best as possible (considering useful technical guidelines discussed in [30,31,83,84]), it must evaluate tasting and sensorial quality of the generated aerosol by incorporating end users into the experimental protocol. An upgraded standard would not only be helpful to avoid some of the shortcomings in the studies we reviewed, but would be highly beneficial to all stakeholders: consumers, regulators, health professionals, governments and the vaping and tobacco industries.

Emerging "fourth generation" disposable pod devices provide another interesting avenue for future research. Their ease of usage and maintenance, together with their inexpensive pricing, explain the increasing prevalence of these devices in the vapor market [85], with justified concern for their increasing popularity among teenagers [86,87]. While there is already research on their flavorings [88] and organic byproducts in their aerosol emissions [89], a proper analysis of metal content in these emissions requires a thorough examination of their coils, plastic and metallic parts (solders, wires). Further laboratory testing of these devices is essential to provide informed safety guidelines to consumers, health professionals and regulators.

As future work we also aim at replicating some of the reviewed studies to verify the existence of overheating, testing also the same devices under more realistic conditions, as well as the compliance with the parameters of the optimal regime defined by Soulet et al. [31,32]. We also aim at reviewing laboratory studies on non-metallic trace compounds: organic byproducts [65,90], carbon monoxide [40,91,92] and free radicals [93–98], whose presence in EC aerosol emissions is also dependent on increasing device power and coil temperature in analogous manner as with metals. We believe the present review contributes to improve testing standards that are consistent with normal device usage and essential to assess objectively the public health impact of vaping products.

Supplementary Materials: The following supporting information can be downloaded at: https://www.mdpi.com/article/10.3390/toxics10090510/s1.

Author Contributions: Conceptualization, R.A.S. and S.S.; methodology, R.A.S. and S.S.; software, R.A.S. and S.S.; validation, R.A.S. and S.S.; formal analysis, R.A.S. and S.S.; investigation, R.A.S. and S.S.; resources, R.A.S. and S.S.; writing-original draft preparation, R.A.S. and S.S.; writing-review and editing, R.A.S. and S.S.; visualization, R.A.S. and S.S.; supervision, R.A.S. and S.S. All authors have read and agreed to the published version of the manuscript.

Funding: R.A.S. received no external funding. S.S. is employed by Ingésciences. Ingésciences had received funding from région Nouvelle Aquitaine. Ingésciences has never received funding from the tobacco industry and its third parties.

Institutional Review Board Statement: Not applicable.

Informed Consent Statement: Not applicable.

Data Availability Statement: Not applicable.

Conflicts of Interest: R.A.S. declares no conflict of interest. S.S. declares that Ingésciences is completely independent of the tobacco industry and its third parties.

Abbreviations

The following abbreviations and units are used in this manuscript:

EC	Electronic Cigarette
HPHC	Harmful and Potentially Harmful Compounds
CO	Carbon Monoxide
ROS	Reactive Oxygen Species
CORESTA	Cooperation Centre for Scientific Research Relative to Tobacco
MTL	Mouth to Lung
DTL	Direct to Lung
TPD	Tobacco Product Directive
MEV	Mass of E-liquid Vaporized
PDE-ICH	Permissible Daily Exposure (International Council for Harmonization of Technical Requirements for Pharmaceuticals for Human Use)
MRL-ATSDR	Minimal Risk Level (Agency for Toxic Substances Disease Registry)
PEL-NIOSH	Permissible Exposure Level (National Institute of Occupational Safety and Health)
PEL-OSHA	Permissible Exposure Level (Occupational Safety and Health Agency)
NOAEL	No Observed Adverse Effect Level
PG	Propylene glycol
VG	Vegetable glycerine (glycerol)
ICP-MS	Inductively Coupled Plasma Mass Spectroscopy
ICP-OES	Induced Coupled Plasma Optical Emissions Spectroscopy
FDA	Food and Drug Agency,
PMTA	Pre-Market Tobacco Autorization
BLOD	Below Detection Limit
BLOQ	Below Quantification Limit
NDFB	Not Different From Blanks
EMA	European Medicine Agency
ADA	American Dentist Association
pg	picogram
ng	nanogram
µg	microgram
mg	milligram
g	gram
mL	milliliter
L	Litter
cm	centimeter
m	meter
h	hour
min	minute
s	second
Ω	Ohm
W	Watt
V	Volt
kPa	kilopascal

References

1. Amos, A.; Arnott, D.; Aveyard, P.; Bauld, L.; Bogdanovica, I.; Britton, J.; Chenoweth, M.; Collin, J.; Dockrell, M.; Hajek, P.; et al. *Nicotine without Smoke: Tobacco Harm Reduction*; Royal College of Physicians: London, UK, 2016.
2. Daynard, R. *Public Health Consequences of E-Cigarettes: A Consensus Study Report of the National Academies of Sciences, Engineering, and Medicine*; National Academy Press: Washington, DC, USA, 2018.
3. McNeill, A.; Brose, L.S.; Calder, R.; Bauld, L.; Robson, D. Evidence review of e-cigarettes and heated tobacco products 2018. *Rep. Comm. Public Health England. Lond. Public Health Engl.* **2018**, *6*. Available online: https://www.gov.uk/government/publications/e-cigarettes-and-heated-tobacco-products-evidence-review (accessed on 8 February 2022).

4. Pisinger, C.; Døssing, M. A systematic review of health effects of electronic cigarettes. *Prev. Med.* **2014**, *69*, 248–260. [CrossRef] [PubMed]
5. Na, C.J.; Jo, S.H.; Kim, K.H.; Sohn, J.R.; Son, Y.S. The transfer characteristics of heavy metals in electronic cigarette liquid. *Environ. Res.* **2019**, *174*, 152–159. [CrossRef] [PubMed]
6. Zervas, E.; Matsouki, N.; Kyriakopoulos, G.; Poulopoulos, S.; Ioannides, T.; Katsaounou, P. Transfer of metals in the liquids of electronic cigarettes. *Inhal. Toxicol.* **2020**, *32*, 240–248. [CrossRef] [PubMed]
7. Potter, N.A.; Meltzer, G.Y.; Avenbuan, O.N.; Raja, A.; Zelikoff, J.T. Particulate matter and associated metals: A link with neurotoxicity and mental health. *Atmosphere* **2021**, *12*, 425. [CrossRef]
8. Jaishankar, M.; Tseten, T.; Anbalagan, N.; Mathew, B.B.; Beeregowda, K.N. Toxicity, mechanism and health effects of some heavy metals. *Interdiscip. Toxicol.* **2014**, *7*, 60. [CrossRef] [PubMed]
9. Zhao, D.; Aravindakshan, A.; Hilpert, M.; Olmedo, P.; Rule, A.M.; Navas-Acien, A.; Aherrera, A. Metal/metalloid levels in electronic cigarette liquids, aerosols, and human biosamples: A systematic review. *Environ. Health Perspect.* **2020**, *128*, 036001. [CrossRef]
10. Olmedo, P.; Goessler, W.; Tanda, S.; Grau-Perez, M.; Jarmul, S.; Aherrera, A.; Chen, R.; Hilpert, M.; Cohen, J.E.; Navas-Acien, A.; et al. Metal concentrations in e-cigarette liquid and aerosol samples: The contribution of metallic coils. *Environ. Health Perspect.* **2018**, *126*, 027010. [CrossRef]
11. Zhao, D.; Navas-Acien, A.; Ilievski, V.; Slavkovich, V.; Olmedo, P.; Adria-Mora, B.; Domingo-Relloso, A.; Aherrera, A.; Kleiman, N.J.; Rule, A.M.; et al. Metal concentrations in electronic cigarette aerosol: Effect of open-system and closed-system devices and power settings. *Environ. Res.* **2019**, *174*, 125–134. [CrossRef]
12. Zhao, D.; Ilievski, V.; Olmedo, P.; Domingo-Relloso, A.; Rule, A.M.; Kleiman, N.J.; Navas-Acien, A.; Holpert, M. Effects of e-liquid flavor, nicotine content, and puff duration on metal emissions from electronic cigarettes. *Environ. Res.* **2022**, *204*, 112270. [CrossRef] [PubMed]
13. Liu, Q.; Huang, C.; Le, X.C. Arsenic species in electronic cigarettes: Determination and potential health risk. *J. Environ. Sci.* **2020**, *91*, 168–176. [CrossRef]
14. Halstead, M.; Gray, N.; Gonzalez-Jimenez, N.; Fresquez, M.; Valentin-Blasini, L.; Watson, C.; Pappas, R.S. Analysis of toxic metals in electronic cigarette aerosols using a novel trap design. *J. Anal. Toxicol.* **2020**, *44*, 149–155. [CrossRef] [PubMed]
15. Gray, N.; Halstead, M.; Valentin-Blasini, L.; Watson, C.; Pappas, R.S. Toxic metals in liquid and aerosol from pod-type electronic cigarettes. *J. Anal. Toxicol.* **2022**, *46*, 69–75. [CrossRef]
16. Kapiamba, K.F.; Hao, W.; Adom, S.; Liu, W.; Huang, Y.W.; Wang, Y. Examining metal contents in primary and secondhand aerosols released by electronic cigarettes. *Chem. Res. Toxicol.* **2022**, *35*, 954–962. [CrossRef] [PubMed]
17. Chen, X.; Bailey, P.C.; Yang, C.; Hiraki, B.; Oldham, M.J.; Gillman, I.G. Targeted characterization of the chemical composition of juul systems aerosol and comparison with 3r4f reference cigarettes and iqos heat sticks. *Separations* **2021**, *8*, 168.
18. Williams, M.; Li, J.; Talbot, P. Effects of model, method of collection, and topography on chemical elements and metals in the aerosol of tank-style electronic cigarettes. *Sci. Rep.* **2019**, *9*, 13969. [CrossRef] [PubMed]
19. Kim, S.A.; Smith, S.; Beauchamp, C.; Song, Y.; Chiang, M.; Giuseppetti, A.; Frikhtbein, S.; Ian Shaffer, I.; Wilhide, J.; Routkevitch, D.; et al. Cariogenic potential of sweet flavors in electronic-cigarette liquids. *PLoS ONE* **2018**, *13*, e0203717.
20. Beauval, N.; Antherieu, S.; Soyez, M.; Gengler, N.; Grova, N.; Howsam, M.; Hardy, E.M.; Fischer, M.; Appenzeller, B.M.; Goossens, J.F.; et al. Chemical evaluation of electronic cigarettes: Multicomponent analysis of liquid refills and their corresponding aerosols. *J. Anal. Toxicol.* **2017**, *41*, 670–678. [CrossRef]
21. Palazzolo, D.L.; Crow, A.P.; Nelson, J.M.; Johnson, R.A. Trace metals derived from electronic cigarette (ECIG) generated aerosol: Potential problem of ECIG devices that contain nickel. *Front. Physiol.* **2017**, *7*, 663. [CrossRef]
22. Williams, M.; Bozhilov, K.; Ghai, S.; Talbot, P. Elements including metals in the atomizer and aerosol of disposable electronic cigarettes and electronic hookahs. *PLoS ONE* **2017**, *12*, e0175430. [CrossRef]
23. Williams, M.; To, A.; Bozhilov, K.; Talbot, P. Strategies to reduce tin and other metals in electronic cigarette aerosol. *PLoS ONE* **2015**, *10*, e0138933. [CrossRef]
24. Williams, M.; Villarreal, A.; Bozhilov, K.; Lin, S.; Talbot, P. Metal and silicate particles including nanoparticles are present in electronic cigarette cartomizer fluid and aerosol. *PLoS ONE* **2013**, *8*, e57987.
25. Mikheev, V.B.; Brinkman, M.C.; Granville, C.A.; Gordon, S.M.; Clark, P.I. Real-time measurement of electronic cigarette aerosol size distribution and metals content analysis. *Nicotine Tob. Res.* **2016**, *18*, 1895–1902. [CrossRef]
26. Goniewicz, M.L.; Knysak, J.; Gawron, M.; Kosmider, L.; Sobczak, A.; Kurek, J.; Prokopowicz, A.; Jablonska-Czapla, M.; Rosik-Dulewska, C.; Havel, C.; et al. Levels of Selected Carcinogens and Toxicants in Vapour from Electronic Cigarettes. *Tob. Control.* **2014**, *23*, 133–139. Available online: http://xxx.lanl.gov/abs/https://tobaccocontrol.bmj.com/content/23/2/133.full.pdf (accessed on 17 February 2022). [CrossRef]
27. CORESTA Recommended Method No 81, June 2015. Routine Analytical Machine for E-cigarette Aerosol Generation and Collection – Definitions and Standard Conditions. Available online: https://www.coresta.org/routine-analytical-machine-e-cigarette-aerosol-generation-and-collection-definitions-and-standard (accessed on 12 May 2022).
28. Marian, C.; O'Connor, R.J.; Djordjevic, M.V.; Rees, V.W.; Hatsukami, D.K.; Shields, P.G. Reconciling human smoking behavior and machine smoking patterns: Implications for understanding smoking behavior and the impact on laboratory studies. *Cancer Epidemiol. Biomarkers Prev.* **2009**, *18*, 3305–3320. [CrossRef]

29. Tobin, M.J.; Schneider, A.W.; Sackner, M.A. Breathing pattern during and after smoking cigarettes. *Clin. Sci.* **1982**, *63*, 473–483. [CrossRef]
30. Soulet, S.; Duquesne, M.; Pairaud, C.; Toutain, J. Highlighting specific features to reduce chemical and thermal risks of electronic cigarette use through a technical classification of devices. *Appl. Sci.* **2021**, *11*, 5254. [CrossRef]
31. Soulet, S.; Duquesne, M.; Toutain, J.; Pairaud, C.; Mercury, M. Impact of vaping regimens on electronic cigarette efficiency. *Int. J. Environ. Res. Public Health* **2019**, *16*, 4753. [CrossRef]
32. Soulet, S.; Duquesne, M.; Toutain, J.; Pairaud, C.; Lalo, H. Influence of coil power ranges on the e-liquid consumption in vaping devices. *Int. J. Environ. Res. Public Health* **2018**, *15*, 1853. [CrossRef]
33. Floyd, E.; Greenlee, S.; Oni, T.; Sadhasivam, B.; Queimado, L. The effect of flow rate on a third-generation Sub-Ohm tank electronic nicotine delivery system, comparison of CORESTA flow rates to more realistic flow rates. *Int. J. Environ. Res. Public Health* **2021**, *18*, 7535. [CrossRef]
34. Gillman, I.; Kistler, K.; Stewart, E.; Paolantonio, A. Effect of variable power levels on the yield of total aerosol mass and formation of aldehydes in e-cigarette aerosols. *Regul. Toxicol. Pharmacol.* **2016**, *75*, 58–65. [CrossRef]
35. Farsalinos, K.E.; Gillman, G. Carbonyl emissions in e-cigarette aerosol: A systematic review and methodological considerations. *Front. Physiol.* **2018**, *8*, 1119. [CrossRef] [PubMed]
36. Zelinkova, Z.; Wenzl, T. Influence of battery power setting on carbonyl emissions from electronic cigarettes. *Tob. Induc. Dis.* **2020**, *18*, 1. [CrossRef]
37. Geiss, O.; Ivana, B.; Barrero-Moreno, J. Correlation of volatile carbonyl yields emitted by e-cigarettes with the temperature of the heating coil and the perceived sensorial quality of the generated vapours. *Int. J. Hyg. Environ. Health* **2015**, *219*, 1268–1277.
38. Beauval, N.; Verriele, M.; Garat, A.; Fronval, I.; Dusautoir, R.; Anthérieu, S.; Garçon, G.; Lo-Guidice, J.M.; Allorge, D.; Locoge, N. Influence of puffing conditions on the carbonyl composition of e-cigarette aerosols. *Int. J. Hyg. Environ. Health* **2019**, *222*, 136–146. [CrossRef] [PubMed]
39. Li, Y.; Burns, A.E.; Tran, L.N.; Abellar, K.A.; Poindexter, M.; Li, X.; Madl, A.K.; Pinkerton, K.E.; Nguyen, T.B. Impact of e-liquid composition, coil temperature, and puff topography on the aerosol chemistry of electronic cigarettes. *Chem. Res. Toxicol.* **2021**, *34*, 1640–1654. [CrossRef]
40. Son, Y.; Bhattarai, C.; Samburova, V.; Khlystov, A. Carbonyls and carbon monoxide emissions from electronic cigarettes affected by device type and use patterns. *Int. J. Environ. Res. Public Health* **2020**, *17*, 2767. [CrossRef] [PubMed]
41. Visser, W.F.; Krüsemann, E.J.; Klerx, W.N.; Boer, K.; Weibolt, N.; Talhout, R. Improving the analysis of e-cigarette emissions: Detecting human "dry puff" conditions in a laboratory as validated by a panel of experienced vapers. *Int. J. Environ. Res. Public Health* **2021**, *18*, 11520. [CrossRef]
42. Aherrera, A.; Olmedo, P.; Grau-Perez, M.; Tanda, S.; Goessler, W.; Jarmul, S.; Chen, R.; Cohen, J.E.; Rule, A.M.; Navas-Acien, A. The association of e-cigarette use with exposure to nickel and chromium: A preliminary study of non-invasive biomarkers. *Environ. Res.* **2017**, *159*, 313–320. [CrossRef]
43. Prokopowicz, A.; Sobczak, A.; Szdzuj, J.; Grygoyć, K.; Kośmider, L. Metal concentration assessment in the urine of cigarette smokers who switched to electronic cigarettes: A pilot study. *Int. J. Environ. Res. Public Health* **2020**, *17*, 1877. [CrossRef]
44. Olmedo, P.; Rodrigo, L.; Grau-Pérez, M.; Hilpert, M.; Navas-Acién, A.; Téllez-Plaza, M.; Pla, A.; Gil, F. Metal exposure and biomarker levels among e-cigarette users in Spain. *Environ. Res.* **2021**, *202*, 111667. [CrossRef]
45. Sussman, R.A.; Golberstein, E.; Polosa, R. Modeling aerial transmission of pathogens (including the SARS-CoV-2 Virus) through aerosol emissions from e-cigarettes. *Appl. Sci.* **2021**, *11*, 6355. [CrossRef]
46. Higenbottam, T.; Feyeraband, C.; Clark, T. Cigarette smoke inhalation and the acute airway response. *Thorax* **1980**, *35*, 246–254. [CrossRef] [PubMed]
47. Prasad, K. A review of electronic cigarette use behaviour studies. *Beitr. Tab. Int. Contrib. Tob. Res.* **2018**, *28*, 81–92.
48. Robinson, R.; Hensel, E.; Morabito, P.; Roundtree, K. Electronic cigarette topography in the natural environment. *PLoS ONE* **2015**, *10*, e0129296.
49. Robinson, R.; Hensel, E.; Roundtree, K.; Difrancesco, A.; Nonnemaker, J.; Lee, Y. Week long topography study of young adults using electronic cigarettes in their natural environment. *PLoS ONE* **2016**, *11*, e0164038. [CrossRef]
50. Dautzenberg, B.; Bricard, D. Real-time characterization of e-cigarettes use: The 1 million puffs study. *J. Addict. Res. Ther* **2015**, *6*, 4172. [CrossRef]
51. Kośmider, L.; Jackson, A.; Leigh, N.; O'connor, R.; Goniewicz, M.L. Circadian puffing behavior and topography among e-cigarette users. *Tob. Regul. Sci.* **2018**, *4*, 41–49. [CrossRef]
52. Dawkins, L.; Cox, S.; Goniewicz, M.; McRobbie, H.; Kimber, C.; Doig, M.; Kośmider, L. 'Real-world' compensatory behaviour with low nicotine concentration e-liquid: Subjective effects and nicotine, acrolein and formaldehyde exposure. *Addiction* **2018**, *113*, 1874–1882. [CrossRef]
53. Cox, S.; Goniewicz, M.L.; Kosmider, L.; McRobbie, H.; Kimber, C.; Dawkins, L. The time course of compensatory puffing with an electronic cigarette: Secondary analysis of real-world puffing data with high and low nicotine concentration under fixed and adjustable power settings. *Nicotine Tob. Res.* **2021**, *23*, 1153–1159. [CrossRef]
54. Cox, S.; Kośmider, L.; McRobbie, H.; Goniewicz, M.; Kimber, C.; Doig, M.; Dawkins, L. E-cigarette puffing patterns associated with high and low nicotine e-liquid strength: Effects on toxicant and carcinogen exposure. *BMC Public Health* **2016**, *16*, 999. [CrossRef]

55. ICH Guideline Q3D (R1) on Elemental Impurities. 2019. Available online: https://www.ema.europa.eu/en/documents/scientific-guideline/international-conference-harmonisation-technical-requirements-registration-pharmaceuticals-human-use_en-32.pdf (accessed on 10 February 2022).
56. E-Cigarettes and E-Liquids—Limits for Chemicals Basis for Discussion. Technical Report. 2019. Available online: https://www.anec.eu/images/Publications/position-papers/Chemicals/ANEC-PT-2019-CEG-005.pdf (accessed on 11 February 2022).
57. Agency for Toxic Substances and Disease Registry. Available online: https://wwwn.cdc.gov/TSP/substances/ToxHealthReferences.aspx (accessed on 11 February 2022).
58. Pocket Guide to Chemical Hazards, The National Institute for Occupational Safety and Health (NIOSH). 2016. Available online: https://www.cdc.gov/niosh/npg/pgintrod.html (accessed on 11 February 2022).
59. Soulet, S.; Duquesne, M.; Toutain, J.; Pairaud, C.; Lalo, H. Experimental Method of Emission Generation Calibration Based on Reference Liquids Characterization. *Int. J. Environ. Res. Public Health* **2019**, *16*, 2262. [CrossRef] [PubMed]
60. Zhao, T.; Shu, S.; Guo, Q.; Zhu, Y. Effects of design parameters and puff topography on heating coil temperature and mainstream aerosols in electronic cigarettes. *Atmos. Environ.* **2016**, *134*, 61–69. [CrossRef]
61. Robinson, R.J.; Eddingsaas, N.C.; DiFrancesco, A.G.; Jayasekera, S.; Hensel Jr, E.C. A framework to investigate the impact of topography and product characteristics on electronic cigarette emissions. *PLoS ONE* **2018**, *13*, e0206341. [CrossRef] [PubMed]
62. Talih, S.; Salman, R.; Karam, E.; El-Hourani, M.; El-Hage, R.; Karaoghlanian, N.; El-Hellani, A.; Saliba, N.; Shihadeh, A. Hot Wires and Film Boiling: Another Look at Carbonyl Formation in Electronic Cigarettes. *Chem. Res. Toxicol.* **2020**, *33*, 2172–2180. [CrossRef]
63. Olmedo, P.; Navas-Acien, A.; Hess, C.; Jarmul, S.; Rule, A. A direct method for e-cigarette aerosol sample collection. *Environ. Res.* **2016**, *149*, 151–156. [CrossRef]
64. Hess, C.A.; Olmedo, P.; Navas-Acien, A.; Goessler, W.; Cohen, J.E.; Rule, A.M. E-cigarettes as a source of toxic and potentially carcinogenic metals. *Environ. Res.* **2017**, *152*, 221–225. [CrossRef] [PubMed]
65. Yan, B.; Zagorevski, D.; Ilievski, V.; Kleiman, N.J.; Re, D.B.; Navas-Acien, A.; Hilpert, M. Identification of newly formed toxic chemicals in E-cigarette aerosols with Orbitrap mass spectrometry and implications on E-cigarette control. *Eur. J. Mass Spectrom.* **2021**, 14690667211040207. [CrossRef]
66. Farsalinos, K.E.; Rodu, B. Metal emissions from e-cigarettes: A risk assessment analysis of a recently-published study. *Inhal. Toxicol.* **2018**, *30*, 321–326. [CrossRef]
67. Le Petit Vapoteur. 2020. Available online: https://www.lepetitvapoteur.com/fr/resistance-clearomiseur/2820-resistance-tfv8-baby.html (accessed on 18 May 2022).
68. Grégory, D.; Parmentier, E.A.; Irene, T.; Ruth, S. Tracing the composition of single e-cigarette aerosol droplets in situ by laser-trapping and Raman scattering. *Sci. Rep.* **2020**, *10*, 1–8.
69. Talih, S.; Balhas, Z.; Salman, R.; Karaoghlanian, N.; Shihadeh, A. "Direct dripping": A high-temperature, high-formaldehyde emission electronic cigarette use method. *Nicotine Tob. Res.* **2016**, *18*, 453–459. [CrossRef]
70. St. Helen, G.; Havel, C.; Dempsey, D.A.; Jacob III, P.; Benowitz, N.L. Nicotine delivery, retention and pharmacokinetics from various electronic cigarettes. *Addiction* **2016**, *111*, 535–544. [CrossRef] [PubMed]
71. Pappas, R.S.; Gray, N.; Halstead, M.; Valentin-Blasini, L.; Watson, C. Toxic metal-containing particles in aerosols from pod-type electronic cigarettes. *J. Anal. Toxicol.* **2021**, *45*, 337–347. [CrossRef] [PubMed]
72. Williams, M.; Talbot, P. Design features in multiple generations of electronic cigarette atomizers. *Int. J. Environ. Res. Public Health* **2019**, *16*, 2904. [CrossRef]
73. Williams, M.; Talbot, P. Variability among electronic cigarettes in the pressure drop, airflow rate, and aerosol production. *Nicotine Tob. Res.* **2011**, *13*, 1276–1283. [CrossRef] [PubMed]
74. Farsalinos, K.E.; Voudris, V.; Poulas, K. Are metals emitted from electronic cigarettes a reason for health concern? A risk-assessment analysis of currently available literature. *Int. J. Environ. Res. Public Health* **2015**, *12*, 5215–5232. [CrossRef]
75. Morton-Bermea, O.; Garza-Galindo, R.; Hernández-Álvarez, E.; Amador-Mu noz, O.; Garcia-Arreola, M.E.; Ordo nez-Godínez, S.L.; Beramendi-Orosco, L.; Santos-Medina, G.L.; Miranda, J.; Rosas-Pérez, I. Recognition of the importance of geogenic sources in the content of metals in PM2. 5 collected in the Mexico City Metropolitan Area. *Environ. Monit. Assess.* **2018**, *190*, 1–18. [CrossRef]
76. Assessment of Within-package and Lot-to-Lot Variability Associated with Quartz Collection Pads in the Determination of Metals in Aerosol. Available online: https://www.coresta.org/abstracts/assessment-within-package-and-lot-lot-variability-associated-quartz-collection-pads (accessed on 5 August 2022).
77. Pappas, R.S.; Fresquez, M.R.; Martone, N.; Watson, C.H. Toxic metal concentrations in mainstream smoke from cigarettes available in the USA. *J. Anal. Toxicol.* **2014**, *38*, 204–211. [CrossRef]
78. Gaur, S.; Agnihotri, R. Health effects of trace metals in electronic cigarette aerosols a systematic review. *Biol. Trace Elem. Res.* **2019**, *188*, 295–315. [CrossRef]
79. Fowles, J.; Barreau, T.; Wu, N. Cancer and non-cancer risk concerns from metals in electronic cigarette liquids and aerosols. *Int. J. Environ. Res. Public Health* **2020**, *17*, 2146. [CrossRef] [PubMed]
80. Hubbs, A.F.; Cummings, K.J.; McKernan, L.T.; Dankovic, D.A.; Park, R.M.; Kreiss, K. Comment on Farsalinos et al.,"Evaluation of electronic cigarette liquids and aerosol for the presence of selected inhalation toxins". *Nicotine Tob. Res.* **2015**, *17*, 1288–1289. [CrossRef]

81. Farsalinos, K.E.; Kistler, K.A.; Gillman, G.; Voudris, V. Why WE Consider The Niosh-Proposed Safety Limits For Diacetyl And Acetyl Propionyl Appropriate In The Risk Assessment Of Electronic Cigarette Liquid Use: A response to Hubbs et al. *Nicotine Tob. Res.* **2015**, *17*, 1290–1291. [CrossRef] [PubMed]
82. Directive 2014/40/EU of the European Parliament and of the Council of 3 April 2014 on the Approximation of the Laws, Regulations and Administrative Provisions of the Member States Concerning the Manufacture, Presentation and Sale of Tobacco and Related Products. Directive 2001/37/EC (OJ L 127, 29.4.2014, p. 56). 2014. Available online: https://eur-lex.europa.eu/legal-content/EN/TXT/PDF/?uri=CELEX:32014L0040 (accessed on 8 May 2022).
83. No. 28—Technical Guide for Setting Method LOD and LOQ Values for the Determination of Metals in E-Liquid and E-Vapour Aerosol by ICP-MS November 2020 Ref. EVAP-210-CTG-2. Available online: https://www.coresta.org/technical-guide-setting-method-lod-and-loq-values-determination-metals-e-liquid-and-e-vapour-aerosol (accessed on 7 August 2022).
84. EVAP. Available online: https://www.coresta.org/groups/e-vapour (accessed on 7 August 2022).
85. Galimov, A.; Leventhal, A.; Meza, L.; Unger, J.B.; Huh, J.; Baezconde-Garbanati, L.; Sussman, S.Y. Prevalence of disposable pod use and consumer preference for e-cigarette product characteristics among vape shop customers in Southern California: A cross-sectional study. *BMJ Open* **2021**, *11*, e049604. [CrossRef] [PubMed]
86. Park-Lee, E.; Ren, C.; Sawdey, M.D.; Gentzke, A.S.; Cornelius, M.; Jamal, A.; Cullen, K.A. Notes from the field: E-cigarette use among middle and high school students—National Youth Tobacco Survey, United States, 2021. *Morb. Mortal. Wkly. Rep.* **2021**, *70*, 1387. [CrossRef] [PubMed]
87. Williams, P.J.; Cheeseman, H.; Arnott, D.; Bunce, L.; Hopkinson, N.S.; Laverty, A. Use of tobacco and e-cigarettes among youth in Great Britain in 2022: Analysis of a cross-sectional survey. *medRxiv* **2022**. [CrossRef]
88. Omaiye, E.E.; Luo, W.; McWhirter, K.J.; Pankow, J.F.; Talbot, P. Disposable Puff bar electronic cigarettes: Chemical composition and toxicity of e-liquids and a synthetic coolant. *Chem. Res. Toxicol.* **2022**, *35*, 1344–1358. [CrossRef]
89. Talih, S.; Salman, R.; Soule, E.; El-Hage, R.; Karam, E.; Karaoghlanian, N.; El-Hellani, A.; Saliba, N.; Shihadeh, A. Electrical features, liquid composition and toxicant emissions from 'pod-mod'-like disposable electronic cigarettes. *Tob. Control.* **2022**, *3*, 667–670. [CrossRef]
90. Tehrani, M.W.; Newmeyer, M.N.; Rule, A.M.; Prasse, C. Characterizing the chemical landscape in commercial e-cigarette liquids and aerosols by liquid chromatography–high-resolution mass spectrometry. *Chem. Res. Toxicol.* **2021**, *34*, 2216–2226. [CrossRef]
91. Casebolt, R.; Cook, S.J.; Islas, A.; Brown, A.; Castle, K.; Dutcher, D.D. Carbon monoxide concentration in mainstream E-cigarette emissions measured with diode laser spectroscopy. *Tob. Control.* **2019**, *29*, 652–655. [CrossRef]
92. El-Hellani, A.; Al-Moussawi, S.; El-Hage, R.; Talih, S.; Salman, R.; Shihadeh, A.; Saliba, N.A. Carbon Monoxide and Small Hydrocarbon Emissions from Sub-ohm Electronic Cigarettes. *Chem. Res. Toxicol.* **2019**, *32*, 312. [CrossRef]
93. Goel, R.; Durand, E.; Trushin, N.; Prokopczyk, B.; Foulds, J.; Elias, R.J.; Richie Jr, J.P. Highly reactive free radicals in electronic cigarette aerosols. *Chem. Res. Toxicol.* **2015**, *28*, 1675–1677. [CrossRef]
94. Bitzer, Z.T.; Goel, R.; Reilly, S.M.; Elias, R.J.; Silakov, A.; Foulds, J.; Muscat, J.; Richie Jr, J.P. Effect of flavoring chemicals on free radical formation in electronic cigarette aerosols. *Free Radic. Biol. Med.* **2018**, *120*, 72–79. [CrossRef] [PubMed]
95. Bitzer, Z.T.; Goel, R.; Reilly, S.M.; Foulds, J.; Muscat, J.; Elias, R.J.; Richie Jr, J.P. Effects of solvent and temperature on free radical formation in electronic cigarette aerosols. *Chem. Res. Toxicol.* **2018**, *31*, 4–12. [CrossRef] [PubMed]
96. Zhao, J.; Zhang, Y.; Sisler, J.D.; Shaffer, J.; Leonard, S.S.; Morris, A.M.; Qian, Y.; Bello, D.; Demokritou, P. Assessment of reactive oxygen species generated by electronic cigarettes using acellular and cellular approaches. *J. Hazard. Mater.* **2018**, *344*, 549–557. [CrossRef] [PubMed]
97. Haddad, C.; Salman, R.; El-Hellani, A.; Talih, S.; Shihadeh, A.; Saliba, N.A. Reactive oxygen species emissions from supra-and sub-ohm electronic cigarettes. *J. Anal. Toxicol.* **2019**, *43*, 45–50. [CrossRef] [PubMed]
98. Son, Y.; Mishin, V.; Laskin, J.D.; Mainelis, G.; Wackowski, O.A.; Delnevo, C.; Schwander, S.; Khlystov, A.; Samburova, V.; Meng, Q. Hydroxyl radicals in e-cigarette vapor and e-vapor oxidative potentials under different vaping patterns. *Chem. Res. Toxicol.* **2019**, *32*, 1087–1095. [CrossRef] [PubMed]

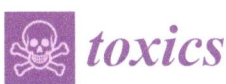

Review

The Effects of E-Cigarette Aerosol on Oral Cavity Cells and Tissues: A Narrative Review

Paweł Szumilas [1], Aleksandra Wilk [2], Kamila Szumilas [3],* and Beata Karakiewicz [1]

1. Department of Social Medicine and Public Health, Pomeranian Medical University, 71-210 Szczecin, Poland; pawel.szumilas@pum.edu.pl (P.S.); beata.karakiewicz@pum.edu.pl (B.K.)
2. Department of Histology and Embryology, Pomeranian Medical University, 70-111 Szczecin, Poland; aleksandra.wilk@pum.edu.pl
3. Department of Physiology, Pomeranian Medical University, 70-111 Szczecin, Poland
* Correspondence: kamila.szumilas@pum.edu.pl

Abstract: A wealth of research has comprehensively documented the harmful effects of traditional cigarette smoking and nicotine on human health. The lower rate of exposure to harmful chemicals and toxic substances offered by alternative electronic smoking devices (e-cigarettes, vaping, etc.) has made these methods of smoking popular, especially among adolescents and young adults, and they are regarded frequently as safer than regular cigarettes. During vaporization of these so-called e-liquids, toxins, carcinogens and various other chemical substances may be released and inhaled by the user. Data on the potential human health effect attendant on exposure to e-vapor are based mainly on animal and in vitro studies. The oral tissues are the first locus of direct interaction with the components of the inhaled vapor. However, the short-term as well as long-term effects of the exposure are not known. The aim of the review is to briefly present data on the effects of the chemical components and toxins of e-cigarette vapor on oral cavity cells and tissues of oral health.

Keywords: e-cigarettes; e-aerosol; chemical components; toxins; microbiome; saliva; oral cavity tissues

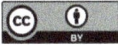

1. Introduction

Despite there being extensive information available on the harmfulness of conventional cigarette smoking, electronic cigarettes (e-cigarettes) are regarded as a safer alternative, which are particularly popular among both adults, young adults and teens, and their use has increased rapidly [1]. Furthermore, waterpipe and cigar smoking are also alternatives to traditional smoking. A very high prevalence of smoking indicates that there is a need for smoking cessation programs, access to effective quitting treatments and mass media campaigns to diminish smoking among the youth [2]. The results from the systematic review and meta analysis performed by O'Brien group (2021) indicated that e-cigarette use in Europe and North America by teenagers correlates with the initiation of conventional smoking [1]. It was observed that vaping can be a reason for relapse into traditional smoking [3]. Moreover, it was found that third-generation electronic cigarettes may cause adverse effects in the oral cavity, and normal e-cigarette use, which involves repeated use of the same atomizer to generate aerosol, may enhance the potential toxic effects of third-generation e-cigarettes [4].

Similar results were observed among eastern European populations; additionally, a higher prevalence of e-cigarettes was recognized among males, adolescents and young adults within populations of countries in this part of the Europe [5]. In Poland, there have been studies aimed at assessing patterns of e-cigarette use and comparing nicotine dependence among cigarette and e-cigarette users in a group of highly educated young adults. The findings from two representative groups suggested that e-cigarettes may have a higher addictive potential than traditional cigarettes among young adults [6]. The next studies performed in five Polish Universities with 7324 participants showed that e-cigarette use among young adults was significantly higher in correlation to the general population [7].

Most traditional cigarette smokers who quit smoking believe e-cigarettes to be less harmful than regular cigarettes. However, the statement that e-cigarette use helps users to quit smoking is highly controversial [8].

The use of e-cigarettes (also known as "vaping") has thus seen an unprecedented increase worldwide [9]. There are four generations of e-cigarettes, all of them are battery-operated devices and cartridge-based products containing fluid with varying levels of nicotine and flavouring and several toxicants as heavy metals [10–12].

While the harmful effects of traditional cigarette smoking on human health is well researched, knowledge of the effects of exposition to e-aerosol is limited, and above all there is a lack of long-term studies. The first contact of the various chemicals inhaled with the e-aerosol takes place in the oral cavity, and conclusions on the effects of this interaction come mainly from animal or in vitro studies. Additionally, conflicting results have been reported, corresponding to the various device and e-liquid combinations and different methods of study [13]. Moreover, together with the increase in EDNS popularity, many accidents were reported connected with burns of patients with various degrees as a result of e-cigarette explosions, including injury of the oral cavity [14,15]. The aim of this review is thus to present the current knowledge of the influence of the toxic and chemical components of e-cigarette aerosols on periodontal tissues and oral health. We aimed to examine articles and reports that we have evaluated, compared and described. MEDLINE, EMBASE, PUBMED, internet websites of research articles and reference lists were searched to identify articles for inclusion. Descriptive analysis was conducted.

2. Chemical Components and Toxins of E-Cigarette Aerosol

Vapes, vaping, vaporizers, vape pens, electronic cigarettes, e-cigarettes and e-cigs are synonyms used to describe electronic nicotine delivery systems (ENDS), which are non-combustible tobacco products. In these products, a solution of "e-liquid" held in a cartridge is heated to a temperature of 100–300 and over to 350 °C depending on the ENDS category, e-liquid composition and power output [16,17] to create an aerosol that is inhaled by the users [18,19]. Standard electronic cigarette liquid is typically composed without/with nicotine (at different doses, from 0 to 24 mg/mL), water, propylene glycol (PG), vegetable glycerin (VG) or glycerol and flavouring constituents [20]. In general, it contains at least three major ingredients: psychoactive agents as nicotine, solvents and flavouring compounds. Nicotine in aqueous solution can be found in three forms as diprotonated, monoprotonated and unprotonated. The content of diprotonated nicotine is low and its presence does not matter much in the e-fluid [21]. Therefore, two of the three forms are taken under consideration. The unprotonated—nicotine freebase is easily vaporized form, and the protonated form—nicotine salt is present in e-liquid as a product of combination of nicotine and different acids, including glycolic, pyruvic, lactic, levulinic, fumaric, succinic, benzoic, salicylic, malic, tartaric and citric acids [22,23]. The unprotonated, freebase nicotine in e-liquid is used in traditional e-cigarettes, while the newer e-cigarette generation called "pod-mods", such as JUUL and others, use the protonated formulation derived from nicotine salts. In the e-fluid of the "pod-mods", nicotine can be found in concentrations 2 to 10 times higher than in traditional e-cigarettes, and in high concentration of 65.2 mg/L [21,22,24].

The main two constituents are present in commercial refill liquid and e-liquid, propylene glycol odorless and tasteless, and vegetable glycerin with a warm, sweet taste that are used as a solvent in e-liquid. The ratio of PG and VG content is perceived by the producers and users of e-cigarettes as an important determinant of their sensory characteristics [25]. Together with the propylene glycol, glycerol and nicotine, the e-liquid also contains various flavors [18]. The flavoring compounds have different names and aromas, such as strawberry, root beer, chai tea, chocolate, fresh watermelon, black currant, forest berries, cherry, and grape; this variety of flavors is one of the main factors that increases attraction for new users, especially for adolescents [26].

During e-liquid heating, aerosol is formed and the main components PG and VG can be disintegrated into hazardous toxic substances. The content and amount of which depend on the type of the device, brands and the smoking parameters. There are toxicants, such as carbonyls, formaldehyde, acetaldehyde, acrolein, crotonaldehyde, epoxides and glycidol in aerosol after the thermal decomposition of PG and VG. The products that are produced during the heating of fluid were divided into three groups: (i) thermal decomposition products derived from PG and VG; (ii) products that originated from other compounds; and (iii) products formed directly [18].

The study of Khlystov and Samburova (2016) with various e-cigarette brands indicated that during the heating of the flavouring compounds, the formation of aldehydes dominated, and these included formaldehyde, acetaldehyde and acrolein [26]. Other research has supported these results, with an emphasis on their potentially harmful effects for human health [27,28]. Nevertheless, multiple potentially harmful components, toxic metals and trace elements, e.g., aluminium, lead, mercury, zinc, carbonyls, epoxides, policyclic aromatic hydroxycarbons (PAHs) and pesticides were found in e-liquids and aerosols [29–33]. New methods used to estimate toxic metal-containing particles in e-aerosols of various pod-type systems are permitted to detect metal-containing particles such as chromium, zinc, iron, cooper, tin, and lead in various concentrations [34]. Recently, Tehrani et al. (2021) performed nontarget and quantitative analyses of e-liquids containing nicotine and generated e-aerosols from four of e-cigarettes: one disposable, two pod and one tank/mod to identify earlier unknown compounds. The liquid chromatography-high-resolution mass spectrometry (LC–HRMS) and chemical fingerprinting techniques used in the study permitted to observe that the number of detected compounds increased significantly in e-aerosol compared to e-liquid in three tested types of e-cigarettes [35].

It has also been showed that aerosols produced during the heating of e-liquids contain reactive oxygen species (ROS) and can produce oxidative stress through the presence of free radicals, NO [36,37] and carbonyls [38]. It can be suggested that falvoring chemicals and nicotine play an important role in the production of ROS [39–41], and the amount and proportions vary from product to product [42]. Nevertheless, the studies also showed that the levels of free radicals are lower in e-fluid and the gas phase of aerosol and heat-not-burn products compared to traditional cigarettes, and contain fewer toxic substances at lower concentrations [43]. An exposure of tissues to free radicals can result in damage to the proliferation, survival and inflammation pathways in cells [36].

It is well-documented that cigarette smoking is considered as a risk factor for inflammatory airway diseases and chronic obstructive disease [44,45]. The components of cigarette smoke can affect transcriptome alteration through chromatin remodelling and DNA methylation in the cells of the respiratory system. These changes are essential on the level of DNA and of specific genes [46]. The use of e-cigarettes can also be expected to have similar harmful effects. These inhaled substances are also classified as toxic and hazardous, particularly for the respiratory system, where they can disturb the oxidative–antioxidative balance (free radicals, irritants) [11,20,47]. e-cigarette aerosols may be expected to cause genotoxicity and immunotoxicity, but to lesser degrees than cigarette smoke. Some of the chemical substances detected in the fluid/aerosol of e-cigarettes or in heat-non-burn products are listed in Agents Classified by the IARC Monographs (Table 1) as cancerogenic to humans (group 1), probably carcinogenic to humans (group 2A) and possibly carcinogenic to humans (group 2B) [48].

Table 1. Agents that can be found in e-aerosol, e-fluid and released from metallic coils [48].

CAS Number	Component	Group
75–07-0	Acetaldehyd	2B
107–02-8	Acreolin	2A
50–00-0	Formaldehyde	1
7439–92-1	Lead	2B

CAS (Chemical Abstracts Service).

Therefore, the need to use modern analytical, reliable and validated methods to quantify both toxic metals and other chemicals inhaled by users of various generations of e-cigarettes, especially the long-term effects of exposition to the compounds, are not fully known. A variety of components seem to indicate that vaping should not be treated as a safe alternative method compared to traditional smoking.

3. Effect of E-Cigarettes Aerosol on Oral Cavity

It is known that both environmental and civilizational factors can affect human health and can impact the functions of tissues and organs. One factor is cigarette smoking and its harmful effects on human health are well documented. Although the content of various chemical compounds and trace elements in e-aerosol are described to be lower than in cigarette smoke, long-term exposure to aerosol can have a negative effect on oral cavity health [16]. However, there is an increasing amount of data on the risks of e-cigarette use compared to the benefits. Vaping, an alternative that simulates tobacco smoking, involves the inhalation of aerosols created by heating of e-cigarette fluid, often considered less harmful [49,50]. The National Academy of Sciences, Engineering and Medicine published in 2018 a report reviewing the evidence for the adverse effects of e-cigarettes in the course of oral cavity and respiratory system diseases [49].

The tissues of the oral cavity are those first exposed to the inhaled e-aerosol and they interact directly with its toxins and chemical components. Research on potential oral health changes following e-cigarette exposure is limited and there is some controversy about the safety of e-cigarette use [51], and daily vaping is associated with poor oral health [25].

Experimental studies are not able to fully reflect real conditions because regular electronic cigarette users may draw more puffs a day than in experiment laboratory studies [52,53]. To evaluate the effects of e-aerosol exposure on the human oral cavity, the development and severity of periodontal disease should be taken into consideration, such as bleeding from gingival tissue after probing, the assessment of the amount of plaque (plaque index), the quantification of the gingival crevice as a marker of periodontitis and the potential effects on the lining of epithelial cells and the oral microbiome [49,50].

3.1. Oral Microenvironment

The maintenance of homeostasis and functionality of the oral cavity are created by saliva, the fluid secretory product of major and minor salivary glands. There are three major paired salivary glands located outside the mouth and their secretion is transported via ducts opening in the oral cavity. The minor salivary glands are located in the mucosa and submucosa of the oral wall. Saliva with a unique composition plays protective and digestive functions, containing water, electrolytes and various protein and signaling molecules [54].

One pilot cross-sectional study was performed with volunteers to assess the effect of e-cigarette use on biomarkers of inflammation, oxidative stress, anti-inflammatory lipid mediators, tissue injury and repair and growth factors in saliva and gingival crevicular fluid. The obtained results were compared between four groups of participants as e-cigarette users (EC), non-smokers, cigarette smokers and both e-cigarette and cigarette (dual) smokers. There was significant increase between levels of myeloperoxidase and matrix metaloproteinase-9 in EC vs. non-smokers, and between dual smokers and EC in inflammatory mediators as receptor for advanced glycation end products, myeloperoxidase and recombinant human uteroglobin/CC10 [55].

The changes in antioxidant capacity of saliva in e-cigarette users and cigarette smokers comparing to non-smokers were observed in a study by Cichońska et al. (2021) [56]. The uric acid, hypoxanthine, xanthine, TAOS (total antioxidant status) and TEAC (Trolox equivalent antioxidant capacity) were determined in the samples of saliva patients. The antioxidant capacity of saliva was affected in the e-cig users in a similar degree as in cigarette smokers when compared to the saliva of non-smokers [56]. The impaired antioxidant function of saliva can stimulate the formation of free radicals and reactive oxygen species (ROS), which play a role in the progression of periodontitis and destruction of tissue [57].

3.2. Oral Microbiome

The microorganisms, harboring over 700 species, that reside in the human oral cavity are described as the oral microbiome, oral microflora or oral microbiota [58]. The microorganisms play an important role in the maintenance of the proper environment in the oral cavity and encompasses oral niches, such as teeth surface, tongue, cheeks, subgingival and supragingival plaque, palates, tonsils and salivary [59,60]. A dysbiosis, an imbalance in the microbial ecosystem, can produce changes in their functional composition and can result in pathological conditions [59,61–63]. The flavoring compounds of e-liquids have various aromas and tastes, and some chemical components, such as saccharides and sucralose are added to provide a sweet taste [64], they may selectively disrupt the homeostasis of the oral microbiome and can be associated with a variety of oral diseases, such as periodontitis and caries. There is evidence that e-cigarette use is associated with a compositional and functional shift in the oral microbiome, with an increase in opportunistic pathogens and virulence traits [65].

The study of salivary microbial communes performed by Pushalkar et al. (2020) revealed the alterations in the content and differences in oral microbiota of e-cigarette users compared to those who have never smoked. They included significantly altered beta-diversity in species and the most abundant species of bacteria *Porphyromonas* and *Veillonella* in e-cigarette users. Additionally, levels of cytokines (IL-6 i IL-1β) were increased. The dysbiosis in microbiome was related to elevated proinflammatory cytokines release and increased inflammation, which clearly indicated that e-cigarette users are more prone to infection processes in the oral cavity [66]. Alterations in bacterial taxonomic composition were also found in buccal samples and the samples of saliva in e-cigarette users. The saliva of the users presented a significantly higher alpha diversity, which declined together with decreased use of e-cigarettes. The most abundant bacteria genera in buccal samples was *Streptococcus* in both e-cigarette users and non-smoking/non-vaping, whereas *Prevotella* was the most abundant in the saliva samples also for both tested groups. When cohorts in aggregate were tested, the buccal samples of e-cigarette users were rich in *Veillonella* and *Haemophilus* species [67].

The salivary malondialdehyde (MDA), total salivary mucins (SM) and buccal smear cells of the micronuclei (MN) were analyzed in patients of three groups: e-cigarette with/without nicotine content users and a non-smoking group as in Menicagli et al. (2020) studies. A significantly higher concentration of malondialdehyse, the final product of polyunsaturated fatty acids peroxidation [68], frequently recognized as a marker of oxidative stress [69], was observed in e-cigarette users compared to the control group. The highest, statistically significant amount of salivary mucin was noted in those smoking e-cigarettes with nicotine. Analysis of the presence of micronuclei in buccal smear cells is used as a biomarker of genotoxicity in smokers to predicting the effects of carcinogens [70]. In the studies, the micronuclei were detected in exfoliated buccal cells of e-cigarette users. However, within the e-cigarette users, there were volunteers with a higher MN score, but who have a higher age ($\geq$39 years). All of the phenomenon could be associated with the free radicals formation and to damage the normal cellular metabolism [71].

There are reports that e-cigarettes can induce changes in epithelial cells on the molecular level that result in the deregulation of gene expression. Tommasi et al. (2019) performed whole transcriptome profile analysis of oral epithelial cells obtained from central and distal regions of the inside of each cheek of volunteers who were e-cigarette users, cigarette smokers and control non-smokers or non-vapers. Analysis of the global transcriptome profile showed the deregulation of number a key genes and molecular pathways in the oral epithelial cells. Functional pathway analysis of differentially expressed genes indicated that in both e-cigarette users and smokers the genes were mainly associated with cancer within disease and disorders. In both experimental groups, differentially expressed genes were predominantly associated with "cancer". The canonical Wnt/Ca+ pathway in e-cigarette users and the non-canonical integrin signaling pathway in smokers were the most disrupted pathways [72]. The result showed that e-cigarette use leads to the deregulation expression of key genes and molecular pathways in oral epithelial cells that are directly exposed to carcinogens.

To explain the effects of e-cigarettes on oral cavity, a prospective cross-sectional study was conducted to evaluate the prevalence and characteristics of oral mucosal lesions in former smokers and e-cigarette users. There were no significant differences in prevalence of oral mucosal lesions between the two groups. However, more frequent symptoms and the prevalence of mucosal lesions, such as nicotine stomatitis, hairy tongue and angular cheilitis were identified among e-cigarettes users [73].

The lamina propria of the lips, cheeks, floor of mouth and the ventral surface of the tongue is lined by stratified squamous nonkeratinized epithelium. The mucosa of the regions in oral cavity is very thin and well vascularized, and it is an attractive route for the administration of drugs and other therapeutic agents. A pilot study was performed by Reuther et al. (2016) to assess the possible effect of e-cigarette use on blood flow in the buccal mucosa as a consequence of postoperative patients' questions about whether to continuing smoking or to switch to vaping. The laser Doppler technique was used to measure the flow of buccal mucosal blood in 10 volunteers showed that e-cigarettes produced a temporary rise in capillary perfusion, which can suggest the better absorption of medicines. However, the results are needed to confirm that e-vapor can improve healing time after oral and maxillofacial operations [74].

The presented data suggest that vaping disrupts both oral microenvironment and ora microbiome.

4. Injury of Oral Cavity as Effect of E-Cigarettes Explosion

One of the complications of e-cigarette use is their malfunctions; spontaneous failure and intra-oral explosion can result in several serious oral injuries, such as oral hard and soft tissue injuries [14,75,76]. Examples of cases of two male patients' injuries after the explosion of the e-cigarette in the mouth included intraoral burns, luxation injuries and alveolar fracture [77], and the other, a fracture, tearing out and dislocation of the front teeth, premaxillary fractures and permanent cuts to the upper lip, the mucosa of the lips, gums, tongue and hard palate [15]. The majority of reported electronic cigarette-related oral injuries have been serious and have frequently required the intervention of a plastic surgeon. The injuries included tooth fracture and tooth avulsion, jaw fracture, dentoalveolar fracture, haematoma formation, traumatic ulceration and tattooing, intra-oral burns and subsequent necrosis, palate perforation with extension into the nasal cavity and extensive soft tissue deficits [78–80]. Recently, a case report of 19-year-old boy was presented with maxillofacial injury after an e-cigarette battery-related explosion in his mouth, as a warning to the public. Significant hard and soft tissue injuries of the oral cavity, in particular the anterior left maxilla were observed. Additionally, there were epidermal burns to the facial area, including the lips and upper chest; the upper lip sustained minimal soft tissue damage [81].

Therefore, to promote the awareness of this phenomenon, wide discussion, especially among adolescent and young adult of e-cigarette users, should be carried out regarding the risk of spontaneous failure and explosion of e-cigarettes. Dental professionals have an important role to play in educating patients about not only the potential harm and the health consequences of e-cigarette use, but also risk of intra-oral explosion of e-cigarettes.

5. Conclusions

The study indicates that exposure to e-cigarette aerosol that contains various ingredients, toxicants and carcinogens can exert harmful effects and induce changes in human oral health, inducing disbiosis, inflammation, cytotoxicity and genotoxicity, contributing to in periodontal diseases. The mechanisms of action of the chemical substances in e-aerosols (vapors) include changes on the biochemical, cellular and molecular levels. However, there is a need for extensive research to assess the actual effects of e-aerosol on oral cavity tissues as well as to evaluate the short-term and long-term use of e-cigarettes and related products. These data illustrate the need for the monitoring of the conditions of different tissues and organs of the e-cigarette users. The obtained results may be important for both adolescents and young adults.

Author Contributions: Conceptualization: P.S. and K.S.; methodology: P.S. and A.W.; software: P.S. and K.S.; validation: P.S., B.K., A.W. and K.S.; formal analysis: P.S.; investigation: K.S.; resources: A.W., B.K.; data curation: P.S. and K.S.; writing (preparation of the original draft): P.S.; writing (review and editing): K.S. and B.K.; visualization: A.W.; supervision: B.K. and K.S.; project administration: K.S. All authors have read and agreed to the published version of the manuscript.

Funding: This research received no external funding.

Institutional Review Board Statement: Not applicable.

Informed Consent Statement: Not applicable.

Data Availability Statement: Data available in a publicly accessible repository.

Conflicts of Interest: The authors declare no conflict of interest.

References

1. O'Brien, D.; Long, J.; Quigley, J.; Lee, C.; McCarthy, A.; Kavanagh, P. Association between electronic cigarette use and tobacco cigarette smoking initiation in adolescents: A systematic review and meta-analysis. *BMC Public Health* **2021**, *21*, 954. [CrossRef]
2. Alolabi, H.; Alchallah, M.O.; Mohsen, F.; Shibani, M.; Ismail, H.; Alzabibi, M.A.; Sawaf, B. Prevalence and behavior regarding cigarette and water pipe smoking among Syrian undergraduates. *Heliyon* **2020**, *6*, e05423. [CrossRef]
3. Adermark, L.; Galanti, M.R.; Ryk, C.; Gilljam, H.; Hedman, L. Prospective association between use of electronic cigarettes and use of conventional cigarettes: A systematic review and meta-analysis. *ERJ Open Res.* **2021**, *7*, 7–18. [CrossRef] [PubMed]
4. Ureña, J.F.; Ebersol, L.A.; Silakov, A.; Elias, R.J.; Lambert, J.D. Impact of Atomizer Age and Flavor on In Vitro Toxicity of Aerosols from a Third-Generation Electronic Cigarette against Human Oral Cells. *Chem. Res. Toxicol.* **2020**, *33*, 2527–2537. [CrossRef] [PubMed]
5. Kapan, A.; Stefanac, S.; Sandner, I.; Haider, S.; Grabovac, I.; Dorner, T.E. Use of Electronic Cigarettes in European Populations: A Narrative Review. *Int. J. Environ. Res. Public Health* **2020**, *17*, 1971. [CrossRef] [PubMed]
6. Jankowski, M.; Krzystanek, M.; Zejda, J.E.; Majek, P.; Lubanski, J.; Lawson, J.A.; Brozek, G. E-Cigarettes are More Addictive than Traditional Cigarettes-A Study in Highly Educated Young People. *Int. J. Environ. Res. Public Health* **2019**, *16*, 2279. [CrossRef]
7. Jankowski, M.; Minarowski, Ł.; Mróz, R.M.; Guziejko, K.; Mojsak, D.; Poznański, M.; Zielonka, T.M.; Rachel, M.; Kornicki, K.; Pepłowska, P.; et al. E-cigarette use among young adults in Poland: Prevalence and characteristics of e-cigarette users. *Adv. Med. Sci.* **2020**, *65*, 437–441. [CrossRef]
8. Zwar, N.A. Smoking cessation. *Aust. J. Gen. Pract.* **2020**, *49*, 474–481. [CrossRef]
9. Marcham, C.L.; Springston, J.P. Electronic cigarettes in the indoor environment. *Rev. Environ. Health* **2019**, *34*, 105–124. [CrossRef]
10. Bals, R.; Boyd, J.; Esposito, S.; Foronjy, R.; Hiemstra, P.S.; Jiménez-Ruiz, C.A.; Katsaounou, P.; Lindberg, A.; Metz, C.; Schober, W.; et al. Electronic cigarettes: A task force report from the European Respiratory Society. *Eur. Respir J.* **2019**, *53*, 1801151. [CrossRef]
11. Clapp, P.W.; Pawlak, E.A.; Lackey, J.T.; Keating, J.E.; Reeber, S.L.; Glish, G.L.; Jaspers, I. Flavored e-cigarette liquids and cinnamaldehyde impair respiratory innate immune cell function. *Am. J. Physiol. Lung Cell Mol. Physiol.* **2017**, *313*, L278–L292. [CrossRef] [PubMed]
12. Almeida-da-Silva, C.L.C.; Matshik Dakafay, H.; O'Brien, K.; Montierth, D.; Xiao, N.; Ojcius, D.M. Effects of electronic cigarette aerosol exposure on oral and systemic health. *Biomed. J.* **2021**, *44*, 252–259. [CrossRef] [PubMed]
13. Ramôa, C.P.; Eissenberg, T.; Sahingur, S.E. Increasing popularity of waterpipe tobacco smoking and electronic cigarette use: Implications for oral healthcare. *J. Periodontal. Res.* **2017**, *52*, 813–823. [CrossRef] [PubMed]

14. Toy, J.; Dong, F.; Lee, C.; Zappa, D.; Le, T.; Archambeau, B.; Culhane, J.T.; Neeki, M.M. Alarming increase in electronic nicotine delivery systems-related burn injuries: A serious unregulated public health issue. *Am. J. Emerg. Med.* **2017**, *35*, 1781–1782. [CrossRef] [PubMed]
15. Brooks, J.K.; Kleinman, J.W.; Brooks, J.B.; Reynolds, M.A. Electronic cigarette explosion associated with extensive intraoral injuries. *Dent. Traumatol.* **2017**, *33*, 149–152. [CrossRef]
16. Ebersole, J.; Samburova, V.; Son, Y.; Cappelli, D.; Demopoulos, C.; Capurro, A.; Pinto, A.; Chrzan, B.; Kingsley, K.; Howard, K.; et al. Harmful chemicals emitted from electronic cigarettes and potential deleterious effects in the oral cavity. *Tob. Induc. Dis.* **2020**, *18*, 41. [CrossRef]
17. Zervas, E.; Matsouki, N.; Kyriakopoulos, G.; Poulopoulos, S.; Ioannides, T.; Katsaounou, P. Transfer of metals in the liquids of electronic cigarettes. *Inhal. Toxicol.* **2020**, *32*, 240–248. [CrossRef]
18. Uchiyama, S.; Noguchi, M.; Sato, A.; Ishitsuka, M.; Inaba, Y.; Kunugita, N. Determination of Thermal Decomposition Products Generated from E-Cigarettes. *Chem. Res. Toxicol.* **2020**, *33*, 576–583. [CrossRef]
19. Klein, M.D.; Sokol, N.A.; Stroud, L.R. Electronic Cigarettes: Common Questions and Answers. *Am. Fam. Physician.* **2019**, *100*, 227–235.
20. Geiss, O.; Bianchi, I.; Barahona, F.; Barrero-Moreno, J. Characterisation of mainstream and passive vapours emitted by selected electronic cigarettes. *Int. J. Hyg. Environ. Health* **2015**, *218*, 169–180. [CrossRef]
21. Shao, X.M.; Friedman, T.C. Pod-mod vs. conventional e-cigarettes: Nicotine chemistry, pH, and health effects. *J. Appl. Physiol.* **2020**, *128*, 1056–1058. [CrossRef] [PubMed]
22. Overbeek, D.L.; Kass, A.P.; Chiel, L.E.; Boyer, E.W.; Casey, A.M.H. A review of toxic effects of electronic cigarettes/vaping in adolescents and young adults. *Crit. Rev. Toxicol.* **2020**, *50*, 531–538. [CrossRef] [PubMed]
23. Harvanko, A.M.; Havel, C.M.; Jacob, P.; Benowitz, N.L. Characterization of Nicotine Salts in 23 Electronic Cigarette Refill Liquids. *Nicotine Tob. Res.* **2020**, *22*, 1239–1243. [CrossRef] [PubMed]
24. Goniewicz, M.L.; Boykan, R.; Messina, C.R.; Eliscu, A.; Tolentino, J. High exposure to nicotine among adolescents who use Juul and other vape pod systems ('pods'). *Tob. Control.* **2019**, *28*, 676–677. [CrossRef] [PubMed]
25. Smith, T.T.; Heckman, B.W.; Wahlquist, A.E.; Cummings, K.M.; Carpenter, M.J. The Impact of E-liquid Propylene Glycol and Vegetable Glycerin Ratio on Ratings of Subjective Effects, Reinforcement Value, and Use in Current Smokers. *Nicotine Tob. Res.* **2020**, *22*, 791–797. [CrossRef] [PubMed]
26. Khlystov, A.; Samburova, V. Flavoring Compounds Dominate Toxic Aldehyde Production during e-Cigarette Vaping. *Environ. Sci. Technol.* **2016**, *50*, 13080–13085. [CrossRef]
27. Samburova, V.; Bhattarai, C.; Strickland, M.; Darrow, L.; Angermann, J.; Son, Y.; Khlystov, A. Aldehydes in Exhaled Breath during e-Cigarette Vaping: Pilot Study Results. *Toxics* **2018**, *6*, 46. [CrossRef]
28. Beauval, N.; Verriele, M.; Garat, A.; Fronval, I.; Dusautoir, R.; Antherieu, S.; Garcon, G.; Lo-Guidice, J.M.; Allorge, D.; Locoge, N. Influence of puffing conditions on the carbonyl composition of e-cigarette aerosols. *Int. J. Hyg. Environ. Health* **2019**, *222*, 136–146. [CrossRef]
29. Mara, A.; Langasco, I.; Deidda, S.; Caredda, M.; Meloni, P.; Deroma, M.; Pilo, M.I.; Spano, N.; Sanna, G. ICP-MS Determination of 23 Elements of Potential Health Concern in Liquids of e-Cigarettes. Method Development, Validation, and Application to 37 Real Samples. *Molecules* **2021**, *26*, 6680. [CrossRef]
30. Gonzalez-Jimenez, N.; Gray, N.; Pappas, R.S.; Halstead, M.; Lewis, E.; Valentin-Blasini, L.; Watson, C.; Blount, B. Analysis of Toxic Metals in Aerosols from Devices Associated with Electronic Cigarette, or Vaping, Product Use Associated Lung Injury. *Toxics* **2021**, *9*, 240. [CrossRef]
31. Landmesser, A.; Scherer, M.; Scherer, G.; Sarkar, M.; Edmiston, J.S.; Niessner, R.; Pluym, N. Assessment of the potential vaping-related exposure to carbonyls and epoxides using stable isotope-labeled precursors in the e-liquid. *Arch. Toxicol.* **2021**, *95*, 2667–2676. [CrossRef] [PubMed]
32. Beauval, N.; Antherieu, S.; Soyez, M.; Gengler, N.; Grova, N.; Howsam, M.; Hardy, E.M.; Fischer, M.; Appenzeller, B.M.R.; Goossens, J.F.; et al. Chemical Evaluation of Electronic Cigarettes: Multicomponent Analysis of Liquid Refills and their Corresponding Aerosols. *J. Anal. Toxicol.* **2017**, *41*, 670–678. [CrossRef] [PubMed]
33. Halstead, M.; Gray, N.; Gonzalez-Jimenez, N.; Fresquez, M.; Valentin-Blasini, L.; Watson, C.; Pappas, R.S. Analysis of Toxic Metals in Electronic Cigarette Aerosols Using a Novel Trap Design. *J. Anal. Toxicol.* **2020**, *44*, 149–155. [CrossRef]
34. Pappas, R.S.; Gray, N.; Halstead, M.; Valentin-Blasini, L.; Watson, C. Toxic Metal-Containing Particles in Aerosols from Pod-Type Electronic Cigarettes. *J. Anal. Toxicol.* **2021**, *45*, 337–347. [CrossRef] [PubMed]
35. Tehrani, M.W.; Newmeyer, M.N.; Rule, A.M.; Prasse, C. Characterizing the Chemical Landscape in Commercial E-Cigarette Liquids and Aerosols by Liquid Chromatography-High-Resolution Mass Spectrometry. *Chem. Res. Toxicol.* **2021**, *34*, 2216–2226. [CrossRef] [PubMed]
36. Bitzer, Z.T.; Goel, R.; Reilly, S.M.; Elias, R.J.; Silakov, A.; Foulds, J.; Muscat, J.; Richie, J.P., Jr. Effect of flavoring chemicals on free radical formation in electronic cigarette aerosols. *Free Radic. Biol. Med.* **2018**, *120*, 72–79. [CrossRef]
37. Bitzer, Z.T.; Goel, R.; Reilly, S.M.; Foulds, J.; Muscat, J.; Elias, R.J.; Richie, J.P., Jr. Effects of Solvent and Temperature on Free Radical Formation in Electronic Cigarette Aerosols. *Chem. Res. Toxicol.* **2018**, *31*, 4–12. [CrossRef]
38. Sleiman, M.; Logue, J.M.; Montesinos, V.N.; Russell, M.L.; Litter, M.I.; Gundel, L.A.; Destaillats, H. Emissions from Electronic Cigarettes: Key Parameters Affecting the Release of Harmful Chemicals. *Environ. Sci. Technol.* **2016**, *50*, 9644–9651. [CrossRef]

39. Shein, M.; Jeschke, G. Comparison of Free Radical Levels in the Aerosol from Conventional Cigarettes, Electronic Cigarettes, and Heat-Not-Burn Tobacco Products. *Chem. Res. Toxicol.* **2019**, *32*, 1289–1298. [CrossRef]
40. Bitzer, Z.T.; Goel, R.; Trushin, N.; Muscat, J.; Richie, J.P., Jr. Free Radical Production and Characterization of Heat-Not-Burn Cigarettes in Comparison to Conventional and Electronic Cigarettes. *Chem. Res. Toxicol.* **2020**, *33*, 1882–1887. [CrossRef]
41. Yogeswaran, S.; Muthumalage, T.; Rahman, I. Comparative Reactive Oxygen Species (ROS) Content among Various Flavored Disposable Vape Bars, including Cool (Iced) Flavored Bars. *Toxics* **2021**, *9*, 235. [CrossRef]
42. Barhdadi, S.; Mertens, B.; van Bossuyt, M.; van de Maele, J.; Anthonissen, R.; Canfyn, M.; Courselle, P.; Rogiers, V.; Deconinck, E.; Vanhaecke, T. Identification of flavouring substances of genotoxic concern present in e-cigarette refills. *Food Chem. Toxicol.* **2021**, *147*, 111864. [CrossRef] [PubMed]
43. Margham, J.; McAdam, K.; Cunningham, A.; Porter, A.; Fiebelkorn, S.; Mariner, D.; Digard, H.; Proctor, C. The Chemical Complexity of e-Cigarette Aerosols Compared With the Smoke From a Tobacco Burning Cigarette. *Front. Chem.* **2021**, *9*, 743060. [CrossRef] [PubMed]
44. Tantisuwat, A.; Thaveeratitham, P. Effects of smoking on chest expansion, lung function, and respiratory muscle strength of youths. *J. Phys. Ther. Sci.* **2014**, *26*, 167–170. [CrossRef] [PubMed]
45. Hikichi, M.; Mizumura, K.; Maruoka, S.; Gon, Y. Pathogenesis of chronic obstructive pulmonary disease (COPD) induced by cigarette smoke. *J. Thorac. Dis.* **2019**, *11*, S2129–S2140. [CrossRef] [PubMed]
46. Kopa, P.N.; Pawliczak, R. Effect of smoking on gene expression profile-overall mechanism, impact on respiratory system function, and reference to electronic cigarettes. *Toxicol. Mech. Methods* **2018**, *28*, 397–409. [CrossRef] [PubMed]
47. Rowell, T.R.; Reeber, S.L.; Lee, S.L.; Harris, R.A.; Nethery, R.C.; Herring, A.H.; Glish, G.L.; Tarran, R. Flavored e-cigarette liquids reduce proliferation and viability in the CALU3 airway epithelial cell line. *Am. J. Physiol. Lung Cell Mol. Physiol.* **2017**, *313*, L52–L166. [CrossRef] [PubMed]
48. Samet, J.M.; Chiu, W.A.; Cogliano, V.; Jinot, J.; Kriebel, D.; Lunn, R.M.; Beland, F.A.; Bero, L.; Browne, P.; Fritschi, L.; et al. The IARC Monographs: Updated Procedures for Modern and Transparent Evidence Synthesis in Cancer Hazard Identification. *J. Natl. Cancer Inst.* **2020**, *112*, 30–37. [CrossRef]
49. Stratton, K.; Kwan, L.Y.; Eaton, D.L. *Public Health Consequences of E-Cigarettes*; The National Academies Press: Washington, DC, USA, 2018; pp. 455–460.
50. Grana, R.; Benowitz, N.; Glantz, S.A. E-cigarettes: A scientific review. *Circulation* **2014**, *129*, 1972–1986. [CrossRef]
51. Ralho, A.; Coelho, A.; Ribeiro, M.; Paula, A.; Amaro, I.; Sousa, J.; Marto, C.; Ferreira, M.; Carrilho, E. Effects of Electronic Cigarettes on Oral Cavity: A Systematic Review. *J. Evid. Based Dent. Pract.* **2019**, *19*, 101318. [CrossRef]
52. Etter, J.F. Electronic cigarettes: A survey of users. *BMC Public Health* **2010**, *10*, 231. [CrossRef]
53. Etter, J.F.; Bullen, C. Electronic cigarette: Users profile, utilization, satisfaction and perceived efficacy. *Addiction* **2011**, *106*, 2017–2028. [CrossRef] [PubMed]
54. Porcheri, C.; Mitsiadis, T.A. Physiology, Pathology and Regeneration of Salivary Glands. *Cells* **2019**, *8*, 976. [CrossRef] [PubMed]
55. Ye, D.; Gajendra, S.; Lawyer, G.; Jadeja, N.; Pishey, D.; Pathagunti, S.; Lyons, J.; Veazie, P.; Watson, G.; McIntosh, S.; et al. Inflammatory biomarkers and growth factors in saliva and gingival crevicular fluid of e-cigarette users, cigarette smokers, and dual smokers: A pilot study. *J. Periodontol.* **2020**, *91*, 1274–1283. [CrossRef] [PubMed]
56. Cichońska, D.; Król, O.; Słomińska, E.M.; Kochańska, B.; Świetlik, D.; Ochocińska, J.; Kusiak, A. Influence of Electronic Cigarettes on Antioxidant Capacity and Nucleotide Metabolites in Saliva. *Toxics* **2021**, *9*, 263. [CrossRef] [PubMed]
57. Sczepanik, F.S.C.; Grossi, M.L.; Casati, M.; Goldberg, M.; Glogauer, M.; Fine, N.; Tenenbaum, H.C. Periodontitis is an inflammatory disease of oxidative stress: We should treat it that way. *Periodontology 2000* **2020**, *84*, 45–68. [CrossRef]
58. Dewhirst, F.E.; Chen, T.; Izard, J.; Paster, B.J.; Tanner, A.C.; Yu, W.H.; Lakshmanan, A.; Wade, W.G. The human oral microbiome. *J. Bacteriol.* **2010**, *192*, 5002–5017. [CrossRef]
59. Willis, J.R.; Gabaldón, T. The Human Oral Microbiome in Health and Disease: From Sequences to Ecosystems. *Microorganisms* **2020**, *8*, 308. [CrossRef]
60. Radaic, A.; Kapila, Y.L. The oralome and its dysbiosis: New insights into oral microbiome-host interactions. *Comput. Struct. Biotechnol. J.* **2021**, *19*, 1335–1360. [CrossRef]
61. Bourgeois, D.; Inquimbert, C.; Ottolenghi, L.; Carrouel, F. Periodontal Pathogens as Risk Factors of Cardiovascular Diseases, Diabetes, Rheumatoid Arthritis, Cancer, and Chronic Obstructive Pulmonary Disease-Is There Cause for Consideration? *Microorganisms* **2019**, *7*, 424. [CrossRef]
62. Gare, J.; Kanoute, A.; Meda, N.; Viennot, S.; Bourgeois, D.; Carrouel, F. Periodontal Conditions and Pathogens Associated with Pre-Eclampsia: A Scoping Review. *Int. J. Environ. Res. Public Health* **2021**, *18*, 7194. [CrossRef]
63. Siqueira, J.F., Jr.; Rôças, I.N. The Oral Microbiota in Health and Disease: An Overview of Molecular Findings. *Methods Mol. Biol.* **2017**, *1537*, 127–138. [PubMed]
64. Kubica, P.; Wasik, A.; Kot-Wasik, A.; Namieśnik, J. An evaluation of sucrose as a possible contaminant in e-liquids for electronic cigarettes by hydrophilic interaction liquid chromatography-tandem mass spectrometry. *Anal. Bioanal. Chem.* **2014**, *406*, 3013–3018. [CrossRef]
65. Kumar, P.S.; Clark, P.; Brinkman, M.C.; Saxena, D. Novel Nicotine Delivery Systems. *Adv. Dent. Res.* **2019**, *30*, 11–15. [CrossRef] [PubMed]

66. Pushkalkar, S.; Paul, B.; Li, Q.; Yang, J.; Vasconcelos, R.; Makwana, S.; González, J.M.; Shah, S.; Xie, C.; Janal, M.N.; et al. Electronic Cigarette Aerosol Modulates the Oral Microbiome and Increases Risk of Infection. *iScience* **2020**, *23*, 100884. [CrossRef] [PubMed]
67. Chopyk, J.; Bojanowski, C.M.; Shin, J.; Moshensky, A.; Fuentes, A.L.; Bonde, S.S.; Chuki, D.; Pride, D.T.; Crotty, A.L.E. Compositional Differences in the Oral Microbiome of E-cigarette Users. *Front Microbiol.* **2021**, *12*, 599664. [CrossRef]
68. Gaweł, S.; Wardas, M.; Niedworok, E.; Wardas, P. Malondialdehyde (MDA) as a lipid peroxidation marker. *Wiad. Lek.* **2004**, *57*, 453–455.
69. Cherian, D.A.; Peter, T.; Narayanan, A.; Madhavan, S.S.; Achammada, S.; Vynat, G.P. Malondialdehyde as a Marker of Oxidative Stress in Periodontitis Patients. *J. Pharm. Bioallied. Sci.* **2019**, *11*, S297–S300. [CrossRef]
70. Upadhyay, M.; Verma, P.; Sabharwal, R.; Subudhi, S.K.; Jatol-Tekade, S.; Naphade, V.; Choudhury, B.K.; Sahoo, P.D. Micronuclei in Exfoliated Cells: A Biomarker of Genotoxicity in Tobacco Users. *Niger J. Surg.* **2019**, *25*, 52–59.
71. Menicagli, R.; Marotta, O.; Serra, R. Free radical production in the smoking of e-cigarettes and their possible effects in human health. *Int. J. Prev. Med.* **2020**, *11*, 53.
72. Tommasi, S.; Caliri, A.W.; Caceres, A.; Moreno, D.E.; Li, M.; Chen, Y.; Siegmund, K.D.; Besaratinia, A. Deregulation of Biologically Significant Genes and Associated Molecular Pathways in the Oral Epithelium of Electronic Cigarette Users. *Int. J. Mol. Sci.* **2019**, *20*, 738. [CrossRef] [PubMed]
73. Bardellini, E.; Amadori, F.; Conti, G.; Majorana, A. Oral mucosal lesions in electronic cigarettes consumers versus former smokers. *Acta Odontol. Scand.* **2018**, *76*, 226–228. [CrossRef] [PubMed]
74. Reuther, W.J.; Hale, B.; Matharu, J.; Blythe, J.N.; Brennan, P.A. Do you mind if I vape? Immediate effects of electronic cigarettes on perfusion in buccal mucosal tissue—A pilot study. *Br. J. Oral Maxillofac. Surg.* **2016**, *54*, 338–341. [CrossRef] [PubMed]
75. Seitz, C.M.; Kabir, Z. Burn injuries caused by e-cigarette explosions: A systematic review of published cases. *Tob. Prev. Cessat.* **2018**, *4*, 32. [CrossRef]
76. Yang, I.; Sandeep, S.; Rodriguez, J. The oral health impact of electronic cigarette use: A systematic review. *Crit Rev. Toxicol.* **2020**, *50*, 1–31. [CrossRef]
77. Harrison, R.; Hicklin, D., Jr. Electronic cigarette explosions involving the oral cavity. *J. Am. Dent. Assoc.* **2016**, *147*, 891–896. [CrossRef]
78. Rogér, J.M.; Abayon, M.; Elad, S.; Kolokythas, A. Oral Trauma and Tooth Avulsion Following Explosion of E-Cigarette. *J. Oral. Maxillofac. Surg.* **2016**, *74*, 1181–1185. [CrossRef]
79. Sultan, A.S.; Jessri, M.; Farah, C.S. Electronic nicotine delivery systems: Oral health implications and oral cancer risk. *J. Oral Pathol. Med.* **2021**, *50*, 316–322. [CrossRef]
80. Bestman, E.G.; Brooks, J.K.; Mostoufi, B.; Bashirelahi, N. What every dentist needs to know about electronic cigarettes. *Gen. Dent.* **2021**, *69*, 31–35.
81. La Valle, A.; O'Connor, R.; Brooks, A.; Freij, R. Maxillofacial injury related to an exploding e-cigarette. *BMJ Case Rep.* **2021**, *14*, e239677. [CrossRef]

MDPI
St. Alban-Anlage 66
4052 Basel
Switzerland
Tel. +41 61 683 77 34
Fax +41 61 302 89 18
www.mdpi.com

Toxics Editorial Office
E-mail: toxics@mdpi.com
www.mdpi.com/journal/toxics

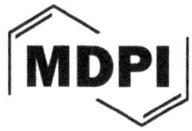